Current Updates on Interventional Cardiac Electrophysiology

Current Updates on Interventional Cardiac Electrophysiology

Editor

Tong Liu

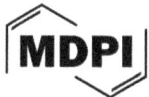

Basel • Beijing • Wuhan • Barcelona • Belgrade • Novi Sad • Cluj • Manchester

Editor
Tong Liu
Second Hospital of Tianjin
Medical University
Tianjin, China

Editorial Office
MDPI
St. Alban-Anlage 66
4052 Basel, Switzerland

This is a reprint of articles from the Special Issue published online in the open access journal *Journal of Clinical Medicine* (ISSN 2077-0383) (available at: https://www.mdpi.com/journal/jcm/special_issues/Interventional_Cardiac_Electrophysiology).

For citation purposes, cite each article independently as indicated on the article page online and as indicated below:

Lastname, A.A.; Lastname, B.B. Article Title. *Journal Name* **Year**, *Volume Number*, Page Range.

ISBN 978-3-0365-8458-4 (Hbk)
ISBN 978-3-0365-8459-1 (PDF)
doi.org/10.3390/books978-3-0365-8459-1

© 2023 by the authors. Articles in this book are Open Access and distributed under the Creative Commons Attribution (CC BY) license. The book as a whole is distributed by MDPI under the terms and conditions of the Creative Commons Attribution-NonCommercial-NoDerivs (CC BY-NC-ND) license.

Contents

About the Editor vii

Yibo Ma, Miaoyang Hu, Lanyan Guo, Jian Xu, Jie Li, Qun Yan, et al.
Clinical Influence of Ethanol Infusion in the Vein of Marshall on Left Atrial Appendage Occlusion: Results of Feasibility and Safety during Implantation and at 60-Day Follow-Up
Reprinted from: *J. Clin. Med.* **2023**, *12*, 1960, doi:10.3390/jcm12051960 1

Shuyu Jin, Weidong Lin, Xianhong Fang, Hongtao Liao, Xianzhang Zhan, Lu Fu, et al.
High-Power, Short-Duration Ablation under the Guidance of Relatively Low Ablation Index Values for Paroxysmal Atrial Fibrillation: Long-Term Outcomes and Characteristics of Recurrent Atrial Arrhythmias
Reprinted from: *J. Clin. Med.* **2023**, *12*, 971, doi:10.3390/jcm12030971 13

Hongda Zhang, Lei Ding, Lijie Mi, Kuo Zhang, Zihan Jiang, Sixian Weng, et al.
Vein of Marshall Collateralization during Ethanol Infusion in Atrial Fibrillation: Solution for Effective Myocardium Staining
Reprinted from: *J. Clin. Med.* **2023**, *12*, 309, doi:10.3390/jcm12010309 29

Yibo Ma, Lanyan Guo, Jie Li, Haitao Liu, Jian Xu, Hui Du, et al.
Iatrogenic Atrial Septal Defect after Intracardiac Echocardiography-Guided Left Atrial Appendage Closure: Incidence, Size, and Clinical Outcomes
Reprinted from: *J. Clin. Med.* **2023**, *12*, 160, doi:10.3390/jcm12010160 37

**Chin-Yu Lin, Fa-Po Chung, Nwe Nwe, Yu-Cheng Hsieh, Cheng-Hung Li,
Yenn-Jiang Lin, et al.**
Impact of Amiodarone Therapy on the Ablation Outcome of Ventricular Tachycardia in Arrhythmogenic Right Ventricular Cardiomyopathy
Reprinted from: *J. Clin. Med.* **2022**, *11*, 7265, doi:10.3390/jcm11247265 49

Feng Hu, Minhua Zang, Lihui Zheng, Wensheng Chen, Jinrui Guo, Zhongpeng Du, et al.
The Impact of COVID-19 Pandemic on the Clinical Practice Patterns in Atrial Fibrillation: A Multicenter Clinician Survey in China
Reprinted from: *J. Clin. Med.* **2022**, *11*, 6469, doi:10.3390/jcm11216469 61

Hong-Wei Tan, Wei-Dong Gao, Xin-Hua Wang, Zhi-Song Chen and Xue-Bo Liu
A Four-Stepwise Electrocardiographic Algorithm for Differentiation of Ventricular Arrhythmias Originated from Left Ventricular Outflow Tract
Reprinted from: *J. Clin. Med.* **2022**, *11*, 6398, doi:10.3390/jcm11216398 75

Lei Ding, Hongda Zhang, Fengyuan Yu, Lijie Mi, Wei Hua, Shu Zhang, et al.
Angiographic Characteristics of the Vein of Marshall in Patients with and without Atrial Fibrillation
Reprinted from: *J. Clin. Med.* **2022**, *11*, 5384, doi:10.3390/jcm11185384 87

Lingping Xu, Yixin Zhao, Yichao Duan, Rui Wang, Junlong Hou, Jing Wang, et al.
Clinical Efficacy of Catheter Ablation in the Treatment of Vasovagal Syncope
Reprinted from: *J. Clin. Med.* **2022**, *11*, 5371, doi:10.3390/jcm11185371 99

Lei Wang, Shipeng Dang, Shuangxiong Chen, Jin-Yu Sun, Ru-Xing Wang and Feng Pan
Deep-Learning-Based Detection of Paroxysmal Supraventricular Tachycardia Using Sinus-Rhythm Electrocardiograms
Reprinted from: *J. Clin. Med.* **2022**, *11*, 4578, doi:10.3390/jcm11154578 111

Binhao Wang, Bin He, Guohua Fu, Mingjun Feng, Xianfeng Du, Jing Liu, et al.
Safety and Efficacy of Left Atrial Catheter Ablation in Patients with Left Atrial Appendage Occlusion Devices
Reprinted from: *J. Clin. Med.* **2022**, *11*, 3110, doi:10.3390/jcm11113110 . . . . **121**

Fei Tong and Zhijun Sun
Strategies for Safe Implantation and Effective Performance of Single-Chamber and Dual-Chamber Leadless Pacemakers
Reprinted from: *J. Clin. Med.* **2023**, *12*, 2454, doi:10.3390/jcm12072454 . . . . **131**

Filippo Toriello, Massimo Saviano, Andrea Faggiano, Domitilla Gentile, Giovanni Provenzale, Alberto Vincenzo Pollina, et al.
Cardiac Implantable Electronic Devices Infection Assessment, Diagnosis and Management: A Review of the Literature
Reprinted from: *J. Clin. Med.* **2022**, *11*, 5898, doi:10.3390/jcm11195898 . . . . **151**

Wenfeng Shangguan, Gang Xu, Xin Wang, Nan Zhang, Xingpeng Liu, Guangping Li, et al.
Stereotactic Radiotherapy: An Alternative Option for Refractory Ventricular Tachycardia to Drug and Ablation Therapy
Reprinted from: *J. Clin. Med.* **2022**, *11*, 3549, doi:10.3390/jcm11123549 . . . . **169**

Feng Li, Lei Zhang, Li-Da Wu, Zhi-Yuan Zhang, Huan-Huan Liu, Zhen-Ye Zhang, et al.
Do Elderly Patients with Atrial Fibrillation Have Comparable Ablation Outcomes Compared to Younger Ones? Evidence from Pooled Clinical Studies
Reprinted from: *J. Clin. Med.* **2022**, *11*, 4468, doi:10.3390/jcm11154468 . . . . **179**

About the Editor

Tong Liu

Dr. Tong Liu graduated from Tianjin Medical University in 2000, and received his PhD in 2006. He received training in electrophysiology research at the Heart Institute, Cedars-Sinai Medical Center, Los Angeles, from 2009 to 2010. He has a particular interest in cardiac electrophysiology, and for the past decade he has focused on research on atrial fibrillation. He is now a Committee Member of the Chinese Society of Pacing and Electrophysiology (CSPE) and Youth Committee Member of Chinese Society of Cardiology (CSC). His work was supported by grants from the National Natural Science Foundation of China (30900618, 81270245, 81570298, 81970270, 82170327). He is the Editor in Chief of *Current Cardiology Reviews*, and is also on the editorial boards of *Journal of Clinical Medicine*, *Cardiovascular Diagnosis and Therapy*, *PACE*, *BMC Cardiovascular Disorders*, *International Journal of Arrhythmia*, and *Cardio-Oncology*, and serves as a peer-reviewer for more than 50 scientific journals. He has published over 500 articles in peer-reviewed medical journals.

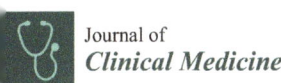

Article

Clinical Influence of Ethanol Infusion in the Vein of Marshall on Left Atrial Appendage Occlusion: Results of Feasibility and Safety during Implantation and at 60-Day Follow-Up

Yibo Ma [1,†], Miaoyang Hu [1,†], Lanyan Guo [1], Jian Xu [1], Jie Li [1], Qun Yan [1], Huani Pang [1], Jinshui Wang [2], Ping Yang [3] and Fu Yi [1,*]

1. Department of Cardiology, Xijing Hospital, Air Force Medical University, Xi'an 710032, China
2. Department of Cardiology, The First Hospital of Hanbin District, Ankang 725000, China
3. Department of Cardiology, Baoji People's Hospital, Baoji 721006, China
* Correspondence: prof_yi@126.com
† These authors contributed equally to this work and share first authorship.

Abstract: Background: Ethanol infusion in the vein of Marshall (EI-VOM) has the advantages of reducing the burden of atrial fibrillation (AF), decreasing AF recurrence, and facilitating left pulmonary vein isolation and mitral isthmus bidirectional conduction block. Moreover, it can lead to prominent edema of the coumadin ridge and atrial infarction. Whether these lesions will affect the efficacy and safety of left atrial appendage occlusion (LAAO) has not yet been reported. Objectives: To explore the clinical outcome of EI-VOM on LAAO during implantation and after 60 days of follow-up. Methods: A total of 100 consecutive patients who underwent radiofrequency catheter ablation combined with LAAO were enrolled in this study. Patients who also underwent EI-VOM at the same period of LAAO were assigned to group 1 ($n = 26$), and those who did not undergo EI-VOM were assigned to group 2 ($n = 74$). The feasibility outcomes included intra-procedural LAAO parameters and follow-up LAAO results involving device-related thrombus, a peri-device leak (PDL), and adequate occlusion (defined as a PDL ≤ 5 mm). Safety outcomes were defined as the composites of severe adverse events and cardiac function. Outpatient follow-up was performed 60 days post-procedure. Results: Intra-procedural LAAO parameters, including the rate of device reselection, rate of device redeployment, rate of intra-procedural PDLs, and total LAAO time, were comparable between groups. Furthermore, intra-procedural adequate occlusion was achieved in all patients. After a median of 68 days, 94 (94.0%) patients received their first radiographic examination. Device-related thrombus was not detected in the follow-up populations. The incidence of follow-up PDLs was similar between the two groups (28.0% vs. 33.3%, $p = 0.803$). The incidence of adequate occlusion was comparable between groups (96.0% vs. 98.6%, $p = 0.463$). In group 1, none of the patients experienced severe adverse events. Ethanol infusion significantly reduced the right atrial diameter. Conclusions: The present study showed that undergoing an EI-VOM procedure did not impact the operation or effectiveness of LAAO. Combining EI-VOM with LAAO was safe and effective.

Keywords: atrial fibrillation; vein of Marshall; left atrial appendage occlusion; peri-device leak; cardiac computed tomography angiography

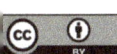

1. Introduction

Atrial fibrillation (AF), one of the most common arrhythmias, can lead to a variety of disabling and fatal complications, particularly stroke and systemic embolism [1]. Left atrial appendage occlusion (LAAO), a nonpharmacological treatment for thromboprophylaxis, has been proven to be non-inferior to warfarin or novel oral anticoagulants in high-risk AF populations [2–4]. Because both LAAO and radiofrequency catheter ablation (RFCA) are percutaneous interventional procedures and need to be performed in a catheterization laboratory, many operators combine both procedures in a single procedure to not only achieve long-term stroke prevention without lifeline anticoagulation but also to acquire effective rhythm control. Previous studies have shown that combining LAAO and RFCA can reduce procedure costs without affecting the long-term efficacy of the individual procedures, and their combination does not increase the incidence of procedure-related complications [5,6].

RFCA alone may be insufficient to achieve ideal rhythm control in persistent AF patients because electrical pulmonary vein isolation (PVI) is difficult to achieve, and the benefits of additional linear ablation or complex fractionated electrogram ablation are unclear [1,7,8]. Moreover, ethanol infusion in the vein of Marshall (EI-VOM) is a novel treatment for persistent AF. It has the advantage of eliminating AF triggers, facilitating a PVI and bidirectional peri-mitral block, achieving local denervation, and cutting the pathological conduction branches [9]. In addition, EI-VOM in combination with RFCA can lead to better rhythm control in patients with persistent AF without excessive complications compared to RFCA alone [10]. In a single-arm study, it was shown that EI-VOM combined with RFCA significantly improved left atrial function [11]. Thus, EI-VOM should be a potential therapeutic measure.

It should be noted that EI-VOM can generate prominent edema of the coumadin ridge and lead to atrial infarction. Whether these lesions will affect the efficacy and safety of LAAO has not yet been reported. Several concerns need to be addressed: (1) whether EI-VOM affects implantation of the closure device; (2) whether EI-VOM leads to a greater leak; and (3) whether patients will experience more clinical adverse events. To address these concerns, this study was developed to explore the clinical influence of EI-VOM on LAAO during implantation and after 60 days of follow-up.

2. Materials and Methods

2.1. Study Populations

This study was a single-center, retrospective cohort study. One hundred consecutive patients who underwent a one-step procedure (RFCA combined with LAAO) were included from February 2020 to August 2022 at the First Affiliated Hospital of Air Force Medical University. Patients were enrolled if they met the following criteria: (1) age between 18 and 85 years; (2) finished at least 60 days of radiographic follow-up; and (3) intracardiac echocardiography-guided LAAO. Exclusion criteria were as follows (1) valvular AF, including but not limited to moderate or severe mitral stenosis; (2) alcohol allergy; (3) a left atrial diameter of greater than 65 mm. This study adhered to the principles of the Declaration of Helsinki and was approved by the institutional ethics committee of the First Affiliated Hospital of Air Force Medical University. Each patient signed an informed written consent form before the procedure.

2.2. Procedure

2.2.1. Ethanol Infusion in the Vein of Marshall

EI-VOM was performed as previously described [9–11]. Firstly, a 6F guide catheter was advanced into the coronary sinus to obtain a venogram and to identify the opening of the vein of Marshall (VOM) (Figure 1A). If found, an angiography wire was advanced through the 6F catheter and into the VOM, and subsequently, an OTW balloon (2 mm * 8 mm) was advanced over the wire and positioned in the ostium of the VOM. A second coronary sinus venogram was performed after the balloon was inflated to reveal the anatomy of the VOM (Figure 1B). Next, the balloon was positioned on the distal part of the VOM. After the inflation of the balloon, the first ethanol injection was performed. Finally, the balloon was deflated and returned to the proximal end of the VOM, during which inflation and ethanol injection were repeated approximately 4 times. Contrast infiltration indicated procedure success (Figure 1C). After EI-VOM, RFCA and electrophysiological studies were performed.

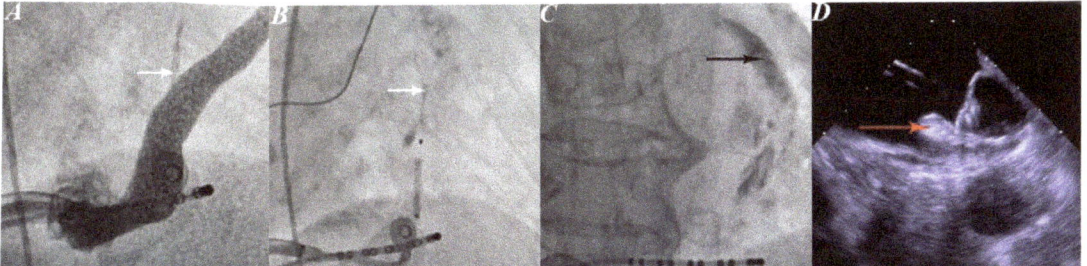

Figure 1. Steps of the procedure. Panel (**A**) VOM (white arrow) in Coronary sinus venogram. Panel (**B**) Vein of Marshall venogram was performed after the balloon was inflated to reveal the anatomy of the VOM (white arrow). Panel (**C**) Contrast infiltration (black arrow). Panel (**D**) Watchman closure implantation. Prominent edema of the coumadin ridge (red arrow) in the echocardiographic image. VOM, vein of Marshall.

2.2.2. Left Atrial Appendage Occlusion

Intracardiac echocardiography (ICE)-guided LAAO was performed as previously described [12]. In brief, the radiofrequency catheter was replaced with a device delivery sheath. An ICE probe was advanced into the left atrium along with the device delivery sheath through the same atrial septal puncture hole. Left atrial appendage (LAA) morphology was first acquired to confirm that the device that was selected before the procedure was appropriate. Then, the closure device was implanted under the guidance of ICE. During occlusion, prominent edema of the coumadin ridge was seen (Figure 1D). Both a Watchman device (Boston Scientific) and a LACbes device (PushMed, Shanghai, China) were used as alternatives. If occlusion was appropriate, the closure device was released. At the end of the LAAO procedure, hemostasis was ensured by manual compression.

2.3. Clinical Outcomes and Follow-Up

In this study, clinical outcomes included feasibility and safety outcomes. The feasibility outcomes included intra-procedural LAAO parameters and follow-up LAAO results. Intra-procedural LAAO parameters included the successful implantation of the first selected device, device redeployment, intra-procedural peri-device leak (PDL), intra-procedural adequate occlusion (defined as a PDL ≤ 5 mm), and total LAAO procedure time (defined as the duration from the first angiography to device release). Follow-up LAAO results included device-related thrombus (DRT), PDL, and adequate occlusion. The safety outcome in this study was the composite of severe adverse events (SAEs) within 30 days [5,13,14]. SAEs included death, ischemic or hemorrhagic stroke, systemic embolism, transient ischemia attack, air or device embolism, pericardial tamponade requiring drainage, and major bleeding requiring transfusion. Changes in cardiac function before and after EI-VOM served as an additional safety outcome. Patients were treated with novel oral anticoagulants post-procedure, and additional single antiplatelet therapy was prescribed to patients who recently underwent coronary revascularization. Reporting on clinical outcomes occurred during periprocedural care until 60 days of follow-up post-procedure.

2.4. Computed Tomography Assessment

Cardiac computed tomography angiography (CCTA) was preferred in detecting DRT or PDL, the details of which have been previously described [15]. A second-generation, dual-source Computed Tomography scanner (Somatom Definition Flash, Siemens Healthcare) was used to show the closure device, LAA, and other adjacent structures. First, a non-contrast Computed Tomography scan was performed. Then, a volume of 50 mL contrast medium was injected, and a region of interest was selected. Once ideal scan acquisition timing was achieved, an arterial phase scan was executed. A venous phase scan (delayed imaging) was performed 30–60 s after the start of the arterial phase scan. The image data was stored on a DVD-R and evaluated by both imaging experts and cardiologists. Finally, the results were integrated. In case the patient refused to receive a CCTA examination, TEE was used as an alternative.

DRT was detected on the arterial and venous phase images and distinguished from the metal artifact on non-contrast images. LAA patency was observed on the venous phase images and defined as LAA density $\geq$ 100 Hounsfield units or $\geq$ 150% of that measured at the same site for the arterial phase [13]. If LAA patency was present, PDL was defined as the passage of contrast medium along the margins of the closure device (Figure 2).

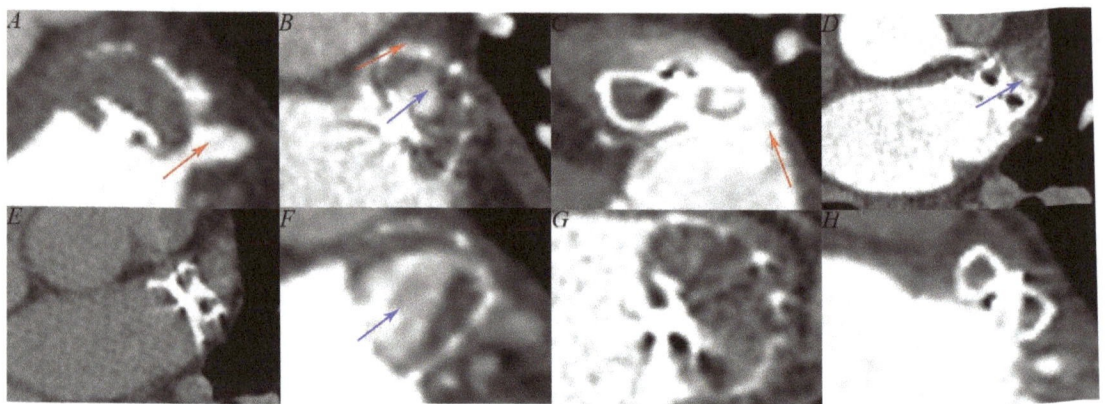

Figure 2. The patterns of left atrial appendage patency. Panel (**A**) Peri-device leak (red arrow) only in Watchman device. Panel (**B**) Peri-device leak (red arrow) with an intra-device leak (blue arrow) in Watchman device. Panel (**C**) Peri-device leak (red arrow) only in LACbes device. Panel (**D**) Intra-device leak (blue arrow) only in LACbes device. Panel (**E**) No contrast image of panel (**D**). Panel (**F**) Intra-device leak only in Watchman device (blue arrow). Panel (**G**) Non-patency left atrial appendage in Watchman device. Panel (**H**) Non-patency left atrial appendage in LACbes device.

2.5. Statistical Analysis

Statistical analysis was performed using R 4.2.0 (Robert Gentleman & Ross Ihaka, Auckland, New Zealand) and SPSS Statistics 26.0 (IBM SPSS Inc., Chicago, USA). Normality distribution was examined by the Shapiro-Wilk test. Continuous variables with a normal distribution are described as the mean $\pm$ standard deviation and were compared using a 1-way analysis of variance or paired t-test. Non-normally distributed continuous variables are expressed as the median with interquartile range (IQR) and were compared using the Mann-Whitney U test. Categorical variables are described as counts (percentages) and were compared using the Chi-square test or Fisher's exact probability test according to positive rates. A 2-sided p-value $\leq$ 0.05 was considered statistically significant.

3. Results

3.1. Baseline Characteristics

A total of 100 consecutive patients were enrolled in this study, with 26 patients in group 1 (underwent EI-VOM) and 74 patients in group 2 (did not undergo EI-VOM), respectively. Baseline characteristics were consistent between the two groups. The mean age was 64.1 $\pm$ 9.0 years, and the majority were male. The medians of the CHA_2DS_2-VASc score and HASBLED score were 3.0 (IQR: 2.0, 4.0) and 2.0 (IQR: 1.0, 3.0), respectively. In both groups, most patients had persistent AF. Twenty-three patients (23.0%) had a history of cardiac embolism, and 15 patients (15.0%) had a history of non-cardiac stroke. The details of the baseline characteristics are listed in Table 1.

Table 1. Patient characteristics at baseline.

	Group 1 (n = 26)	Group 2 (n = 74)	p-Value
Demographics			
Male sex	14 (53.8)	51 (68.9)	0.232
Age, years	65.4 ± 10.4	63.8 ± 8.6	0.553
BMI, kg/m^2	25.0 ± 2.8	25.5 ± 3.1	0.447
AF overview			
CHA$_2$DS$_2$-VASc score	3.0 (2.0, 4.0)	3.0 (2.0, 4.0)	0.674
HASBLED score	2.0 (1.0, 3.0)	2.0 (1.0, 3.0)	0.794
AF pattern			0.353
Paroxysmal	8 (30.8)	32 (43.2)	–
Non-paroxysmal	18 (69.2)	42 (56.8)	–
AF duration, months	24.0 (5.0, 48.0)	12.0 (4.0, 36.0)	0.544
Comorbidities			
Heart failure	8 (30.8)	20 (27.0)	0.801
Hypertension	13 (50.0)	42 (56.8)	0.648
Type II diabetes	5 (19.2)	15 (20.3)	1.000
Previous stroke/TIA/SE	11 (42.3)	27 (36.5)	0.643
Coronary heart disease	6 (23.1)	25 (33.8)	0.460
Bleeding tendency	6 (23.1)	16 (21.6)	1.000
Echocardiographic index			
Left atrial diameter, mm	46.2 ± 6.0	44.7 ± 5.6	0.247
Left ventricular ejection fraction, %	56.5 ± 5.9	55.9 ± 5.9	0.651

BMI = body mass index; AF = atrial fibrillation; TIA = transient ischemic attack; SE = systemic embolism.

3.2. Intra-Procedural Left Atrial Appendage Occlusion Parameters

Periprocedural characteristics are summarized in Table 2. The majority morphology of the LAA was cauliflower, and the orifice diameter and depth of LAA were comparable between groups. Most patients in both groups chose a Watchman device.

Table 2. Periprocedural characteristics and feasibility.

	Group 1 (n = 26)	Group 2 (n = 74)	p-Value
Periprocedural characteristics			
LAA morphology			0.346
Cauliflower	20 (76.9)	53 (71.6)	–
Chicken wing	2 (7.7)	10 (13.5)	–
Reversed chicken wing	3 (11.5)	2 (2.7)	–
Windsock	1 (3.8)	7 (9.5)	–
Cactus	0 (0.0)	2 (2.7)	–
LAA ostia diameter, mm	22.9 ± 4.0	23.0 ± 3.8	0.942
LAA depth, mm	23.6 ± 4.7	24.1 ± 3.1	0.571 [1]
Device			0.073
Watchman	18 (69.2)	64 (86.5)	–
LACbes	8 (30.8)	10 (13.5)	–
Periprocedural feasibility			
LAAO time, min	24.0 (14.0, 34.0)	20.0 (16.0, 28.0)	0.553
LAAO success	26 (100.0)	74 (100.0)	1.000
Device reselection	1 (3.8)	5 (6.8)	1.000
Redeployment	7 (26.9)	33 (44.6)	0.162
Incidence of PDL	5 (19.2)	13 (17.6)	1.000
<3 mm jet size	3 (11.5)	7 (9.5)	0.717
3–5 mm jet size	2 (7.7)	6 (8.1)	1.000
Mean size, mm	2.4 ± 1.1	2.6 ± 0.7	0.559

[1] Patients who underwent LACbes implantation were excluded when evaluating the mean depth. LAA = left atrial appendage; LAAO = left atrial appendage occlusion; PDL = peri-device leak.

All intra-procedural LAAO parameters were comparable (Table 2). One patient (3.8%) in group 1 and five patients (6.8%) in group 2 underwent at least two different device implantation attempts (p = 1.000). Seven patients (26.9%) in group 1 and 33 patients (44.6%) in group 2 had their devices redeployed before final release (p = 0.162). Adequate intra-procedural device deployment was achieved in all patients, and ICE and fluoroscopy confirmed that five (19.2%) and 13 (17.6%) patients had PDLs < 5 mm in groups 1 and 2, respectively (p = 1.000). Three patients (11.5%) in group 1 and seven patients (7.7%)

in group 2 had <3 mm intra-procedural PDLs (*p* = 0.717); two patients (9.5%) in group 1 and six patients (8.1%) in group 2 had 3–5 mm intra-procedural PDLs (*p* = 1.000). The procedure time spent on LAAO in groups 1 and 2 was 24.0 (IQR: 14.0, 34.0) min and 20.0 (16.0, 28.0) min, respectively (*p* = 0.553).

3.3. Follow-Up Left Atrial Appendage Occlusion Results

After a median of 68 (IQR: 59, 89) days, 25 patients (96.2%) in group 1 and 69 patients (93.2%) in group 2 received their first radiographic examinations (Table 3). A total of 66 patients (70.2%) received a CCTA examination. More patients in group 1 chose CCTA as their follow-up examination (88.5% vs. 58.1%, *p* = 0.005). Follow-up results were comparable between the two groups: DRT or suspicious DRT was not found in the follow-up cohort; seven (28.0%) and 23 (33.3%) patients had PDLs in groups 1 and 2, respectively (*p* = 0.803); two patients (8.0%) in group 1 and 11 patients (15.9%) in group 2 had < 3 mm PDLs (*p* = 0.502); four patients (16.0%) in group 1 and 11 patients (15.9%) in group 2 had 3–5 mm PDLs (*p* = 1.000); and 24 patients (96.0%) in group 1 and 68 patients (98.6%) in group 2 achieved adequate occlusion (*p* = 0.463). The LAA patency in patients who received CCTA follow-up was also evaluated (Figure 3). A total of 31 patients (52.2%) had patency LAA, with 11 patients (51.3%) in group 1 and 21 patients (52.3%) in group 2 (Fisher exact test, *p* = 1.000).

Table 3. Follow-up feasibility.

	Group 1 (*n* = 25)	Group 2 (*n* = 69)	*p*-Value
Time to review, days	69.0 (60.0, 87.0)	67.0 (57.0, 88.0)	0.827
Radiographic examination			0.005
CCTA follow-up	23 (88.5)	43 (58.1)	–
TEE follow-up	2 (11.5)	26 (35.1) [1]	–
DRT or suspicious DRT	0 (0.0)	0 (0.0)	1.000
Adequate occlusion	24 (96.0)	68 (98.6)	0.463
PDL	7 (28.0)	23 (33.3)	0.803
<3 mm jet size	2 (8.0)	11 (15.9)	0.502
3–5 mm jet size	4 (16.0)	11 (15.9)	1.000

[1] One patient received both TEE and CCTA. CCTA = cardiac computed tomography angiography; TEE = transesophageal echocardiography; DRT = device-related thrombus; PDL = peri-device leak.

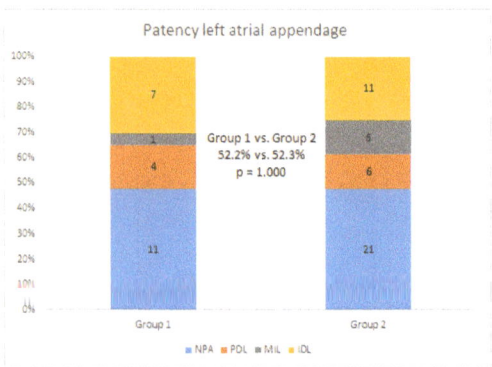

Figure 3. Follow-up results in patients who received cardiac computed tomography angiography. NPA = no patency left atrial appendage; PDL = peri-device leak; MIL = mixed leak; IDL = intra-device leak.

3.4. Safety Outcomes

In group 1, none of the patients experienced SAEs. In group 2, one patient (1.4%) experienced major bleeding. The patient improved after the transfusion.

Cardiac function was evaluated in 25 follow-up patients before and after EI-VOM, and the results are presented in Figure 4. After 2 months of follow-up, the post-procedural right atrial diameter was significantly reduced (42.5 ± 5.4 vs. 40.0 ± 5.9, $p = 0.02$), while the left atrial diameter (46.3 ± 6.1 vs. 45.0 ± 4.7, $p = 0.23$) and left ventricular ejection fraction (56.7 ± 5.9 vs. 56.2 ± 5.0, $p = 0.64$) did not significantly different between pre-procedure and post-procedure.

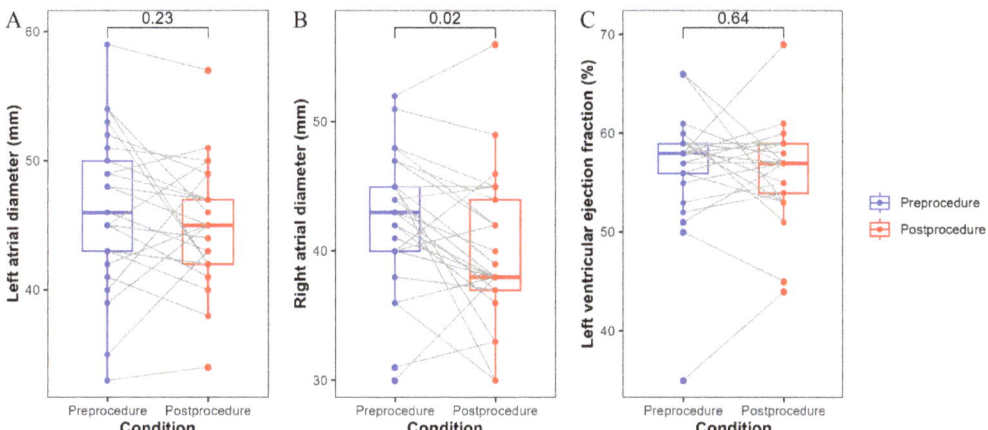

Figure 4. Cardiac function pre- and post-ethanol infusion. Panel (**A**) Changes in the left atrial diameter; Panel (**B**) Changes in the right atrial diameter; Panel (**C**) Changes in the left ventricular ejection fraction. Variables were compared using the paired *t*-test.

4. Discussion

In this study, the clinical influence of EI-VOM on LAAO was reported during implantation and after 60 days of follow-up. The following was found: (1) EI-VOM did not make the LAAO procedure more difficult because all intra-procedural LAAO parameters were comparable between the two groups; (2) group-to-group differences in follow-up LAAO results were comparable; and (3) in group 1, none of the patients experienced SAEs. Taken together, these results show that combining EI-VOM with LAAO is feasible and safe.

4.1. Intra-Procedural Feasibility

Electrophysiologists face the same challenges, whether performing the one-step procedure or a combination of EI-VOM, RFCA, and LAAO. For the one-step procedure, the main problem operators face is edema of the coumadin ridge [6]. Phillips et al. reported their 5-year single-center experience with the one-step procedure. Although coumadin ridge edema was common, adequate occlusion was achieved in all patients, thereby suggesting that edema did not affect the LAAO operation [16]. In fact, many studies have reported that the one-step procedure did not decrease adequate occlusion rates when compared to LAAO alone [6]. It is worth noting that the coumadin ridge is the corresponding endocardial structure of the ligament of Marshall, so EI-VOM combined with RFCA could lead to more severe edema than RFCA alone (Figure 2D). However, in our study, we demonstrated that EI-VOM did not affect the implantation of the closure device.

In the present study, it was shown that the rate of follow-up PDLs was increased compared to intra-procedural PDLs in both group 1 and group 2. This might be related to the dissipation of the coumadin ridge edema. This indicates that edema of the coumadin ridge has a substantial influence on PDL. Unfortunately, the degree of edema was not measured. So far, no accurate measure of coumadin ridge edema has been published [17]. Attempts at further comparisons of edema pre- and post-procedure or between groups were abandoned in our study. When performing the three-dimensional reconstruction of the left atrial pre-EI-VOM, the ICE probe was placed in the right atrial area. While executing the LAAO operation, the ICE probe was deployed in the left atrium. This resulted in the lack of comparability of measurements pre- and post-procedure. In addition to PVI, ablation targets in our study varied because of differences in the atrial substrate. This resulted in the lack of comparability of measurements between patients. Therefore, the results for intra-procedural feasibility are relatively crude. The development of a standard measure program will be required to further explore what degree of edema will occur and its effects.

4.2. Follow-Up Feasibility

In recent years, several studies have reported the value of CCTA in LAAO procedure follow-up. Zhao et al. reported their single-center experience in detecting incomplete occlusion by CCTA after the one-step procedure [18]. In the SWISS-APERO trial, both TEE and CCTA were used simultaneously as follow-up examinations after LAAO [13] The results of both studies showed that the sensitivity of CCTA in detecting a leak was better than that of TEE. Considering the above, in this study, CCTA was chosen as the primary follow-up examination. CCTA could be detected as a very small PDL, as shown in Figure 2B. Our study revealed that the EI-VOM procedure did not affect the follow-up results for LAAO: DRT or suspicious DRT was not observed in our study; the occlusion rate was adequate, and PDLs were comparable between groups. When considering the degree of PDL, no statistical significance was observed between groups. In addition, adequate occlusion was comparable between groups, and so was patency LAA. As previously mentioned, edema of the coumadin ridge has a substantial influence on PDL. Furthermore, atrial infarction, which was caused by ethanol injection, may also affect the incidence and size of the PDL. The VENUS trial showed that EI-VOM could damage 4.9 ± 3.2 cm^2 of atrial tissue on average [10], which included part of the LAA tissue. LAA infarction might increase the incidence and rate of PDL; it may also prevent the endothelialization of the closure device and even cause acute and delayed cardiac tamponade. One of our primary concerns was whether tissue loss affects the efficacy of the procedure. We are currently providing a possibility that the damage caused by EI-VOM will not increase the incidence and degree of PDL, as well as the incidence of patency LAA.

The PDL in our study was comparable with that presented in previous reports. Zhao et al. reported that the 6-month PDL in the CCTA examination was 39.3% (33/84). The SWISS-APERO trial showed that the total incidence of peri-device leakages (PDL and mixed leak) in the Amulet group and Watchman group were 22.9% (24/105) and 34.0% (34/100), respectively. These results also prove that EI-VOM will not increase the risk of PDL.

4.3. Safety Outcome

As mentioned earlier, safety considerations for atrial infarction were another critical concern. The present study showed that none of the patients experienced pericardial effusion or tamponade. Thus, our results do not indicate an increased risk of pericardial effusion caused by atrial infarction.

In previous studies, the safety of the one-step procedure has been widely reported, and the RECORD real-world study showed that combining catheter ablation, whether using radiofrequency or a cryoballoon, with LAAO did not increase the risk of SAEs [5,6]. The safety of EI-VOM combined with RFCA has also been reported in previous studies. Valderrábano et al. showed that the blood alcohol level after EI-VOM was undetectable at regular doses [19]. The VENUS trial and a real-world study showed that combining EI-VOM with RFCA did not increase the risk of clinical adverse events [10,15]. Chen et al. shared their single-center experience with a one-step procedure. More than 1000 patients were enrolled, and the safety and efficacy were supported. Patients who underwent EI-VOM combined with LAAO were also included. However, these patients were not analyzed separately [20]. Our results showed that combining EI-VOM with LAAO did not increase the risk of clinical adverse events. In group 1, none of the patients experienced

SAEs. Recently, the concept of a same-day discharge after LAAO was proposed, and its effectiveness and safety were preliminarily verified [21,22]. These findings provide a clear direction for our further clinical practice.

In addition, the short-term changes in cardiac function pre- and post-procedure were evaluated. According to the echocardiographic findings, ethanol infusion significantly reduced the right atrial diameter. Derval et al. reported their single-center experience in EI-VOM combined with RFCA; the atrial function also served as an additional feasibility endpoint. Significant improvements in transmitral A-wave and ejection fraction were observed at day 1 and month 12 post-ablation [11]. These improvements may be attributed to better rhythm control. It has been widely verified that EI-VOM combined with RFCA significantly reduced the risk of arrhythmia recurrence compared to RFCA alone [10,23,24]. Further follow-up is needed to determine the long-term improvements in the left atrial diameter and left ventricular ejection fraction.

4.4. Limitations

There were several limitations to this study. The sample size of the study was small, and the ratio of the intervention group (group 1) to the control group (group 2) was 1:3, which may limit the power to detect potential differences. We abandoned EI-VOM for those patients who experienced VOM dissection intra-procedure in order to not increase the risk of pericardial effusion [14]. The use of two completely different types of closure devices may introduce confounding bias.

5. Conclusions

Combining ethanol infusion in the vein of Marshall and left atrial appendage occlusion is feasible and safe. The intra-procedure parameters and follow-up results were comparable with those of the one-step procedure both in our cohort as well as in previous reports. This combination did not increase the risk of clinical adverse events. Furthermore, ethanol infusion significantly reduced the right atrial diameter. Large-scale and long-term prospective clinical follow-up is warranted to further complement our findings.

Author Contributions: Conceptualization, F.Y.; methodology, Y.M. and M.H.; software, L.G.; validation, J.X. and J.L.; formal analysis, L.G.; investigation, H.P. and J.W.; resources, F.Y.; data curation, Q.Y. and P.Y.; writing—original draft preparation, Y.M. and M.H.; writing—review and editing, F.Y. and L.G.; supervision, J.X. and J.L.; project administration, F.Y. All authors have read and agreed to the published version of the manuscript.

Funding: This research was funded by the General program of the National Natural Science Foundation of China, grant number 81970274.

Institutional Review Board Statement: The study was conducted according to the guidelines of the Declaration of Helsinki and approved by the Institutional Review Board of the First Affiliated Hospital of Air Force Military Medical University.

Informed Consent Statement: Informed consent was obtained from all subjects involved in the study.

Data Availability Statement: The datasets used and/or analyzed during the current study can be available from the corresponding author upon reasonable request.

Conflicts of Interest: The authors declare no conflict of interest.

References

1. Hindricks, G.; Potpara, T.; Dagres, N.; Arbelo, E.; Bax, J.J.; Blomström-Lundqvist, C.; Boriani, G.; Castella, M.; Dan, G.A.; Dilaveris, P.E.; et al. 2020 ESC Guidelines for the diagnosis and management of atrial fibrillation developed in collaboration with the European Association for Cardio-Thoracic Surgery (EACTS). *Eur. Heart J.* **2021**, *42*, 373–498. [PubMed]
2. Reddy, V.Y.; Sievert, H.; Halperin, J.; Doshi, S.K.; Buchbinder, M.; Neuzil, P.; Huber, K.; Whisenant, B.; Kar, S.; Swarup, V.; et al. Percutaneous left atrial appendage closure vs warfarin for atrial fibrillation: A randomized clinical trial. *JAMA* **2014**, *312*, 1988–1998. [CrossRef] [PubMed]

3. Holmes, D.R., Jr.; Kar, S.; Price, M.J.; Whisenant, B.; Sievert, H.; Doshi, S.K.; Huber, K.; Reddy, V.Y. Prospective randomized evaluation of the Watchman Left Atrial Appendage Closure device in patients with atrial fibrillation versus long-term warfarin therapy: The PREVAIL trial. *J. Am. Coll. Cardiol.* **2014**, *64*, 1–12. [CrossRef]
4. Osmancik, P.; Herman, D.; Neuzil, P.; Hala, P.; Taborsky, M.; Kala, P.; Poloczek, M.; Stasek, J.; Haman, L.; Branny, M.; et al. Left Atrial Appendage Closure Versus Direct Oral Anticoagulants in High-Risk Patients With Atrial Fibrillation. *J. Am. Coll. Cardiol.* **2020**, *75*, 3122–3135. [CrossRef]
5. Su, F.; Gao, C.; Liu, J.; Ning, Z.; He, B.; Liu, Y.; Xu, Y.; Yang, B.; Li, Y.; Zhang, J.; et al. Periprocedural Outcomes Associated With Use of a Left Atrial Appendage Occlusion Device in China. *JAMA Netw. Open* **2022**, *5*, e2214594. [CrossRef]
6. Chen, M.; Wang, Z.Q.; Wang, Q.S.; Sun, J.; Zhang, P.P.; Feng, X.F.; Li, W.; Yu, Y.; Liu, B.; Mo, B.F.; et al. One-stop strategy for treatment of atrial fibrillation: Feasibility and safety of combining catheter ablation and left atrial appendage closure in a single procedure. *Chin. Med. J.* **2020**, *133*, 1422–1428. [CrossRef]
7. Parameswaran, R.; Al-Kaisey, A.M.; Kalman, J.M. Catheter ablation for atrial fibrillation: Current indications and evolving technologies. *Nat. Rev. Cardiol.* **2021**, *18*, 210–225. [CrossRef]
8. Verma, A.; Jiang, C.Y.; Betts, T.R.; Chen, J.; Deisenhofer, I.; Mantovan, R.; Macle, L.; Morillo, C.A.; Haverkamp, W.; Weerasooriya, R.; et al. Approaches to catheter ablation for persistent atrial fibrillation. *N. Engl. J. Med.* **2015**, *372*, 1812–1822. [CrossRef]
9. Valderrábano, M. Vein of Marshall ethanol infusion in the treatment of atrial fibrillation: From concept to clinical practice. *Heart Rhythm.* **2021**, *18*, 1074–1082. [CrossRef]
10. Valderrábano, M.; Peterson, L.E.; Swarup, V.; Schurmann, P.A.; Makkar, A.; Doshi, R.N.; DeLurgio, D.; Athill, C.A.; Ellenbogen, K.A.; Natale, A.; et al. Effect of Catheter Ablation With Vein of Marshall Ethanol Infusion vs Catheter Ablation Alone on Persistent Atrial Fibrillation: The VENUS Randomized Clinical Trial. *JAMA* **2020**, *324*, 1620–1628. [CrossRef]
11. Derval, N.; Duchateau, J.; Denis, A.; Ramirez, F.D.; Mahida, S.; André, C.; Krisai, P.; Nakatani, Y.; Kitamura, T.; Takigawa, M.; et al. Marshall bundle elimination, Pulmonary vein isolation, and Line completion for ANatomical ablation of persistent atrial fibrillation (Marshall-PLAN): Prospective, single-center study. *Heart Rhythm.* **2021**, *18*, 529–537. [CrossRef] [PubMed]
12. Berti, S.; Pastormerlo, L.E.; Santoro, G.; Brscic, E.; Montorfano, M.; Vignali, L.; Danna, P.; Tondo, C.; Rezzaghi, M.; D'Amico, G.; et al. Intracardiac Versus Transesophageal Echocardiographic Guidance for Left Atrial Appendage Occlusion: The LAAO Italian Multicenter Registry. *JACC Cardiovasc. Interv.* **2018**, *11*, 1086–1092. [CrossRef] [PubMed]
13. Galea, R.; De Marco, F.; Meneveau, N.; Aminian, A.; Anselme, F.; Gräni, C.; Huber, A.T.; Teiger, E.; Iriart, X.; Bosombo, F.B.; et al. Amulet or Watchman Device for Percutaneous Left Atrial Appendage Closure: Primary Results of the SWISS-APERO Randomized Clinical Trial. *Circulation* **2022**, *145*, 724–738. [CrossRef] [PubMed]
14. Kamakura, T.; Derval, N.; Duchateau, J.; Denis, A.; Nakashima, T.; Takagi, T.; Ramirez, F.D.; André, C.; Krisai, P.; Nakatani, Y.; et al. Vein of Marshall Ethanol Infusion: Feasibility, Pitfalls, and Complications in Over 700 Patients. *Circ. Arrhythmia Electrophysiol.* **2021**, *14*, e010001. [CrossRef] [PubMed]
15. Korsholm, K.; Berti, S.; Iriart, X.; Saw, J.; Wang, D.D.; Cochet, H.; Chow, D.; Clemente, A.; De Backer, O.; Jensen, J.M.; et al. Expert Recommendations on Cardiac Computed Tomography for Planning Transcatheter Left Atrial Appendage Occlusion. *JACC Cardiovasc. Interv.* **2020**, *13*, 277–292. [CrossRef] [PubMed]
16. Phillips, K.P.; Walker, D.T.; Humphries, J.A. Combined catheter ablation for atrial fibrillation and Watchman®left atrial appendage occlusion procedures: Five-year experience. *J. Arrhythmia* **2016**, *32*, 119–126. [CrossRef] [PubMed]
17. Gasperetti, A.; Fassini, G.; Tundo, F.; Zucchetti, M.; Dessanai, M.; Tondo, C. A left atrial appendage closure combined procedure review: Past, present, and future perspectives. *J. Cardiovasc. Electrophysiol.* **2019**, *30*, 1345–1351. [CrossRef]
18. Zhao, M.Z.; Chi, R.M.; Yu, Y.; Wang, Q.S.; Sun, J.; Li, W.; Zhang, P.P.; Liu, B.; Feng, X.F.; Zhao, Y.; et al. Value of detecting peri-device leak and incomplete endothelialization by cardiac CT angiography in atrial fibrillation patients post Watchman LAAC combined with radiofrequency ablation. *J. Cardiovasc. Electrophysiol.* **2021**, *32*, 2655–2664. [CrossRef]
19. Valderrábano, M.; Liu, X.; Sasaridis, C.; Sidhu, J.; Little, S.; Khoury, D.S. Ethanol infusion in the vein of Marshall: Adjunctive effects during ablation of atrial fibrillation. *Heart Rhythm.* **2009**, *6*, 1552–1558. [CrossRef]
20. Chen, M.; Sun, J.; Wang, Q.S.; Zhang, P.P.; Li, W.; Zhang, R.; Mo, B.F.; Yu, Y.C.; Cai, X.; Yang, M.; et al. Long-term outcome of combined catheter ablation and left atrial appendage closure in atrial fibrillation patients. *Int. J. Cardiol.* **2022**, *368*, 41–48. [CrossRef]
21. Tan, B.E.; Boppana, L.K.T.; Abdullah, A.S.; Chuprun, D.; Shah, A.; Rao, M.; Bhatt, D.L.; Depta, J.P. Safety and Feasibility of Same-Day Discharge After Left Atrial Appendage Closure With the WATCHMAN Device. *Circ. Cardiovasc. Interv.* **2021**, *14*, e009669. [CrossRef] [PubMed]
22. Kawamura, I.; Kuno, T.; Sahashi, Y.; Tanaka, Y.; Passman, R.; Briasoulis, A.; Malik, A.H. Thirty-day readmission rate of same-day discharge protocol after left atrial appendage occlusion: A propensity score-matched analysis from the National Readmission Database. *Heart Rhythm.* **2022**, *19*, 1819–1825. [CrossRef] [PubMed]

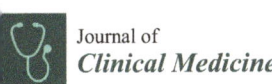

Article

High-Power, Short-Duration Ablation under the Guidance of Relatively Low Ablation Index Values for Paroxysmal Atrial Fibrillation: Long-Term Outcomes and Characteristics of Recurrent Atrial Arrhythmias

Shuyu Jin [1,2,†], Weidong Lin [2,†], Xianhong Fang [2], Hongtao Liao [2], Xianzhang Zhan [2], Lu Fu [2], Junrong Jiang [2], Xingdong Ye [2], Huiyi Liu [2], Yanlin Chen [2], Sijia Pu [2,3], Shulin Wu [2], Hai Deng [1,2,*] and Yumei Xue [1,2,*]

1. The Second School of Clinical Medicine, Southern Medical University, Guangzhou 510515, China
2. Guangdong Provincial People's Hospital (Guangdong Academy of Medical Sciences), Southern Medical University, Guangzhou 510080, China
3. School of Medicine, South China University of Technology, Guangzhou 510006, China
* Correspondence: doctordh@hotmail.com (H.D.); xymgdci@163.com (Y.X.)
† These authors contributed equally to this work.

Abstract: Objective: The purpose of this study was to evaluate the difference in effectiveness and safety of high-power, short-duration (HPSD) radiofrequency catheter ablation (RFA) guided by relatively low ablation index (AI) values and conventional RFA in paroxysmal atrial fibrillation (PAF) patients. Methods: The HPSD RFA strategy (40–50 W, AI 350–400 for anterior, 320–350 for posterior wall; $n = 547$) was compared with the conventional RFA strategy (25–40 W, without AI; $n = 396$) in PAF patients who underwent their first ablation. Propensity-score matching analyses were used to compare the outcomes of the two groups while controlling for confounders. Results: After using propensity-score matching analysis, the HPSD group showed a higher early recurrence rate (22.727% vs. 13.636%, $p = 0.003$), similar late recurrence rate, and comparable safety ($p = 0.604$) compared with the conventional group. For late recurrent atrial arrhythmia types, the rate of regular atrial tachycardia was significantly higher in the HPSD group ($p = 0.013$). Additionally, the rate of chronic pulmonary vein reconnection and non-pulmonary vein triggers during repeat procedures was similar in both groups. Conclusions: For PAF patients, compared with the conventional RFA strategy, the HPSD RFA strategy at relatively low AI settings had a higher early recurrence rate, similar long-term success rate, and comparable safety.

Keywords: paroxysmal atrial fibrillation; high-power; short-duration; radiofrequency ablation; ablation index; pulmonary vein reconnection; non-pulmonary vein triggers

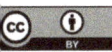

1. Introduction

With global population aging and chronic disease survival rates increasing, both the incidence and prevalence of atrial fibrillation (AF) show a tendency of deterioration [1]. In the 2020 European Society of Cardiology (ESC) guidelines, catheter ablation to improve symptoms of AF recurrences was given a Class I recommendation for AF refractory to medical therapy [2]. Pulmonary vein isolation (PVI), acting as the cornerstone of AF radiofrequency catheter ablation (RFA) [3,4], aims to produce continuous, transmural, and durable lesions around the pulmonary veins (PVs). The ablation index (AI) is a novel marker of lesion quality during RFA that is strongly correlated with lesion depth, width, and volume [5]. Compared with conventional applications (20–35 W at the posterior wall, 35–40 W in the other segments, 10–30 s), the high-power, short-duration (HPSD) ablation strategy is characterized by higher radiofrequency power (≥40 W) and shorter duration (5–15 s). In vitro and in vivo models demonstrated that the HPSD RFA strategy made transmural lesions broader and shallower, with fewer steam pops than the conventional

RFA strategy at proper settings [6]. Multiple studies have been conducted to investigate the efficacy and safety of the HPSD strategy. However, whether the HPSD strategy is more effective than the conventional strategy is still debated. Compared to the conventional strategy, Kewcharoen J et al. [7] reported that the HPSD strategy was not associated with increased freedom from atrial tachyarrhythmia at the 12-month follow-up, but other studies [8,9] showed that the HPSD strategy had higher freedom from atrial arrhythmia. Pulmonary vein reconnection (PVR) and non-PV triggers could be the dominant mechanism of paroxysmal AF (PAF) recurrence [10,11]. Furthermore, age, gender, left atrial (LA) size, deterioration of the left ventricular diastolic dysfunction, posterior wall isolation, and CHA_2DS_2-VASc scores have been found to be independent risk factors associated with AF recurrence after RFA [12–14]. Meanwhile, animal studies indicate that the HPSD settings can create more durable lesions [15,16], which may reduce the rate of chronic PVR. However, little data regarding chronic PVR patterns and non-PV triggers in repeat procedures have been published comparing the HPSD and conventional RFA settings. Therefore, in this study, we sought to compare the effectiveness and safety of the HPSD RFA settings guided by relatively low AI values with the conventional RFA settings for PAF. In addition, we evaluated the sites of chronic PVR and non-PV triggers in patients of both groups who underwent repeat ablation in order to provide further guidance for RFA.

2. Methods

2.1. Study Population

In this single-center prospective cohort study, we investigated 1176 PAF patients who underwent RFA at Guangdong Provincial People's Hospital from July 2019 to March 2021 and followed them prospectively. All the patients signed a written informed consent form for ablation procedures. All the participants met the following criteria: (1) included patients' age $\geq$ 18; (2) patients with PAF refractory to medical therapy and undergoing initial catheter ablation. The exclusion criteria were as follows: (1) previous cardiac surgeries or/and AF ablations; (2) a history of rheumatic valvular disease and ischemic heart disease; (3) LA diameter > 55 mm; (4) patients who failed to complete the procedure due to complications.

All the ablation procedures were performed by nine doctors with over 300 ablation experiences each. Anti-arrhythmia drugs (AADs) were stopped five half-lives prior to ablation. All the patients were required to uninterruptedly take non-vitamin K oral anticoagulants (NOACs) for at least 3 weeks prior to the ablation procedure. LA thrombus was excluded by transesophageal echocardiography or PV computed tomography (CT) within 72 h before the procedure. NOACs were suspended once on the morning of the procedure and recovered 4 h after the procedure.

2.2. Ethics Statement

The registry was approved by the ethics committee of Guangdong Provincial People's Hospital (No. GDREC2019568H, approved on 23 September 2019) and local institutional review boards. Written informed consent was obtained from all individual participants included in the study.

2.3. Ablation Procedure

All the patients underwent RFA under conscious sedation with fentanyl. Under local anesthesia, the right femoral vein was punctured three times, a 7F vascular sheath was put in place, and two 8.5F SL1 vascular sheaths were delivered. A diagnostic decapolar catheter (Triguy™ Steerable Decapolar Mapping Catheter; APT Medical, Shenzhen, China) was placed in the coronary sinus. Intravenous heparin was continuously administered to maintain an activated coagulation time (ACT) at 300 to 350 s during the procedure. After two successful transseptal punctures, three-dimensional mapping of the LA was obtained using a multielectrode catheter (PentaRay Nav Catheter or Lasso; Biosense-Webster Inc., Diamond Bar, CA, USA) with the guidance of the CARTO three-dimensional mapping system (Biosense Webster Inc., Diamond Bar, CA, USA). Then, an open-irrigated, 3.5 mm cooled-tip catheter (Thermocool SMART TOUCH® Uni-Directional Catheter or Thermocool SMART TOUCH® SF Uni-Directional Navigation Catheter; Biosense Webster Inc., Diamond Bar, CA, USA) was used for ablation. All accepted bilateral PVI, non-PV triggers, and additional linear ablations were performed at the operators' discretion. If there was an absence of isolation, touch-up ablation was performed until complete PVI was achieved. Ibutilide or/and electrical cardioversion was/were administered when the AF rhythm remained unconverted during ablation.

In the HPSD group guided by AI, PVI was performed at 40–50 W targeting AI values of 350–400 in the anterior, 350–380 at the superior and inferior wall of the PV, and 320–350 at the posterior wall of the LA with a CF of 5–15 g, irrigation flow rate of 15–30 mL/min per site (ST catheter at 30 mL/min; STSF catheter at 15 mL/min; specific sites adjusted according to operators' experience), and an inter-lesion distance (ILD) of 4 mm. For additional ablation, in the HPSD group, the output power of the mitral isthmus and posterior wall isolation were 40–50 W with AI values of 350–400, that of the tricuspid isthmus was 35 W, and that of the coronary sinus was 25 W. While in the conventional group without the guidance of AI, the power setting of PVs was limited to 35 W at the anterior wall, 25–35 W at the posterior wall, and 35–40 W in the other segments. RF applications did not last more than 30 s, and every single RF delivery was performed with 10 to 20 g CF.

For recurrent patients who underwent repeat ablation procedures, the appropriate three-dimensional mapping system was selected according to the type of recurrent arrhythmia, which included an Ensite Velocity system (Abbott, St. Paul, MN, USA), a Rhythmia™ system (Boston Scientific, Marlborough, MA, USA), and a CARTO system.

2.4. Follow-Up

Patients were evaluated at 1, 3, and 6 months, followed by 6-month intervals up to one year, by electrocardiogram (ECG) or 24 h Holter and when symptoms were reported. Atrial arrhythmia recurrence was defined as any symptomatic or asymptomatic atrial arrhythmia lasting > 30 s after ablation. Recurrence within 3 months after the first ablation was defined as early recurrence, and recurrence after 3 months was defined as late recurrence. For patients suffering from recurrent atrial arrhythmias, repeat procedures were considered after 3 months.

Oral anticoagulants were continued for 3 months after ablation procedure unless uncontrolled bleeding or invasive procedures appeared. Long-term use of anticoagulants depended on CHA_2DS_2-VASc scores. AADs were appropriately selected according to operators' discretion after ablation. After excluding the contraindications, AADs (amiodarone or propafenone) were routinely used for 3 months postoperatively, and the decision to continue AADs was based on the patient's Holter results and symptoms 3 months after the procedure. If recurrence occurred during follow-up, the addition of AADs was recommended, and if the AF load was heavy and symptoms were severe, a repeat ablation was recommended.

2.5. Statistical Analysis

Continuous variables are presented as the mean ± standard deviation ($x \pm s$). Data were analyzed using Student's t test for two-group comparisons if normally distributed or the Mann–Whitney U test for non-parametric two-group comparisons. Categorical variables are presented as frequencies and percentages (%), which were analyzed using a chi-squared test or Fisher exact test between two groups. We performed propensity-score matching using the nearest neighbor method without a replacement and a caliper at a 1:1 ratio of the two groups. The variables age, LA diameter, LVEF, left ventricular diastolic dimension, CHA_2DS_2-VASc scores, and ablation strategy were included in the propensity-score matching. The standardized mean differences of all adjusted variables were under 0.02 after propensity-score matching. The time-to-arrhythmia recurrence was estimated using the Kaplan–Meier method and compared using the log-rank test. A two-sided p-

value < 0.05 was considered statistically significant. A multivariable Cox proportional hazards regression analysis was used to investigate any predictors associated with one year AF recurrence. Multifactorial analysis of survival data was performed using Cox regression if the assumption of equal proportional risk was satisfied. If the assumption of equal proportional risk was not satisfied, a non-equal proportional Cox regression analysis was considered to study the effect of prognostic factors. The variables with $p \leq 0.2$ in the univariate Cox regression analysis and age were included in the multivariate Cox regression analysis. Statistical analyses were performed using SPSS 26.0 (IBM, Armonk NY, USA).

3. Results

3.1. Baseline Characteristics of Patients

A total of 1176 PAF patients who underwent their first ablation from July 2019 to March 2021 were included, of whom 29 (2.466%) were lost to follow-up. A total of 943 patients completed at least the one-year follow-up, of whom 547 patients were in the HPSD RFA strategy group and 396 received the conventional RFA strategy. In the HPSD group and conventional group, the average age was 60.005 ± 10.977 and 60.333 ± 11.216 years, with 63.620% and 60.606% of patients being male, respectively. The baseline characteristics were not significantly different between the two groups except LA diameter ($p = 0.002$) and left ventricular diastolic dimension ($p = 0.042$) (Table 1).

Table 1. Baseline characteristics of the study patients.

Variable	HPSD Group (n = 547) (%)	Conventional Group (n = 396) (%)	p Value
Age (year)	60.005 ± 10.977	60.333 ± 11.216	0.654
Male	348 (63.620)	240 (60.606)	0.346
Hypertension	222 (40.585)	161 (40.657)	0.982
Diabetes	76 (13.894)	57 (14.394)	0.828
Stroke	53 (9.689)	39 (9.848)	0.935
Peripheral vascular disease	32 (5.850)	29 (7.323)	0.364
Heart failure (LVEF ≤ 50%)	13 (2.377)	16 (4.040)	0.144
CHA$_2$DS$_2$-VASc scores	2.013 ± 1.767	2.154 ± 1.685	0.217
Smoke	70 (12.797)	47 (11.869)	0.670
Prior PCI	42 (7.678)	31 (7.828)	0.932
LA diameter (mm)	35.901 ± 4.867	36.949 ± 5.387	0.002
LVEF (%)	64.244 ± 6.185	64.108 ± 6.498	0.749
LVDD (mm)	45.266 ± 4.308	45.887 ± 4.842	0.042
AF duration [months, M (P$_{25}$, P$_{75}$)] *	12.000 (5.000–36.000)	12.000 (3.000–48.000)	0.750
Pacemaker implantation during follow-up	2 (0.366)	2 (0.505)	1.000
LAAC	24 (4.388)	16 (4.040)	0.794

AF: atrial fibrillation; CHA$_2$DS$_2$-VASc = congestive heart failure, hypertension, age ≥ 75 years, diabetes mellitus, stroke, vascular disease, age 65–74 years, sex category (female); HPSD: high-power, short-duration; LVEF: left ventricular ejection fraction; LVDD: left ventricular diastolic dimension; LAAC: left atrial appendage closure; LA: left atrial; PCI: percutaneous coronary intervention; *: results are presented as median (interquartile range).

3.2. Procedural Results

PVI was achieved in all patients. Additionally, the ablation strategies were different between the two groups. Superior vena cava isolation was performed in 88 (16.088%) and 58 (14.646%) patients in the HPSD and conventional groups, respectively. The proportion of mitral isthmus ablation (7.130% vs. 1.768%, $p < 0.001$) and epicardial ablation in the coronary sinus (3.473% vs. 0.505%, $p = 0.002$) was significantly higher in the HPSD group than in the conventional group. The proportions of intraoperative use of ibutilide (10.603% vs. 19.192%, $p < 0.001$) and electrical cardioversion (3.839% vs. 8.838%, $p < 0.001$) were higher in the conventional group (Table 2).

Table 2. Procedure characteristics.

Variable	HPSD Group (n = 547) (%)	Conventional Group (n = 396) (%)	p Value
Performed procedure			
SVC isolation	88 (16.088)	58 (14.646)	0.546
LA roof line ablation	61 (11.152)	54 (13.636)	0.250
LA inferior line ablation	16 (2.925)	13 (3.283)	0.627
LA anterior wall line ablation	4 (0.731)	2 (0.505)	0.987
CTI ablation	165 (30.165)	143 (36.111)	0.055
MI ablation	39 (7.130)	7 (1.768)	<0.001
Endocardial ablation in coronary sinus	16 (2.925)	9 (2.273)	0.538
Epicardial ablation in coronary sinus	19 (3.473)	2 (0.505)	0.002
CFAE ablation	8 (1.463)	3 (0.758)	0.492
Intraoperative use of ibutilide	58 (10.603)	76 (19.192)	<0.001
Intraoperative conversion to sinus rhythm with ibutilide	37/58 (63.793)	52/76 (68.421)	0.574
Intraoperative use of electrical cardioversion	21 (3.839)	35 (8.838)	<0.001
Intraoperative conversion to sinus rhythm with electrical cardioversion	21/21 (100.000)	35/35 (100.000)	1.000

CFAE: complex fractionated atrial electrograms; CTI: cavotricuspid isthmus; HPSD: high-power, short-duration; LA: left atrial; MI: mitral isthmus; SVC: superior vena cava.

After using propensity-score matching analysis, new subsets (HPSD and conventional group, n = 308 each) were obtained. No significant differences were observed between the two groups with regard to baseline characteristics and performed procedures (Supplementary materials, Tables S1 and S2).

3.3. Follow-Up Outcomes

The follow-up durations differed between the two groups, so we evaluated the atrial arrhythmia recurrence within 12 months after a single ablation. Propensity-score matching analysis showed that the early recurrence rate in the HPSD group was still significantly higher than in the conventional group (22.727% vs. 13.636%, p = 0.003). For early recurrent atrial arrhythmia types, 54.286% had AF in the HPSD group compared with 52.381% in the conventional group (p = 0.845). Additionally, there was no statistically significant difference in the late recurrence rate after a single procedure between two groups (19.805% vs. 15.584%, p = 0.170). However, for late recurrent atrial arrhythmia types, regular atrial tachycardia was more common in the HPSD group compared with the conventional group (65.574% vs. 41.667%, p = 0.013) (Table 3).

Table 3. Characteristics of recurrent atrial arrhythmias between two groups after a single procedure.

Variable	Pre-Propensity Score Matching			Post-Propensity Score Matching		
	HPSD Group (n = 547) (%)	Conventional Group (n = 396) (%)	p Value	HPSD Group (n = 308) (%)	Conventional Group (n = 308) (%)	p Value
Early recurrence	129 (23.583)	72 (18.182)	0.046	70 (22.727)	42 (13.636)	0.003
AF	81 (62.791)	37 (51.389)	0.115	38 (54.286)	22 (52.381)	0.845
Atrial tachycardia	48 (37.209)	35 (48.611)		32 (45.714)	20 (47.619)	
Late recurrence	107 (19.561)	70 (17.677)	0.465	61 (19.805)	48 (15.584)	0.170
AF	39 (36.449)	34 (48.571)	0.109	21 (34.426)	28 (58.333)	0.013
Atrial tachycardia	68 (63.551)	36 (51.429)		40 (65.574)	20 (41.667)	

AF: atrial fibrillation; HPSD: high-power, short-duration.

In the Kaplan–Meier survival analysis, the early recurrence rate was higher in the HPSD group than in the conventional group (log rank, p = 0.036 before propensity score matching; p = 0.004 after propensity score matching) (Figure 1). Additionally, the rate of freedom from atrial arrhythmia at one year after a single procedure was similar between the two groups (Log rank, p = 0.446 before propensity score matching; p = 0.169 after propensity score matching) (Figure 2). In the multivariate Cox regression analysis, after adjusting for important covariates including sex, age, and LA diameter, LA diameter was associated with late recurrence within a year (hazard ratio (HR) 1.046, 95% confidence interval (CI) 1.016–1.077, $p = 0.003$) (Table 4).

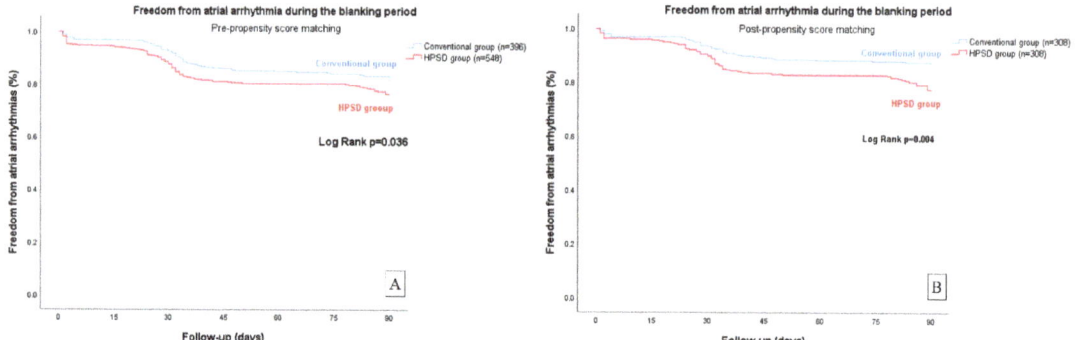

Figure 1. Kaplan–Meier survival analysis of freedom from arrhythmia during the blanking period. (**A**) Freedom from arrhythmia during the blanking period before propensity-score matching; (**B**) Freedom from arrhythmia during the blanking period after propensity-score matching.

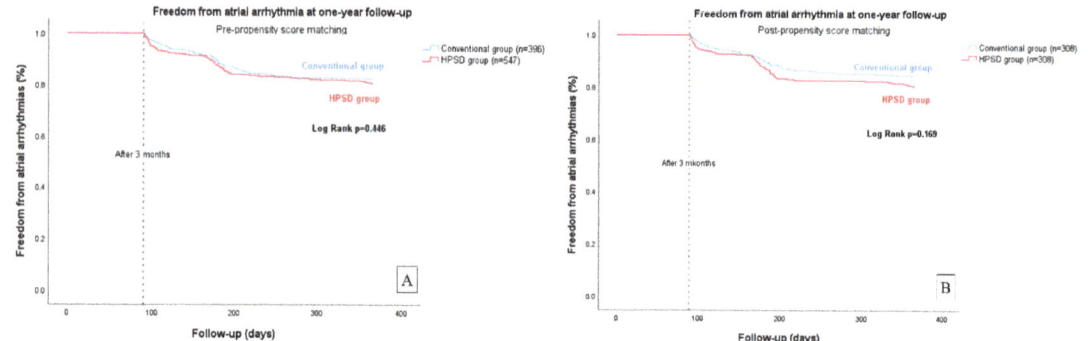

Figure 2. Kaplan–Meier survival analysis of freedom from arrhythmia at one-year follow-up. (**A**) Freedom from arrhythmia at one-year follow-up before propensity-score matching; (**B**) Freedom from arrhythmia at one-year follow-up after propensity-score matching.

3.4. Findings in Repeat Procedures

During 11.19 ± 0.82 months follow-up, a total of 41 patients underwent repeat procedures, including one patient who underwent repeat ablation for atrioventricular nodal reentry tachycardia (AVNRT) and another for LA appendage closure due to high CHA_2DS_2-VASc scores. Eventually, 15 patients in the HPSD group and 24 patients in the conventional group were analyzed. In the conventional group, one patient underwent a third procedure for recurrent regular atrial tachycardia. Superior vena cava isolation was performed in 2 (13.333%) and 5 (20.833%) patients in the HPSD and conventional groups, respectively. Additionally, the proportion of cavotricuspid isthmus ablation was higher in the conventional group than in the HPSD group (6.667% vs. 50.000%, $p = 0.006$). The baseline characteristics and first procedure characteristics of the recurrent patients are shown in Tables 5 and 6.

The spatial distribution of chronic PVR differed between the two groups. In the HPSD group, chronic PVR occurred in 9 out of 15 (60.000%) patients, including 5 left superior PVs, 4 left inferior PVs, 7 right superior PVs, and 5 right inferior PVs. In the conventional group, 18 out of 24 (75.000%) patients had chronic PVR during redo procedures, with 9 left superior PVs, 8 left inferior PVs, 13 right superior PVs, and 12 right inferior PVs.

There was no significant difference in the rate of chronic PVR between the two groups ($p = 0.478$). Additionally, the two groups had similar rates of non-PV triggers (40.000% vs. 29.167%, $p = 0.361$). In terms of PV triggers, there were 5/15 (33.333%) recurrences with a total of 5 sites in the HPSD group and 8/24 (33.333%) recurrences with a total of 15 sites in the conventional group. Meanwhile, for non-PV triggers, there were 6/15 (40.000%) recurrences with a total of 6 sites in the HPSD group and 7/24 (29.167%) recurrences with a total of 13 sites in the conventional group (Table 7). The non-PV trigger sites were located in the Marshall vein, the epicardial surface of the LA roof, the cavotricuspid isthmus, the mitral isthmus, the right atrial free wall, the mitral annulus, the superior vena cava, and the coronary sinus. The specific trigger sites are detailed in Figure 3 and Supplementary Materials Table S3.

Table 4. Cox regression analysis for one-year atrial arrhythmia recurrence.

Variable	Univariate		Multivariate	
	HR (95% CI)	p Value	HR (95% CI)	p Value
Age (year)	1.000 (0.987–1.014)	0.952	0.996 (0.982–1.010)	0.576
Male	0.798 (0.592–1.076)	0.139	0.736 (0.539–1.006)	0.055
Hypertension	0.892 (0.658–1.208)	0.459		
Stroke	1.069 (0.843–1.356)	0.582		
Peripheral vascular disease	1.047 (0.583–1.881)	0.879		
Heart failure (LVEF $\leq$ 50%)	0.470 (0.066–3.353)	0.451		
CHA$_2$DS$_2$-VASc scores	0.978 (0.897–1.066)	0.612		
Smoke	0.834 (0.518–1.343)	0.456		
Prior PCI	0.949 (0.540–1.669)	0.856		
LA diameter (mm)	1.043 (1.013–1.073)	0.005	1.046 (1.016–1.077)	0.003
LVEF (%)	1.007 (0.983–1.032)	0.579		
LVDD (mm)	0.997 (0.964–1.030)	0.848		
AF duration (months)	0.999 (0.996–1.003)	0.774		
HPSD ablation	0.999 (0.996–1.003)	0.774		

AF: atrial fibrillation; CHA$_2$DS$_2$-VASc = congestive heart failure, hypertension, age $\geq$ 75 years, diabetes mellitus, stroke, vascular disease, age 65–74 years, sex category (female); CI: confidence intervals; HPSD: high-power, short-duration; HR: hazard ratio; LVEF: left ventricular ejection fraction; LVDD: left ventricular diastolic dimension; LA: left atrial; PCI: percutaneous coronary intervention.

Table 5. Baseline characteristics of patients undergoing repeat procedures.

Variable	HPSD Group (n = 15) (%)	Conventional Group (n = 24) (%)	p Value
Age (year)	54.867 ± 9.702	61.125 ± 11.521	0.088
Male	8 (53.333)	12 (50.000)	1.000
Hypertension	3 (20.000)	13 (54.167)	0.049
Diabetes	1 (6.667)	3 (12.500)	1.000
Stroke	0 (0.000)	3 (12.500)	0.271
Peripheral vascular disease	0 (0.000)	4 (16.667)	0.146
Heart failure (LVEF $\leq$ 40%)	0 (0.000)	0 (0.000)	1.000
CHA$_2$DS$_2$-VASc scores	1.333 ± 1.447	2.625 ± 1.789	0.024
Smoke	2 (13.333)	3 (12.500)	1.000
LA diameter (mm)	34.286 ± 3.221	37.833 ± 5.939	0.047
LVEF (%)	63.286 ± 3.950	65.042 ± 3.962	0.195
LVDD (mm)	45.143 ± 3.634	46.000 ± 4.294	0.535
AF duration [months, M (P$_{25}$, P$_{75}$)] *	12 (6.000–72.000)	15 (3.500–57.000)	0.898

AF: atrial fibrillation; HPSD: high-power, short-duration; LVEF: left ventricular ejection fraction; LVDD: left ventricular diastolic dimension; LA: left atrial; *: results are presented as median (interquartile range).

Table 6. First procedure characteristics of patients undergoing repeat procedures.

Variable	HPSD Group (n = 15) (%)	Conventional Group (n = 24) (%)	p Value
Performed procedure			
SVC isolation	2 (13.333)	5 (20.833)	0.686
LA roof line ablation	1 (6.667)	3 (12.500)	1.000
LA inferior line ablation	0 (0.000)	0 (0.000)	1.000
LA anterior wall line ablation	1 (6.667)	0 (0.000)	0.385
CTI ablation	1 (6.667)	12 (50.000)	0.006
MI ablation	0 (0.000)	1 (4.167)	1.000
Endocardial ablation in coronary sinus	0 (0.000)	0 (0.000)	1.000
Epicardial ablation in coronary sinus	1 (6.667)	0 (0.000)	0.385
CFAE ablation	0 (0.000)	1 (4.167)	1.000
Intraoperative use of ibutilide	2 (13.333)	6 (25.000)	0.450
Intraoperative conversion to sinus rhythm with ibutilide	1/2 (50.000)	5/6 (83.333)	0.464
Intraoperative use of electrical cardioversion	1 (6.667)	2 (8.333)	1.000
Intraoperative conversion to sinus rhythm with electrical cardioversion	1/1 (100.00)	2/2 (100.00)	1.000

CFAE: complex fractionated atrial electrograms; CTI: cavotricuspid isthmus; HPSD: high-power, short-duration; LA: left atrial; MI: mitral isthmus; SVC: superior vena cava.

Table 7. Repeat procedure characteristics of recurrent patients.

Variable	HPSD Group (n = 15) (%)	Conventional Group (n = 24) (%)	p Value
Recurrent arrhythmia type			0.907
PAF	7 (46.667)	12 (50.000)	
PeAF	1 (6.667)	2 (8.333)	
Atrial tachycardia	6 (40.000)	7 (29.167)	
AF + Atrial tachycardia	1 (6.667)	3 (12.500)	
PVR during redo procedure	9 (60.000)	18 (75.000)	0.478
Left superior PVR	5 (33.333)	9 (37.500)	1.000
Left inferior PVR	4 (26.667)	8 (33.333)	0.734
Right superior PVR	7 (46.667)	13 (54.167)	0.748
Right inferior PVR	5 (33.333)	12 (50.000)	0.343
Left carina	1 (6.667)	4 (16.667)	0.631
Right carina	1 (6.667)	5 (20.833)	0.376
PV triggers	5 (33.333)	8 (33.333)	1.000
Non-PV triggers	6 (40.000)	7 (29.167)	0.361

AF: atrial fibrillation; HPSD: high-power, short-duration; PV: pulmonary vein; PVR: pulmonary vein reconnection; PAF: paroxysmal atrial fibrillation; PeAF: persistent atrial fibrillation.

The dots indicate the site of the trigger. The red dots represent the HPSD group, and the blue dots represent the conventional group.

3.5. Safety Outcomes

As is shown in Table 8, no significant difference was observed in the incidence rate of complications between two groups ($p = 0.604$). During the perioperative period, in the HPSD group, five patients had pericardial effusion, of which one patient had a reduction in pericardial effusion after conservative treatment, three patients received insertion of a pericardial drain, and one patient required surgical treatment. In the conventional group, three patients who developed pericardial effusion required insertion of a pericardial drain. During the follow-up period, no patients in either group had thromboembolic events or strokes. However, two patients died in the conventional group, one due to cancer progression and the other was unclear.

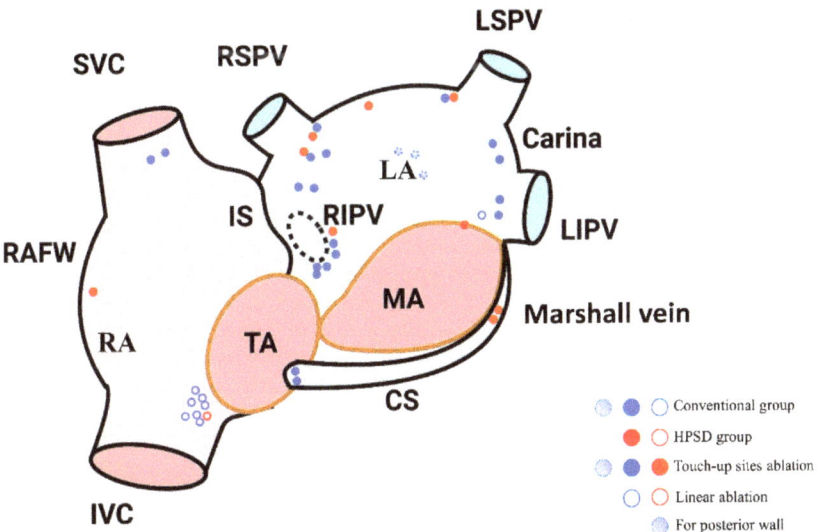

Figure 3. Anteroposterior schematic diagram of trigger sites during repeat procedure for recurrent patients.

Table 8. Complications in the two groups.

Variable	HPSD Group (n = 547) (%)	Conventional Group (n = 396) (%)	p Value
Total complication events	5 (0.914)	5 (1.263)	0.604
During the perioperative period			
Pericardial effusion	5 (0.914)	3 (0.758)	1.000
During the follow-up period			
Strokes	0 (0.000)	0 (0.000)	1.000
Thromboembolic Events	0 (0.000)	0 (0.000)	1.000
Death *	0 (0.000)	2 (0.505)	0.176

HPSD: high-power, short-duration; *: two patients died in the conventional group, one due to cancer progression and the other unknown.

4. Discussion

4.1. Main Findings

This single-center, prospective cohort study demonstrated that the HPSD RFA strategy guided by relatively low AI values had a higher early recurrence rate, a similar late recurrence rate, and comparable safety when compared with the conventional strategy in PAF patients during the one-year follow-up. For recurrent atrial arrhythmia types, the rate of early recurrence types was similar in both groups, but the rate of recurrence with regular atrial tachycardia for late recurrent patients was significantly higher in the HPSD group according to propensity-score matching. Furthermore, no significant difference was found in the rate of chronic PVR and non-PV triggers during repeat procedures in both groups.

4.2. The Success Rate with Different Application Settings

The success rate of AF ablation has risen over the past two decades with the evolution of three-dimensional electroanatomic mapping, contact force sensing catheters, and catheter irrigation [17]. Cryoablation is a promising alternative technique to RFA for treating PAF with encouraging results. Chen YH et al. [18] demonstrated that cryoablation presented comparable long-term AF/atrial tachycardial-free survival and procedure-related adverse events compared with RFA. Meanwhile, cryoablation markedly shortens the procedure time with negligible impact on the fluoroscopy time. However, the HPSD ablation strategies are only applicable when using single point-by-point ablation devices. AI and lesion size index (LSI) are novel ablation quality markers to predict lesion quality that incorporates CF, time, and power in a weighted formula [19]. However, the exact power settings and AI values that result in a high success rate with AF are unclear. Currently, the setting of foreign and domestic mainstream AI is 400–600 for the anterior wall and 400–450 for the posterior wall. However, the results vary from study to study, with similar or slightly higher success rates in the HPSD group with the guidance of AI values than in the conventional group [20–23]. With the targeted AI values of 450–500 for the anterior wall and 350–400 for the posterior wall in two groups, Liu Z et al. demonstrated the HPSD-AI group ($\geq$45 W) had lower recurrence of atrial arrhythmia at 12 months (6.8% vs. 28.3%, $p = 0.011$), higher PV first-pass isolation, shorter ablation times, and fewer patients with anatomical leakages and sites of unreached AI compared with the low power-AI group (<35 W) [24]. O'Brien J et al. [23] illustrated that with a power setting of 50 W and target AI values of 550–600 in the anterior LA region and 400–450 in the posterior LA region, there was no significant difference in the success rate at 12-month follow-up compared with the AI-guided conventional group with a power setting of 35–40 W (80.2% vs. 82.8%, $p = 0.918$). Similarly, for PAF patients, there was no significant difference in the success rate between the HPSD group (40 W) and the conventional group (30 W) at 12 months of follow-up under the same AI-guided ablation (400 for posterior and 500 for anterior wall) in both groups (92% vs. 84%, respectively, $p = 0.22$) [25]. In addition, the measurement of the local impedance might predict optimal lesion formation. A local impedance drop more than 21.80 ohms on the anterior wall and more than 18.30 ohms on the posterior wall significantly increased the probability of creating a successful lesion [26]. Boussoussou M et al. [27] found that LA wall thickness did not influence the first-pass isolation rate during PVI guided by the modified CLOSE protocol (AI 400 on the posterior wall and 500 on the anterior wall, CF 10–40 g). Only the diameter of the right superior PV was associated with the success rate of right-sided first pass isolation, as a wider right superior PV diameter led to an easier first-pass isolation.

However, fewer studies have compared the effectiveness of a HPSD group with a conventional group guided by relatively low AI values. Solimene F et al. [28] reported on 156 AF patients (124 PAF patients and 32 PeAF patients) undergoing AI-guided PVI with target AI values of 400–450 for anterior and 330–350 for posterior LA regions, with 89.2% of patients (91% PAF vs. 78% PeAF) being in the sinus rhythm at 14 $\pm$ 6 months. Okamatsu H et al. [29] investigated 60 AF patients undergoing AI-guided PVI (AI values of 400 at the anterior, 360 at the posterior LA wall, and 260 on the esophagus) randomly assigned to 3 groups (LP group: 30 W at the anterior and 20 W at the posterior wall; MP group: 40 W at the anterior and 30 W at the posterior wall; HP group: 50 W at the anterior, 40 W at the posterior wall and 30 W on the esophagus) and found no significant difference among the groups (100%, 95%, and 95% in LP, MP, and HP groups, respectively, $p = 0.44$).

Additionally, a very high power ablation strategy applied clinically improved procedural efficiency with comparable safety compared with the conventional strategy. Kottmaier M et al. [30] demonstrated that very high power, short-duration (vHPSD) applications with a high power of 70 W for 5–7 s had significantly less arrhythmia recurrence during the one-year follow-up (26.9% vs. 34.9%, $p < 0.013$) with no major complications. Additionally, vHPSD ablation performed by applying 90 W for 4 s during follow-up had more than a 90% success rate with comparable safety [31,32]. A prospective, observational cohort study showed that both HPSD (50 W, AI 500 on the anterior and 400 on the posterior LA wall) and vHPSD RFA settings (90 W/4 s) shorten procedure and RF time and result in a higher rate of first-pass isolation at 9-month AF recurrence rate (10%, 8% and 36%, $p < 0.01$) compared to LPLD RFA settings (30 W, AI 500 on the anterior and 400 on the posterior LA wall). Moreover, the presence of first-pass isolation was associated with a lower AF recurrence rate at 9 months (OR = 0.09, 95% CI 0.04–0.24, $p < 0.01$) [33].

In our study, after using propensity-score matching, compared with the conventional RFA strategy (without AI, 35 W at anterior wall, 25–35 W at the posterior wall, and 35–40 W was applied in the other segments), the HPSD RFA strategy with relatively lower AI values

(40–50 W, AI values of 350–400 for anterior, 350–380 for superior and inferior, and 320–350 for posterior LA wall) had higher early recurrence, similar freedom from atrial arrhythmia, and comparable safety during 12 months of follow-up. Additionally, we are a high-volume electrophysiology center with operators who have over 10 years of AF ablation experience, and there may be no significant difference between the guidance with AI and non-AI ablation. AI is a quantitative metric that may help shorten the learning curve. We used a relatively low AI-guided ablation, which may reflect better long-term outcomes if ablation guided with a relatively high AI is currently available at other centers.

The internal aspect of the LA is relatively smooth, but its wall thickness is not uniform, with an average thickness of 4.5 ± 0.6 mm (range, 3.5–6.5 mm) at the roof, 3.9 ± 0.7 mm (range, 2.5–4.9 mm) at the left lateral wall, and 3.3 ± 1.2 mm (range, 1.5–4.8 mm) at the anterior wall, 2 mm near the vestibule of the mitral annulus, and 4.1 ± 0.7 mm (range, 2.5–5.3 mm) at the posterior wall. The wall thickness of PVs varied from heart to heart. At 0.5 cm away from the junction, the thickness of the left superior PV (LSPV), left inferior PV (LIPV), right superior PV (RSPV), and right inferior PV (RIPV) was 2.8 ± 0.5 mm (range, 1.9–3.5 mm), 1.5 ± 0.4 mm (range, 0.9–2.1 mm), 2.5 ± 0.5 mm (range, 1.8–3.3 mm) and 2.0 ± 0.4 mm (range, 1.5–2.5 mm), respectively. At 0.5 cm away from the junction, the thickness of the LSPV, LIPV, RSPV, and RIPV was 2.3 ± 0.4 mm (range, 1.8–2.8 mm), 1.2 ± 0.3 mm (range, 0.5–1.7 mm), 2.0 ± 0.3 mm (range, 1.5–2.5 mm), and 1.5 ± 0.2 mm (range, 0.9–2.2 mm), respectively. Additionally, the LA posterior wall thickness increased from the most superior to the most inferior measured level, whereas the wall was thinner in the middle and between the inferior venous orifices in those with AF (for AF patients: 2.1 ± 0.9 mm between the superior PVs, 2.2 ± 1.0 mm in the center of the posterior LA wall, and 2.5 ± 1.3 mm between the inferior PVs; for non-AF patients: 2.3 ± 1.0 mm between the superior PVs, 2.6 ± 1.0 mm in the center of the posterior LA wall, and 2.9 ± 1.3 mm between the inferior PVs) [34–36]. The myocardium of the left lateral ridge at its superior level was thicker than at its inferior level (2.8 ± 1.1 (range 1.5–4.2 mm) vs. 1.7 ± 0.8 mm (range 0.5–3.5 mm), respectively, $p < 0.001$) [37]. The minimal distance between the right PV antrum, left PV antrum, LA posterior wall, and esophageal wall was 6.3 ± 2.8 mm (range, 3.4–11.5 mm), 5.6 ± 2.2 mm (range, 3.3–10.5 mm), and 6.2 ± 2.5 mm (range, 3.6–13.5 mm), respectively [38]. The HPSD RFA strategy with a power of 50 W for 7 s (LSI 4.8 ± 0.52) creates wider but shallower lesions that had a diameter of 4.98 ± 0.91 mm and a depth of 2.2 ± 0.76 mm, whereas the conventional RFA strategy with a power of 25 W for 30 s (LSI 4.73 ± 0.59) had a diameter of 4.45 ± 0.74 mm and a depth of 2.8 ± 1.56 mm [39]. Additionally, the HPSD settings for 90 W/4 s in the beating heart of swine produced wider lesions (6.02 ± 0.2 mm vs. 4.43 ± 1.0 mm) and similar depth (3.58 ± 0.3 mm vs. 3.53 ± 0.6 mm) compared with the conventional RFA strategy for 25 W/20 s (CF of two groups range from 5–40 g) [16]. From the anatomy of the LA, the thickness of the posterior wall ranged from 2.5 mm to 5.3 mm [36]. Therefore, using relatively conservative AI values in patients is more consistent with safety principles, while AI values of 320–350 for posterior walls are able to balance effectiveness and safety.

4.3. Characteristics of Recurrent Atrial Arrhythmia

In a recent publication by Vassallo F et al. [40], the HPSD RFA strategy increased the incidence of early recurrence and reduced late recurrence compared with the conventional strategy, while AT or AFL occurring during the blanking period is more common in the HPSD group. However, Bunch et al. [41] reported a similar recurrence of AF at one year and three years between two groups, and a higher rate of AFL at one year and three years was observed in patients treated with the HPSD RFA. In our study, the propensity-score matching analysis showed that a similar recurrence of AF was observed during the blanking period in both groups, while a higher rate of atrial arrhythmia was observed after one year's follow-up in patients treated with the HPSD RFA strategy.

The early recurrence for AF patients was associated with an inflammatory process caused by the 40–50 W power setting used in this ablation protocol [42]. After the blanking period, the spontaneous resolution of the arrhythmias with sinus rhythm conversion may be explained by the decrease in inflammatory responses or the use of AADs. Because the HPSD RFA strategy had relatively low AI values, shallower lesions, and less total energy, transmural damage may not be achieved, resulting in no difference in the late recurrence rate between the two groups. Therefore, further studies are required to explore the most optimal power setting and AI values for RFA to yield greater clinical value.

PVI is the cornerstone of AF ablation, whereas PVR is attributed to catheter instability, tissue edema, and reversible non-transmural injury [43]. Therefore, the continuous and transmural lines are key to the success of ablation. In animal studies, HPSD applications resulted in 100% contiguous lines with all transmural and improved lesions showing lesion-to-lesion consistency compared with conventional applications [15,16]. Recent studies [44–47] have shown different consequences in terms of chronic PVR during the second procedure between two groups. Yavin HD et al. [47] demonstrated that incidence of chronic PVR during the redo procedure was lower in a HPSD group than in a conventional group (16.66% vs. 52.2%, $p = 0.03$), and reconnection sites occurred in the septal aspect of the right PV or the anterior left PV in the HPSD group and in the anterior left PV, septal right PV, and posterior wall in the conventional group. However, Hansom SP et al. [45] reported that the right PV carinal segments had a higher rate of reconnection in HPSD applications compared with conventional applications, but there was no difference in chronic PVR between the two groups.

In our study, there was no difference in the proportion of chronic PVR during repeat procedure between the two groups. Some patients who did not undergo redo procedures had recurrence during the follow-up period. Additionally, areas of chronic PVR were co-located at sites of decreased catheter stability in both groups. Reconnection sites occurred more in right PVs and left carina in both groups. In terms of anatomy, it is more difficult for a catheter to reach right PVs than left PVs. Furthermore, the myocardial thickness of the carina is thicker, and the catheter attachment of the carina is more difficult, and thus the HPSD strategy with conservative AI values and lower energy may lead to non-transmural lesions. Therefore, for all the reasons listed above, we may underestimate the rate of chronic PVR, contributing to chronic PVR in both groups. Non-PV triggers were frequently found in the superior vena cava, LA anterior wall, LA posterior wall, coronary sinus, and vein of Marshall [48]. In our study, since 15% of patients in both groups underwent superior vena cava isolation in the first ablation procedure, the number of patients requiring superior vena cava isolation in the repeat ablation procedure was minimal. Additionally, both groups had similar rates of PV triggers. The proportion of non-PV triggers was relatively high in the HPSD group compared with the conventional group, but there was no significant difference in non-PV triggers between the two groups.

This implies that the relatively low AI values might not have produced transmural injury lesions, while the thicker carina and the difficulty of catheter apposition during the procedure contributed to the chronic PVR in both groups. Furthermore, a limited number of recurrent patients had repeat procedures, and additional lesions were performed during the initial procedure in both groups, which might have reduced the incidence of non-PV triggers. More well-designed and large-scale RCTs are required to confirm these findings.

4.4. Safety Outcomes

Safety during ablation RFA is of worthwhile concern. The primary reason for tissue injury during RFA is thermally mediated, including resistive and conductive heating. It causes irreversible damage to the myocardium once a temperature of approximately 50 °C has been reached [49]. Contrary to the conventional ablation strategy, the HPSD ablation strategy results in higher resistive heating, lower conductive heating, larger lesion diameters, and smaller lesion depths, which may reduce collateral injury to surrounding structures such as the esophagus [16,50]. HPSD ablation with a power setting of 50 W for 6 s will not result in severe esophageal temperature increases when lesions are >20 mm away from a temperature sensor [51]. Via intraoperative esophageal temperature monitoring, or late gadolinium enhancement (LGE) magnetic resonance imaging (MRI) within 24 h post-ablation, it can be seen that the two groups have similar esophageal temperature dynamics and comparable esophageal tissue injury results [52,53]. In addition to the incidence of esophageal injury, the overall complications were very low in the HPSD application performed at 45–50 W, with one death due to an atrioesophageal fistula and 33 cases of cardiac tamponade in 10,284 patients [54]. Similar to other findings, the HPSD RFA strategy with relatively low AI values appears to be as safe as the conventional RFA strategy. Additionally, combined with previous anatomical data on the LA, the thickness of the posterior wall ranges from 2.5 mm to 5.3 mm, and AI values of 320–350 in the posterior wall of the LA may have a positive effect on the prevention of atrioesophageal fistula.

5. Limitations

There are several limitations to our study. First, this study is a single-center study. Additionally, there were variations in the ablation parameters and ablation strategies compared with other centers. Thus, the results need to be further validated by clinical randomized prospective studies. In addition, limited by way of the follow-up, the onset time may not be recorded in time for patients with asymptomatic recurrence, which may underestimate the rate of freedom from atrial arrhythmia. Additionally, not all patients with recurrence underwent electrophysiological examination and a repeat ablation, which may bias the proportion of chronic PVR and non-PV triggers during repeat procedures. Finally, in our study, we lacked data on procedure time, ablation time, and fluoroscopy time, resulting in an inability to compare efficacy between the two groups in many respects. We still need a multicenter, prospective randomized controlled study with uniform ablation strategy to further validate our findings.

6. Conclusions

Compared with the conventional group, the HPSD group with relatively low AI settings had a higher early recurrence rate and a similar late recurrence rate with comparable safety. Additionally, whereas both groups exhibited a similar recurrence rate of AF throughout the blanking period, patients treated with the HPSD RFA strategy experienced a higher rate of atrial arrhythmia after the one-year follow-up. Meanwhile, the rate of chronic PVR and non-PV triggers was similar between the two groups. The HPSD RFA strategy with relatively low AI settings was demonstrated to be a feasible, effective, and safe approach to PAF ablation.

Supplementary Materials: The following supporting information can be downloaded at: https://www.mdpi.com/article/10.3390/jcm12030971/s1; Table S1: Baseline characteristics of the study patients after propensity-score matching; Table S2: Procedure characteristics after propensity-score matching; Table S3: The specific trigger sites in both groups.

Author Contributions: Conceptualization, X.F.; data curation, S.J.; formal analysis, J.J.; funding acquisition, Y.X.; methodology, Y.C. and S.P.; resources, X.Y.; software, L.F. and H.L. (Huiyi Liu); supervision, H.L. (Hongtao Liao), X.Z. and S.W.; writing—original draft, S.J. and W.L.; writing—review and editing, H.D. and Y.X. All authors have read and agreed to the published version of the manuscript.

Funding: This work was supported by the Science and Technology Programs of Guangdong Province (No. 2019B020230004), the Science and Technology Programs of Guangdong Province (No. 2020B1111170011), the Guangdong special funds for science and technology innovation strategy, China (Stability support for scientific research institutions affiliated with Guangdong Province-GDCI 2021), and the Zhongnanshan medical foundation of Guangdong Province (No. 202151).

Institutional Review Board Statement: The study was conducted according to the guidelines of the Declaration of Helsinki of 1975 and approved by the ethics committee of Guangdong Provincial People's Hospital (No. GDREC2019568H, approved on 23 September 2019).

Informed Consent Statement: Informed consent was obtained from all the subjects involved in the study.

Data Availability Statement: The data presented in this study are available on request from the corresponding author.

Conflicts of Interest: The authors declare that the research was conducted in the absence of any commercial or financial relationships that could be construed as a potential conflict of interest.

References

1. Kornej, J.; Börschel, C.S.; Benjamin, E.J.; Schnabel, R.B. Epidemiology of Atrial Fibrillation in the 21st Century: Novel Methods and New Insights. *Circ. Res.* **2020**, *127*, 4–20. [CrossRef] [PubMed]
2. Hindricks, G.; Potpara, T.; Dagres, N.; Arbelo, E.; Bax, J.J.; Blomström-Lundqvist, C.; Boriani, G.; Castella, M.; Dan, G.A.; Dilaveris, P.E.; et al. 2020 ESC Guidelines for the diagnosis and management of atrial fibrillation developed in collaboration with the European Association for Cardio-Thoracic Surgery (EACTS): The Task Force for the diagnosis and management of atrial fibrillation of the European Society of Cardiology (ESC) Developed with the special contribution of the European Heart Rhythm Association (EHRA) of the ESC. *Eur. Heart J.* **2021**, *42*, 373–498. [CrossRef] [PubMed]
3. Haïssaguerre, M.; Jaïs, P.; Shah, D.C.; Takahashi, A.; Hocini, M.; Quiniou, G.; Garrigue, S.; Le Mouroux, A.; Le Métayer, P.; Clémenty, J. Spontaneous initiation of atrial fibrillation by ectopic beats originating in the pulmonary veins. *N. Engl. J. Med.* **1998**, *339*, 659–666. [CrossRef] [PubMed]
4. Kantachuvessiri, A. Pulmonary veins: Preferred site for catheter ablation of atrial fibrillation. *Heart Lung* **2002**, *31*, 271–278. [CrossRef] [PubMed]
5. Kawaji, T.; Hojo, S.; Kushiyama, A.; Nakatsuma, K.; Kaneda, K.; Kato, M.; Yokomatsu, T.; Miki, S. Limitations of lesion quality estimated by ablation index: An in vitro study. *J. Cardiovasc. Electrophysiol.* **2019**, *30*, 926–933. [CrossRef]
6. Winkle, R.A. HPSD ablation for AF high-power short-duration RF ablation for atrial fibrillation: A review. *J. Cardiovasc. Electrophysiol.* **2021**, *32*, 2813–2823. [CrossRef]
7. Kewcharoen, J.; Techorueangwiwat, C.; Kanitsoraphan, C.; Leesutipornchai, T.; Akoum, N.; Bunch, T.J.; Navaravong, L. High-power short duration and low-power long duration in atrial fibrillation ablation: A meta-analysis. *J. Cardiovasc. Electrophysiol.* **2021**, *32*, 71–82. [CrossRef]
8. Chen, C.F.; Wu, J.; Jin, C.L.; Liu, M.J.; Xu, Y.Z. Comparison of high-power short-duration and low-power long-duration radiofrequency ablation for treating atrial fibrillation: Systematic review and meta-analysis. *Clin. Cardiol.* **2020**, *43*, 1631–1640. [CrossRef]
9. Ravi, V.; Poudyal, A.; Abid, Q.U.; Larsen, T.; Krishnan, K.; Sharma, P.S.; Trohman, R.G.; Huang, H.D. High-power short duration vs. conventional radiofrequency ablation of atrial fibrillation: A systematic review and meta-analysis. *Europace* **2021**, *23*, 710–721. [CrossRef]
10. Buist, T.J.; Zipes, D.P.; Elvan, A. Atrial fibrillation ablation strategies and technologies: Past, present, and future. *Clin. Res. Cardiol.* **2021**, *110*, 775–788. [CrossRef]
11. Cherian, T.S.; Callans, D.J. Recurrent Atrial Fibrillation after Radiofrequency Ablation: What to Expect. *Card. Electrophysiol. Clin.* **2020**, *12*, 187–197. [CrossRef] [PubMed]
12. Kisheva, A.; Yotov, Y. Risk factors for recurrence of atrial fibrillation. *Anatol. J. Cardiol.* **2021**, *25*, 338–345. [CrossRef] [PubMed]
13. Kranert, M.; Shchetynska-Marinova, T.; Liebe, V.; Doesch, C.; Papavassiliu, T.; Akin, I.; Borggrefe, M.; Hohneck, A. Recurrence of Atrial Fibrillation in Dependence of Left Atrial Volume Index. *In Vivo* **2020**, *34*, 889–896. [CrossRef]
14. Winkle, R.A.; Mead, R.H.; Engel, G.; Kong, M.H.; Salcedo, J.; Brodt, C.R.; Patrawala, R.A. High-power, short-duration atrial fibrillation ablations using contact force sensing catheters: Outcomes and predictors of success including posterior wall isolation. *Heart Rhythm* **2020**, *17*, 1223–1231. [CrossRef] [PubMed]
15. Barkagan, M.; Contreras-Valdes, F.M.; Leshem, E.; Buxton, A.E.; Nakagawa, H.; Anter, E. High-power and short-duration ablation for pulmonary vein isolation: Safety, efficacy, and long-term durability. *J. Cardiovasc. Electrophysiol.* **2018**, *29*, 1287–1296. [CrossRef]
16. Leshem, E.; Zilberman, I.; Tschabrunn, C.M.; Barkagan, M.; Contreras-Valdes, F.M.; Govari, A.; Anter, E. High-Power and Short-Duration Ablation for Pulmonary Vein Isolation: Biophysical Characterization. *JACC Clin. Electrophysiol.* **2018**, *4*, 467–479. [CrossRef]
17. Parameswaran, R.; Al-Kaisey, A.M.; Kalman, J.M. Catheter ablation for atrial fibrillation: Current indications and evolving technologies. *Nat. Rev. Cardiol.* **2021**, *18*, 210–225. [CrossRef]
18. Chen, Y.H.; Lu, Z.Y.; Xiang, Y.; Hou, J.W.; Wang, Q.; Lin, H.; Li, Y.G. Cryoablation vs. radiofrequency ablation for treatment of paroxysmal atrial fibrillation: A systematic review and meta-analysis. *Europace* **2017**, *19*, 784–794. [CrossRef]
19. Virk, S.A.; Bennett, R.G.; Trivic, I.; Campbell, T.; Kumar, S. Contact Force and Ablation Index. *Card. Electrophysiol. Clin.* **2019**, *11*, 473–479. [CrossRef] [PubMed]
20. Kiliszek, M.; Krzyżanowski, K.; Wierzbowski, R.; Winkler, A.; Smalc-Stasiak, M. The value of the ablation index in patients undergoing ablation for atrial fibrillation. *Kardiol. Pol.* **2020**, *78*, 1015–1019. [CrossRef]
21. Liu, X.; Gui, C.; Wen, W.; He, Y.; Dai, W.; Zhong, G. Safety and Efficacy of High Power Shorter Duration Ablation Guided by Ablation Index or Lesion Size Index in Atrial Fibrillation Ablation: A Systematic Review and Meta-Analysis. *J. Interv. Cardiol.* **2021**, *2021*, 5591590. [CrossRef] [PubMed]

2. Pranata, R.; Vania, R.; Huang, I. Ablation-index guided versus conventional contact-force guided ablation in pulmonary vein isolation—Systematic review and meta-analysis. *Indian Pacing Electrophysiol. J.* **2019**, *19*, 155–160. [CrossRef] [PubMed]
3. O'Brien, J.; Obeidat, M.; Kozhuharov, N.; Ding, W.Y.; Tovmassian, L.; Bierme, C.; Chin, S.H.; Chu, G.S.; Luther, V.; Snowdon, R.L.; et al. Procedural efficiencies, lesion metrics, and 12-month clinical outcomes for Ablation Index-guided 50 W ablation for atrial fibrillation. *Europace* **2021**, *23*, 878–886. [CrossRef]
4. Liu, Z.; Liu, L.F.; Liu, X.Q.; Liu, J.; Wang, Y.X.; Liu, Y.; Liu, X.P.; Yang, X.C.; Chen, M.L. Ablation index-guided ablation with milder targets for atrial fibrillation: Comparison between high power and low power ablation. *Front. Cardiovasc. Med.* **2022**, *9*, 949918. [CrossRef] [PubMed]
5. Zhu, X.; Wang, C.; Chu, H.; Li, W.; Zhou, H.; Zhong, L.; Li, J. Effectiveness and Safety of High-Power Radiofrequency Ablation Guided by Ablation Index for the Treatment of Atrial Fibrillation. *Comput. Math. Methods Med.* **2022**, *2022*, 5609764. [CrossRef]
6. Szegedi, N.; Salló, Z.; Perge, P.; Piros, K.; Nagy, V.K.; Osztheimer, I.; Merkely, B.; Gellér, L. The role of local impedance drop in the acute lesion efficacy during pulmonary vein isolation performed with a new contact force sensing catheter-A pilot study. *PLoS ONE* **2021**, *16*, e0257050. [CrossRef]
7. Boussoussou, M.; Szilveszter, B.; Vattay, B.; Kolossváry, M.; Vecsey-Nagy, M.; Salló, Z.; Orbán, G.; Péter, P.; Katalin, P.; Vivien, N.K.; et al. The effect of left atrial wall thickness and pulmonary vein sizes on the acute procedural success of atrial fibrillation ablation. *Int. J. Cardiovasc. Imaging* **2022**, *38*, 1601–1611. [CrossRef]
8. Solimene, F.; Schillaci, V.; Shopova, G.; Urraro, F.; Arestia, A.; Iuliano, A.; Maresca, F.; Agresta, A.; La Rocca, V.; De Simone, A.; et al. Safety and efficacy of atrial fibrillation ablation guided by Ablation Index module. *J. Interv. Card. Electrophysiol.* **2019**, *54*, 9–15. [CrossRef]
9. Okamatsu, H.; Koyama, J.; Sakai, Y.; Negishi, K.; Hayashi, K.; Tsurugi, T.; Tanaka, Y.; Nakao, K.; Sakamoto, T.; Okumura, K. High-power application is associated with shorter procedure time and higher rate of first-pass pulmonary vein isolation in ablation index-guided atrial fibrillation ablation. *J. Cardiovasc. Electrophysiol.* **2019**, *30*, 2751–2758. [CrossRef]
10. Kottmaier, M.; Popa, M.; Bourier, F.; Reents, T.; Cifuentes, J.; Semmler, V.; Telishevska, M.; Otgonbayar, U.; Koch-Büttner, K.; Lennerz, C.; et al. Safety and outcome of very high-power short-duration ablation using 70 W for pulmonary vein isolation in patients with paroxysmal atrial fibrillation. *Europace* **2020**, *22*, 388–393. [CrossRef]
11. Orbán, G.; Salló, Z.; Perge, P.; Ábrahám, P.; Piros, K.; Nagy, K.V.; Osztheimer, I.; Merkely, B.; Gellér, L.; Szegedi, N. Characteristics of Very High-Power, Short-Duration Radiofrequency Applications. *Front. Cardiovasc. Med.* **2022**, *9*, 941434. [CrossRef] [PubMed]
12. Reddy, V.Y.; Grimaldi, M.; De Potter, T.; Vijgen, J.M.; Bulava, A.; Duytschaever, M.F.; Martinek, M.; Natale, A.; Knecht, S.; Neuzil, P.; et al. Pulmonary Vein Isolation with Very High Power, Short Duration, Temperature-Controlled Lesions: The QDOT-FAST Trial. *JACC Clin. Electrophysiol.* **2019**, *5*, 778–786. [CrossRef] [PubMed]
13. Salló, Z.; Perge, P.; Balogi, B.; Orbán, G.; Piros, K.; Herczeg, S.; Nagy, K.V.; Osztheimer, I.; Ábrahám, P.; Merkely, B.; et al. Impact of High-Power and Very High-Power Short-Duration Radiofrequency Ablation on Procedure Characteristics and First-Pass Isolation During Pulmonary Vein Isolation. *Front. Cardiovasc. Med.* **2022**, *9*, 935705. [CrossRef] [PubMed]
14. Ho, S.Y.; Cabrera, J.A.; Sanchez-Quintana, D. Left atrial anatomy revisited. *Circ. Arrhythmia Electrophysiol.* **2012**, *5*, 220–228. [CrossRef]
15. Platonov, P.G.; Ivanov, V.; Ho, S.Y.; Mitrofanova, L. Left atrial posterior wall thickness in patients with and without atrial fibrillation: Data from 298 consecutive autopsies. *J. Cardiovasc. Electrophysiol.* **2008**, *19*, 689–692. [CrossRef]
16. Ho, S.Y.; Sanchez-Quintana, D.; Cabrera, J.A.; Anderson, R.H. Anatomy of the left atrium: Implications for radiofrequency ablation of atrial fibrillation. *J. Cardiovasc. Electrophysiol.* **1999**, *10*, 1525–1533. [CrossRef]
17. Cabrera, J.A.; Ho, S.Y.; Climent, V.; Sánchez-Quintana, D. The architecture of the left lateral atrial wall: A particular anatomic region with implications for ablation of atrial fibrillation. *Eur. Heart J.* **2008**, *29*, 356–362. [CrossRef]
18. Sánchez-Quintana, D.; Cabrera, J.A.; Climent, V.; Farré, J.; Mendonça, M.C.; Ho, S.Y. Anatomic relations between the esophagus and left atrium and relevance for ablation of atrial fibrillation. *Circulation* **2005**, *112*, 1400–1405. [CrossRef] [PubMed]
19. Enomoto, Y.; Nakamura, K.; Ishii, R.; Toyoda, Y.; Asami, M.; Takagi, T.; Hashimoto, H.; Hara, H.; Sugi, K.; Moroi, M.; et al. Lesion size and adjacent tissue damage assessment with high power and short duration radiofrequency ablation: Comparison to conventional radiofrequency ablation power setting. *Heart Vessel.* **2021**, *36*, 1438–1444. [CrossRef]
20. Vassallo, F.; Meigre, L.L.; Serpa, E.; Cunha, C.; Simoes, A., Jr.; Carloni, H.; Amaral, D.; Meira, K.; Pezzin, F. Changes and impacts in early recurrences after atrial fibrillation ablation in contact force era: Comparison of high-power short-duration with conventional technique-FIRST experience data. *J. Interv. Card. Electrophysiol.* **2021**, *62*, 363–371. [CrossRef]
21. Bunch, T.J.; May, H.T.; Bair, T.L.; Crandall, B.G.; Cutler, M.J.; Mallender, C.; Weiss, J.P.; Osborn, J.S.; Day, J.D. Long-term outcomes after low power, slower movement versus high power, faster movement irrigated-tip catheter ablation for atrial fibrillation. *Heart Rhythm* **2020**, *17*, 184–189. [CrossRef] [PubMed]
22. Ukita, K.; Egami, Y.; Kawamura, A.; Nakamura, H.; Matsuhiro, Y.; Yasumoto, K.; Tsuda, M.; Okamoto, N.; Matsunaga-Lee, Y.; Yano, M.; et al. Clinical impact of very early recurrence of atrial fibrillation after radiofrequency catheter ablation. *J. Cardiol.* **2021**, *78*, 571–576. [CrossRef] [PubMed]
23. Han, S.; Hwang, C. How to Achieve Complete and Permanent Pulmonary Vein Isolation without Complications. *Korean Circ. J.* **2014**, *44*, 291–300. [CrossRef] [PubMed]
24. Kumagai, K.; Toyama, H. High-power, short-duration ablation during Box isolation for atrial fibrillation. *J. Arrhythmia* **2020**, *36*, 899–904. [CrossRef]

45. Hansom, S.P.; Alqarawi, W.; Birnie, D.H.; Golian, M.; Nery, P.B.; Redpath, C.J.; Klein, A.; Green, M.S.; Davis, D.R.; Sheppard Perkins, E.; et al. High-power, short-duration atrial fibrillation ablation compared with a conventional approach: Outcomes and reconnection patterns. *J. Cardiovasc. Electrophysiol.* **2021**, *32*, 1219–1228. [CrossRef]
46. Ejima, K.; Higuchi, S.; Yazaki, K.; Kataoka, S.; Yagishita, D.; Kanai, M.; Shoda, M.; Hagiwara, N. Comparison of high-power and conventional-power radiofrequency energy deliveries in pulmonary vein isolation using unipolar signal modification as a local endpoint. *J. Cardiovasc. Electrophysiol.* **2020**, *31*, 1702–1708. [CrossRef] [PubMed]
47. Yavin, H.D.; Leshem, E.; Shapira-Daniels, A.; Sroubek, J.; Barkagan, M.; Haffajee, C.I.; Cooper, J.M.; Anter, E. Impact of High Power Short-Duration Radiofrequency Ablation on Long-Term Lesion Durability for Atrial Fibrillation Ablation. *JACC Clin Electrophysiol.* **2020**, *6*, 973–985. [CrossRef]
48. Gianni, C.; Mohanty, S.; Trivedi, C.; Di Biase, L.; Natale, A. Novel concepts and approaches in ablation of atrial fibrillation: The role of non-pulmonary vein triggers. *Europace* **2018**, *20*, 1566–1576. [CrossRef]
49. Nath, S.; DiMarco, J.P.; Haines, D.E. Basic aspects of radiofrequency catheter ablation. *J. Cardiovasc. Electrophysiol.* **1994**, *5*, 863–876. [CrossRef]
50. Bourier, F.; Duchateau, J.; Vlachos, K.; Lam, A.; Martin, C.A.; Takigawa, M.; Kitamura, T.; Frontera, A.; Cheniti, G.; Pambrun, T.; et al. High-power short-duration versus standard radiofrequency ablation: Insights on lesion metrics. *J. Cardiovasc. Electrophysiol.* **2018**, *29*, 1570–1575. [CrossRef]
51. Barbhaiya, C.R.; Kogan, E.V.; Jankelson, L.; Knotts, R.J.; Spinelli, M.; Bernstein, S.; Park, D.; Aizer, A.; Chinitz, L.A.; Holmes, D Esophageal temperature dynamics during high-power short-duration posterior wall ablation. *Heart Rhythm* **2020**, *17*, 721–727 [CrossRef] [PubMed]
52. Yavin, H.D.; Bubar, Z.P.; Higuchi, K.; Sroubek, J.; Kanj, M.; Cantillon, D.; Saliba, W.I.; Tarakji, K.G.; Hussein, A.A.; Wazni, O. et al. Impact of High-Power Short-Duration Radiofrequency Ablation on Esophageal Temperature Dynamic. *Circ. Arrhythmia Electrophysiol.* **2021**, *14*, e010205. [CrossRef] [PubMed]
53. Baher, A.; Kheirkhahan, M.; Rechenmacher, S.J.; Marashly, Q.; Kholmovski, E.G.; Siebermair, J.; Acharya, M.; Aljuaid, M.; Morris A.K.; Kaur, G.; et al. High-Power Radiofrequency Catheter Ablation of Atrial Fibrillation: Using Late Gadolinium Enhancement Magnetic Resonance Imaging as a Novel Index of Esophageal Injury. *JACC Clin. Electrophysiol.* **2018**, *4*, 1583–1594. [CrossRef]
54. Winkle, R.A.; Mohanty, S.; Patrawala, R.A.; Mead, R.H.; Kong, M.H.; Engel, G.; Salcedo, J.; Trivedi, C.G.; Gianni, C.; Jais, P.; et al. Low complication rates using high power (45–50 W) for short duration for atrial fibrillation ablations. *Heart Rhythm* **2019**, *16* 165–169. [CrossRef] [PubMed]

Disclaimer/Publisher's Note: The statements, opinions and data contained in all publications are solely those of the individual author(s) and contributor(s) and not of MDPI and/or the editor(s). MDPI and/or the editor(s) disclaim responsibility for any injury to people or property resulting from any ideas, methods, instructions or products referred to in the content.

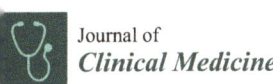

Vein of Marshall Collateralization during Ethanol Infusion in Atrial Fibrillation: Solution for Effective Myocardium Staining

Hongda Zhang [1,†], Lei Ding [1,†], Lijie Mi [1], Kuo Zhang [1], Zihan Jiang [1], Sixian Weng [2], Fengyuan Yu [1] and Min Tang [1,*]

[1] Arrhythmia Center, State Key Laboratory of Cardiovascular Disease, Fuwai Hospital, National Center for Cardiovascular Diseases, Chinese Academy of Medical Sciences & Peking Union Medical College, Beijing 100037, China
[2] National Center for Clinical Laboratories, Institute of Geriatric Medicine, Chinese Academy of Medical Sciences, Beijing Hospital, National Center of Gerontology, Beijing 100037, China
* Correspondence: doctortangmin@yeah.net; Tel.: +86-10-88396965
† These authors contributed equally to this study.

Abstract: Background: The vein of Marshall (VOM) ethanol infusion improves sinus rhythm maintenance in patients with atrial fibrillation (AF). Distal collateral circulation of VOM can be a challenge to effective ethanol infusion. Objective: This study aimed to evaluate the feasibility and efficacy of ethanol infusion in VOM with distal collateral circulation. Methods: Patients with AF scheduled for catheter ablation and VOM ethanol infusion were consecutively enrolled. During the procedure, non-occluded coronary sinus angiography was first performed for VOM identification. After VOM identification, an over-the-wire angioplasty balloon was used for cannulation and occluded angiography of the VOM. Those with distal VOM collateral circulation were included in this study. A method of slower ethanol injection (2 mL over 5 min) plus additional balloon occlusion time for 3 min after each injection was used. Results: Of 162 patients scheduled for VOM ethanol infusion, apparent distal VOM collateral circulation was revealed in seven (4.3%) patients. Five patients had collateral circulation to the left atrium, one to the right superior vena cava, and one to the great cardiac vein. Two patients did not undergo further ethanol infusion because of our inadequate experience during the early stage of the project. Five patients had successful VOM ethanol infusion with manifest localized myocardium staining. Conclusions: Ethanol infusion in VOM with distal collateral circulation can be solved by slow injection of ethanol and enough balloon occlusion time between multiple injections.

Keywords: atrial fibrillation; vein of Marshall; ethanol infusion; collateral circulation; slow injection

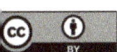

1. Introduction

The vein of Marshall (VOM), a remnant of the left superior vena cava, has been proven to be an arrhythmogenic source in patients with atrial fibrillation (AF) [1–4]. VOM ethanol infusion, in combination with catheter ablation of the pulmonary veins, improves sinus rhythm maintenance in patients with persistent AF [1,2,5]. The VOM can be extremely narrow, and its anatomical variability is substantial [2,6–8]. Identification and cannulation of the VOM require knowledge of fluoroscopic anatomy and different angioplasty tools. VOM ethanol infusion can be technically challenging. There has been a growing body of literature focusing on techniques of VOM ethanol infusion [7,9,10].

Prior studies have reported that VOM can have none or many branches, be a venous plexus, and have collateral circulation to the left atrium, great cardiac vein, coronary sinus, or superior vena cava [2,8]. Collateral circulation of VOM can be a challenge to effective ethanol infusion. In centers with a low volume of VOM ethanol infusion, collateral circulation might prevent inexperienced operators from further ethanol infusion. In cases of ethanol infusion attempts, collateral circulation might weaken the effect of VOM ethanol infusion. This study aimed to evaluate the feasibility and efficacy of ethanol infusion in VOM with distal collateral circulation.

2. Methods

2.1. Patient Selection

Patients with AF who underwent radiofrequency catheter ablation and VOM ethanol infusion in Fuwai Hospital, Beijing, China, between November 2021 and September 2022 were consecutively enrolled. Those with distal VOM collateral circulation were further included in this study. This study was performed in accordance with the Declaration of Helsinki and was approved by the Ethics Committee of Fuwai Hospital. Informed consent was obtained from all participants.

2.2. Procedural Approach

The procedure included pulmonary vein isolation, coronary sinus angiography for VOM identification, VOM cannulation and ethanol infusion, and catheter ablation of the mitral isthmus. The technical details of catheter ablation have been previously reported [7].

After catheter ablation, a guiding catheter (6-F Judkins Right [JR] 4; Medtronic, Minneapolis, MN, USA) was positioned inside the coronary sinus (CS) through an SL1 long sheath (8.5F; St. Jude Medical, Inc., St Paul, MN, USA) or a flexible long sheath (8.5-F, Agilis NxT; Abbott, St Paul, MN, USA) inserted from the right femoral vein. Non-occluded coronary sinus angiography was performed in the right anterior oblique (RAO), the left anterior oblique (LAO), and the LAO cranial views for VOM identification [7]. After VOM identification, an over-the-wire angioplasty balloon positioned in distal VOM was used for cannulation and occluded angiography of the VOM. If there was no distal VOM collateral circulation in either the non-occluded coronary sinus angiography or occluded VOM angiography, ethanol was delivered slowly at 2–3 positions distally to proximally in the VOM. After ethanol infusion, catheter ablation of the mitral isthmus was performed. If there was apparent distal VOM collateral circulation, a method of slower ethanol injection (2 mL over 5 min) plus additional balloon occlusion time for 3 min after each injection was used. Manifest localized myocardium staining was considered successful ethanol infusion.

2.3. Statistical Analysis

Continuous variables are expressed as mean ± standard deviation or median (interquartile range) as appropriate, and categorical variables are shown as ratio or percentage. Data analyses were performed using R software, version 4.2.0 (R Core Team, Vienna, Austria).

3. Results

3.1. Baseline Characteristics

A total of 162 patients were enrolled, and apparent distal VOM collateral circulation was found in 7 (4.3%) patients. The baseline characteristics of these seven patients are displayed in Table 1. They all had persistent AF. Patients had a mean age of 59 ± 7 years old, and 3 (28.6%) were female. The mean left atrium dimension was 43 ± 2.0 mm.

Table 1. Patient characteristics and procedural data.

Patient No.	Age, y	Sex	BMI, kg/m^2	Comorbidities	CHA$_2$DS$_2$-VASc Score	HAS-BLED Score	LA, mm	LVEF, %	Cannulation Success	Ethanol Infusion Success
1	58	Male	23.4	HTN, DM, stroke	4	1	47	68	Yes	No
2	59	Male	23.9	stroke	2	1	41	65	Yes	No
3	65	Male	25.3	HTN, stroke	4	3	43	63	Yes	Yes
4	59	Female	25.4	HTN, CAD	2	1	43	66	Yes	Yes

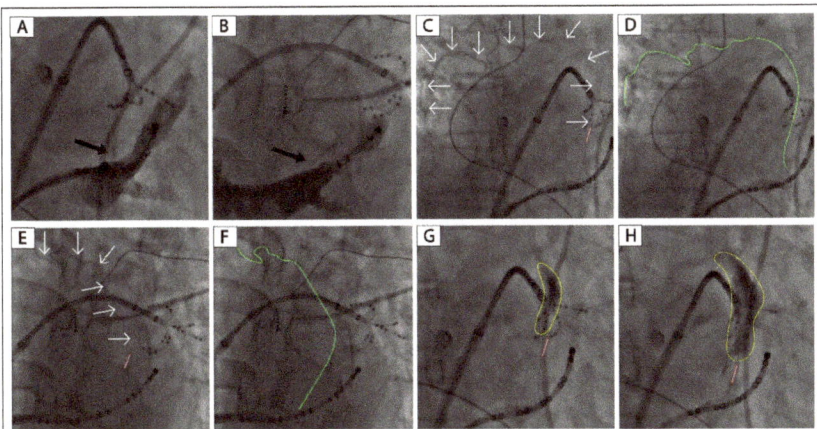

Figure 3. Successful ethanol infusion in a VOM with collateral circulation to the right superior vena cava. (**A,B**): Non-occluded venograms of VOM in the RAO and LAO projection, respectively. C and E: Balloon occluded venograms of VOM in the RAO and LAO projection, respectively. (**D,F**): Highlighted VOM of panels (**C,E**). (**G,H**): Balloon occluded venograms of VOM in the RAO projection after 4 and 8 mL of ethanol infusion, respectively. The black arrow indicates the ostium of VOM. The white arrows and green lines indicate the drainage of the VOM. The tubule outlined in red indicates the angioplasty balloon. The yellow circles indicate localized myocardium staining. VOM, the vein of Marshall; RAO, right anterior oblique; LAO, left anterior oblique.

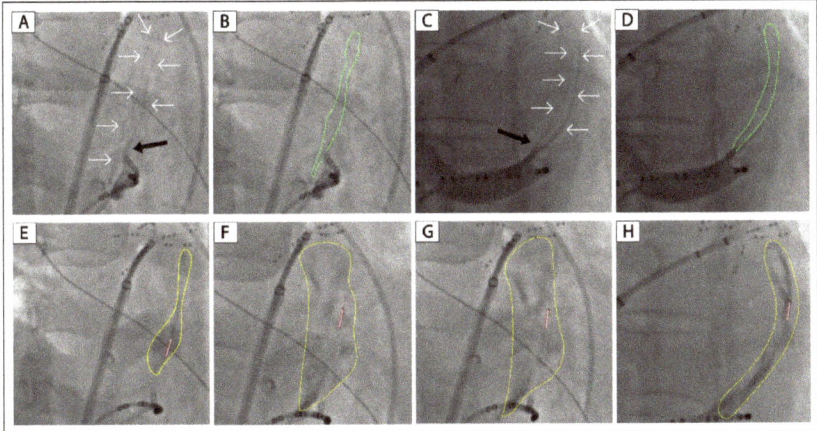

Figure 4. Successful ethanol infusion in a VOM with collateral circulation to the great cardiac vein. (**A,C**): Non-occluded venograms of VOM in the RAO and LAO projection, respectively. (**B,D**): Highlighted VOMs of panels (**A,C**), respectively. (**E–G**): Balloon occluded venograms of VOM in the RAO projection after 2, 4, and 8 mL of ethanol infusion, respectively. (**H**): Balloon occluded venograms of VOM in the LAO projection after 8 mL of ethanol infusion. The black arrow indicates the ostium of VOM. The white arrows and green lines indicate the drainage of the VOM. The tubule outlined in red indicates the angioplasty balloon. The yellow circles indicate localized myocardium staining. VOM, the vein of Marshall; RAO, right anterior oblique; LAO, left anterior oblique.

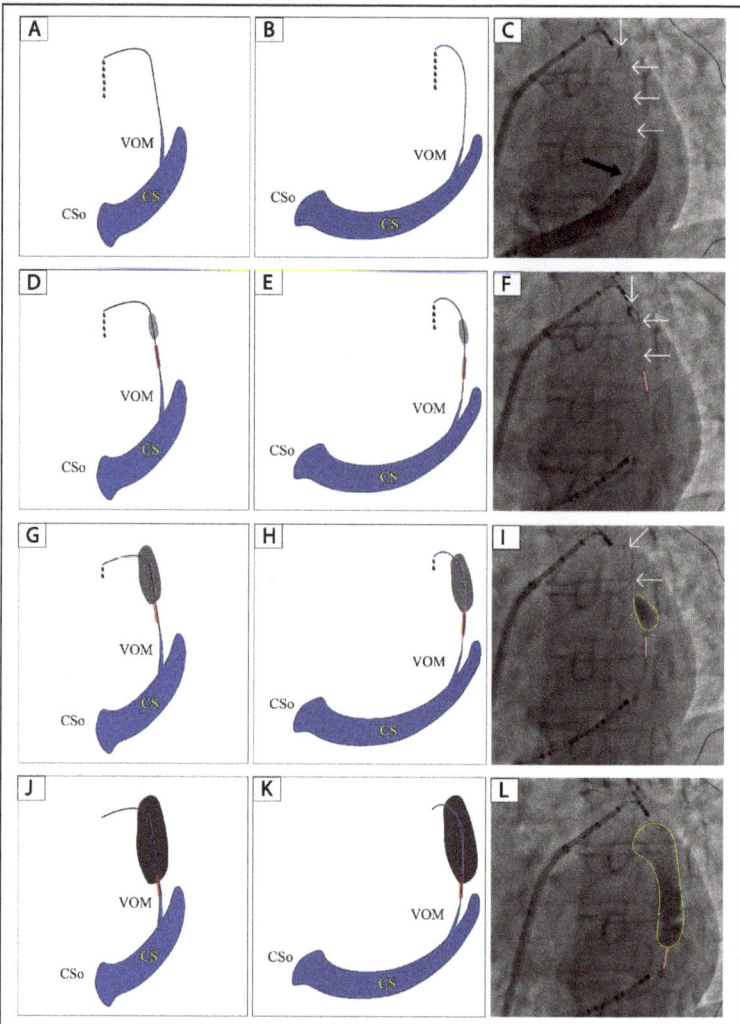

Figure 5. A step-by-step illustration of ethanol infusion in a VOM with collateral circulation. (**A,B**): Schematic diagram of non-occluded venograms of VOM in the RAO and LAO projection, respectively. (**D,G,J**): Schematic diagram of balloon occluded venograms of VOM in the RAO projection after 2, 4, and 8 mL of ethanol infusion, respectively. (**E,H,K**): Schematic diagram of balloon occluded venograms of VOM in the LAO projection after 2, 4, and 8 mL of ethanol infusion, respectively. (**C**): Non-occluded venogram of VOM in the LAO projection. (**F,I,L**): Balloon occluded venograms of VOM in the RAO projection after 2, 4, and 8 mL of ethanol infusion, respectively. The black arrow indicates the ostium of VOM. The white arrows indicate the drainage of the VOM. The tubule outlined in red indicates the angioplasty balloon. The gray and black shadows in Panels (**D,E,G,H,J**) and yellow circles in Panels (**I,L**) indicate localized myocardium staining. The black dots in Panels (**A,B,D,E,G,H**) indicate contrast leakage through the collateral circulation. VOM, the vein of Marshall; RAO, right anterior oblique; LAO, left anterior oblique.

4. Discussion

This study introduces our experience in ethanol infusion in VOM with distal collateral circulation. The results showed that VOM could connect with adjacent vessels or chambers distally and that slow ethanol injection could occlude the anastomosis and facilitate successfully localized myocardium staining.

In this study, only 4.9% of all patients had collateral circulation, which was significantly lower than in previous studies [2]. The main reason for this might be the different angiography methods used in our center, which only identified distal VOM collateral circulation. The first is non-occluded angiography for VOM identification. As we conclude, the key to identifying the VOM is to perform angiography in three fluoroscopic views and at least three positions of the guiding catheter in the coronary sinus lumen from distal to proximal. A balloon occlusion for coronary sinus angiogram is no longer needed in our lab, simplifying the procedure and shortening the procedure time. The second is the different locations of the balloon for occluded VOM angiography. We always advance the balloon as distal as possible rather than in the ostium in the VOM to perform VOM angiography and the first ethanol injection. So, a large proportion of collateral circulation originating from the proximal-to-medium VOM might be missing in our study. Similar to previous studies, the distal collateral connections included the left atrium, great cardiac vein, coronary sinus, and superior vena cava [2,8].

In patients No. 1–2, ethanol infusion was not performed because of our inadequate experience in the early stage of the VOM ethanol infusion project. As shown in Figure 1 and Supplemental Figure S1, these two patients had VOM collateral circulation to the left atrium, like the successful case shown in Figure 2. We believe ethanol infusion could occlude the connections between the distal VOM and the left atrium.

Figures 2–4 and Supplemental Figures S2 and S3 show the successful cases of ethanol infusion with manifest localized staining (Patients No. 3–7). Three had collateral circulation to the left atrium, one to the right superior vena cava, and one to the great cardiac vein. We conclude that the key to successful ethanol infusion in VOM with collateral circulation is the injection speed and the waiting time between multiple injections. In regular cases, we inject 2 mL of ethanol over 1 min and wait 1 min for the next injection. In such cases with collateral circulation, we will increase the injection time to 5 min for 2 mL of ethanol. And the waiting time between injections will be increased to 3 min. The anastomosis between distal VOM and adjacent vessels or chambers could be occluded using this method. The underlying reason might be that the anastomosis is always narrow, and the blood flow through it is slow. We succeeded in all five patients with VOM collateral circulation using this method.

5. Limitations

This study was conducted in a single center with only seven cases with VOM collateral circulation. The rate of VOM collateral circulation was low in our study because of the different methods used for angiography. We only identified distal VOM collateral circulation, which was crucial to ethanol infusion. Multicenter prospective studies with larger sample sizes are warranted in the future.

6. Conclusions

Ethanol infusion in VOM with collateral circulation can be solved by slow injection of ethanol and enough balloon occlusion time between multiple injections.

Supplementary Materials: The following supporting information can be downloaded at: https://www.mdpi.com/article/10.3390/jcm12010309/s1, Figure S1: VOM collateralization in a patient (Patient No. 1) without ethanol infusion attempt; Figure S2: Successful ethanol infusion in a VOM (Patient No. 6) with collateral circulation to the left atrium; Figure S3: Successful ethanol infusion in a VOM (Patient No. 7) with collateral circulation to the left atrium; Figure S4: Voltage maps of the left atrial lateral wall after ethanol infusion.

Author Contributions: Study conception and design: H.Z., L.D., M.T.; Analysis and interpretation of data: H.Z., L.D., M.T.; Drafting of the article: H.Z., L.D., M.T.; Critical revision of the article for intellectual content: H.Z., L.D., L.M., K.Z., Z.J., S.W., F.Y., M.T.; Final approval of the article: H.Z., L.D., L.M., K.Z., Z.J., S.W., F.Y., M.T.; Provision of study materials or patients: M.T.; Statistical expertise: H.Z., M.T.;

Obtaining of funding: H.Z., M.T.; Administrative, technical, or logistic support: H.Z., M.T.; Collection of data: H.Z., L.D. All authors have read and agreed to the published version of the manuscript.

Funding: The study was supported by the National Natural Science Foundation of China (U1913210 and 82000064) and the CAMS Innovation Fund for Medical Sciences (2022-I2M-C&T-B-047). The funding source had no role in the study design; in the collection, analysis, and interpretation of data; in writing the report; and in the decision to submit the article for publication.

Institutional Review Board Statement: The study was conducted in accordance with the Declaration of Helsinki, and approved by the Ethics Committee of Fuwai Hospital (Approval No. 2022-1810 Approval date: 18 September 2022).

Informed Consent Statement: Informed consent was obtained from all subjects involved in the study.

Data Availability Statement: Research data is confidential. Data-sharing requests are required to meet the policies of the hospital and the funder.

Conflicts of Interest: The authors declare that there is no conflict of interest.

Abbreviations

AF	atrial fibrillation
VOM	vein of Marshall
RAO	the right anterior oblique
LAO	the left anterior oblique

References

1. Valderrábano, M.; Peterson, L.E.; Swarup, V.; Schurmann, P.A.; Makkar, A.; Doshi, R.N.; DeLurgio, D.; Athill, C.A.; Ellenbogen, K.A.; Natale, A.; et al. Effect of Catheter Ablation with Vein of Marshall Ethanol Infusion vs Catheter Ablation Alone on Persistent Atrial Fibrillation: The VENUS Randomized Clinical Trial. *JAMA* **2020**, *324*, 1620–1628. [CrossRef] [PubMed]
2. Kamakura, T.; Derval, N.; Duchateau, J.; Denis, A.; Nakashima, T.; Takagi, T.; Ramirez, F.D.; André, C.; Krisai, P.; Nakatani, Y.; et al. Vein of Marshall Ethanol Infusion: Feasibility, Pitfalls, and Complications in Over 700 Patients. *Circ. Arrhythm Electrophysiol.* **2021**, *14*, e010001. [CrossRef] [PubMed]
3. Kim, D.T.; Lai, A.C.; Hwang, C.; Fan, L.T.; Karagueuzian, H.S.; Chen, P.S.; Fishbein, M.C. The ligament of Marshall: A structural analysis in human hearts with implications for atrial arrhythmias. *J. Am. Coll. Cardiol.* **2000**, *36*, 1324–1327. [CrossRef] [PubMed]
4. Doshi, R.N.; Wu, T.J.; Yashima, M.; Kim, Y.H.; Ong, J.J.; Cao, J.M.; Hwang, C.; Yashar, P.; Fishbein, M.C.; Karagueuzian, H.S.; et al. Relation between ligament of Marshall and adrenergic atrial tachyarrhythmia. *Circulation* **1999**, *100*, 876–883. [CrossRef] [PubMed]
5. Derval, N.; Duchateau, J.; Denis, A.; Ramirez, F.D.; Mahida, S.; André, C.; Krisai, P.; Nakatani, Y.; Kitamura, T.; Takigawa, M.; et al. Marshall bundle elimination, Pulmonary vein isolation, and Line completion for ANatomical ablation of persistent atrial fibrillation (Marshall-PLAN): Prospective, single-center study. *Heart Rhythm* **2021**, *18*, 529–537. [CrossRef] [PubMed]
6. Valderrábano, M. Vein of Marshall ethanol infusion in the treatment of atrial fibrillation: From concept to clinical practice. *Heart Rhythm* **2021**, *18*, 1074–1082. [CrossRef] [PubMed]
7. Ding, L.; Zhang, H.; Yu, F.; Mi, L.; Hua, W.; Zhang, S.; Yao, Y.; Tang, M. Angiographic Characteristics of the Vein of Marshall in Patients with and without Atrial Fibrillation. *J. Clin. Med.* **2022**, *11*, 5384. [CrossRef] [PubMed]
8. Valderrabano, M.; Morales, P.F.; Rodriguez-Manero, M.; Lloves, C.; Schurmann, P.A.; Dave, A.S. The Human Left Atrial Venous Circulation as a Vascular Route for Atrial Pharmacological Therapies: Effects of Ethanol Infusion. *JACC Clin. Electrophysiol.* **2017**, *3*, 1020–1032. [CrossRef] [PubMed]
9. Takagi, T.; Derval, N.; Pambrun, T.; Nakatani, Y.; Andre, C.; Ramirez, F.D.; Nakashima, T.; Krisai, P.; Kamakura, T.; Pineau, X.; et al. Optimized Computed Tomography Acquisition Protocol for Ethanol Infusion into the Vein of Marshall. *JACC Clin. Electrophysiol.* **2022**, *8*, 168–178. [CrossRef] [PubMed]
10. Krisai, P.; Pambrun, T.; Nakatani, Y.; Nakashima, T.; Takagi, T.; Kamakura, T.; André, C.; Cheniti, G.; Tixier, R.; Chauvel, R.; et al. How to perform ethanol ablation of the vein of Marshall for treatment of atrial fibrillation. *Heart Rhythm* **2021**, *18*, 1083–1087. [CrossRef] [PubMed]

Disclaimer/Publisher's Note: The statements, opinions and data contained in all publications are solely those of the individual author(s) and contributor(s) and not of MDPI and/or the editor(s). MDPI and/or the editor(s) disclaim responsibility for any injury to people or property resulting from any ideas, methods, instructions or products referred to in the content.

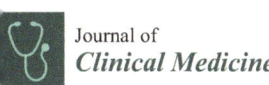

Article

Iatrogenic Atrial Septal Defect after Intracardiac Echocardiography-Guided Left Atrial Appendage Closure: Incidence, Size, and Clinical Outcomes

Yibo Ma [†], Lanyan Guo [†], Jie Li, Haitao Liu, Jian Xu, Hui Du, Yi Wang, Huihui Li and Fu Yi *

Department of Cardiology, Xijing Hospital, Air Force Medical University, Xi'an 710032, China
* Correspondence: yi12fu56@126.com
† These authors contributed equally to this work.

Abstract: Background: The data on iatrogenic atrial septal defect (iASD) after left atrial appendage closure (LAAC), especially intracardiac echocardiography (ICE)-guided LAAC, are limited. Compared with transesophageal echocardiography (TEE)- or digital subtraction angiography (DSA)-guided LAAC, the transseptal puncture (TP) ICE-guided LAAC is more complicated. Whether or not ICE-guided TP increases the chances of iASD is controversial. We investigate the incidence, size, and clinical outcomes of iASD after ICE-guided LAAC. Methods: A total of 177 patients who underwent LAAC were enrolled in this study and were assigned to the ICE-guided group (group 1) and the TEE- or DSA-guided group (group 2). Echocardiography results and clinical performances at months 2 and 12 post-procedure were collected from the electronic outpatient records. Results: A total of 112 and 65 patients were assigned to group 1 and group 2, respectively. The incidence of iASD at follow-up (FU) month 2 was comparable between the groups (21.4% in group 1 vs. 15.4% in group 2, $p = 0.429$). At month 12 of FU, the closure rate of iASD was comparable to that of group 2 (70.6% vs. 71.4%, $p = 1.000$). No right-to-left (RL) shunt was observed among the iASD patients during the FU. Numerically larger iASD were observed in group 1 patients at month 2 of FU (2.8 ± 0.9 mm vs. 2.2 ± 0.8 mm, $p = 0.065$). No new-onset of pulmonary hypertension and iASD-related adverse events were observed. Univariable and multivariable logistic regression analysis showed that ICE-guided LAAC was not associated with the development of iASD (adjusted OR = 1.681; 95%CI, 0.634–4.455; $p = 0.296$). Conclusions: The ICE-guided LAAC procedure does not increase the risk of iASD. Despite the numerically large size of the iASD, it did not increase the risk of developing adverse complications.

Keywords: iatrogenic atrial septal defect; intracardiac echocardiography; left atrial appendage closure; atrial fibrillation; right-to-left shunt

Citation: Ma, Y.; Guo, L.; Li, J.; Liu, H.; Xu, J.; Du, H.; Wang, Y.; Li, H.; Yi, F. Iatrogenic Atrial Septal Defect after Intracardiac Echocardiography-Guided Left Atrial Appendage Closure: Incidence, Size, and Clinical Outcomes. *J. Clin. Med.* **2023**, *12*, 160. https://doi.org/10.3390/jcm12010160

Academic Editor: Andrea Igoren Guaricci

Received: 16 November 2022
Revised: 9 December 2022
Accepted: 20 December 2022
Published: 25 December 2022

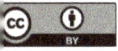

Copyright: © 2022 by the authors. Licensee MDPI, Basel, Switzerland. This article is an open access article distributed under the terms and conditions of the Creative Commons Attribution (CC BY) license (https://creativecommons.org/licenses/by/4.0/).

1. Introduction

Transcatheter left atrial appendage closure (LAAC) has become an effective and safe alternative to oral anticoagulant (OAC) in patients at high risk of atrial fibrillation (AF) and anticoagulation intolerance [1–3]. Transseptal puncture (TP) is performed during the LAAC procedure, providing access for a 12-F closure device delivery sheath to the left atrial appendage (LAA) through the left atrium. The fossa ovalis, the weakest part of the atrial septum, was the most common site for TP in the past. Because acute transseptal shunts were detected in almost all patients post-procedure, this site is currently seldom considered [4]. The most common site for TP is now the posterior and inferior area of the fossa ovalis, which is associated with a lower incidence of immediate left-to-right (LR) shunting and allows for more accurate delivery of the sheath [5]. The reliability of the puncture of the posterior and inferior area of the fossa ovalis is higher than that of puncture of the fossa ovalis.

Transesophageal echocardiography (TEE), intracardiac echocardiography (ICE), and digital subtraction angiography (DSA) were the most commonly used methods for guiding the LAAC procedure. Using ICE to deliver a catheter into the left atrium during the LAAC has unique advantages [6,7]. For instance, compared with the TEE method, it is feasible and safe, and general anesthesia is not needed, which eliminates the usage of contrast, shortening the time in the catheterization room [8]. During the ICE-guided LAAC procedure, more TP operations are performed to construct another access. Whether or not this method can increase the incidence of the iatrogenic atrial septal defect (iASD) remains controversial [8,9]. In addition, a previous report showed that the iASD, especially the right-to-left (RL) shunt iASD, causes acute anoxia and exacerbates pulmonary hypertension in patients who undergo the MitraClip procedure [10]. Considering that most patients who undergo LAAC also have complex underlying complications, the clinical relevance of iASD caused by ICE-guided LAAC should be clarified. Our study compared the incidence, size, and clinical outcomes of iASD after ICE-guided LAAC procedure and TEE- or DSA-guided LAAC.

2. Materials and Methods

2.1. Study Population

This was a single-center retrospective study. AF patients who underwent LAAC at the First Affiliated Hospital of Air Force Military Medical University, Cardiology Department, between March 2019 and December 2021 were enrolled in this study. The indication of LAAC was according to the local guidelines, which can be summarized as patients who are unwilling to receive long-term OAC, have intolerance to anticoagulation, or are at high risk of embolism. The inclusion criteria were: (1) aged 18–85 years old; (2) non-valvular AF confirmed by both echocardiography and standard 12-lead electrocardiogram; and (3) finished at least 2 months of outpatient follow-up (FU). The exclusion criteria included (1) atrial septal defect confirmed by transthoracic echocardiography (TTE), which had then not been corrected by whichever procedure by the time of the LAAC procedure; (2) history of cardiac surgery; and (3) a thicker sheath that advanced into the left atrium at the time of such LAAC procedure, such as cryoballoon ablation (CBA) combined with LAAC. The patients were assigned to the ICE-guided group (group 1) and the TEE- or DSA-guided group (group 2) based on the type of imaging used. The details of the patient enrollment process are shown in Figure 1. The protocol for this study was approved by the ethics board of the First Affiliated Hospital of Air Force Military Medical University. Written informed consent was acquired from all the patients before the procedure.

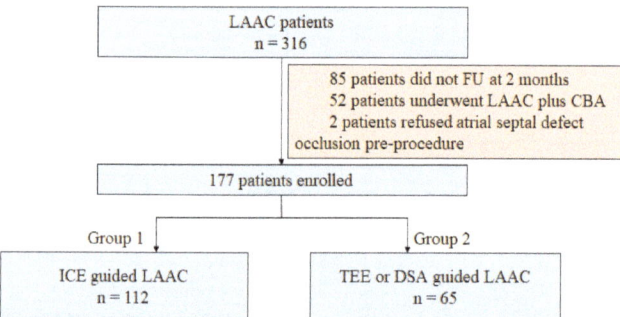

Figure 1. Study flowchart. LAAC = left atrial appendage closure; FU = follow-up; CBA = cryoballoon ablation; ICE = intracardiac echocardiography; TEE = transesophageal echocardiography; DSA = digital subtraction angiography.

2.2. Procedure

2.2.1. ICE-Guided TP Procedure

The ICE-guided LAAC was performed as previously described [11]. The intracardiac images for reconstructing the three-dimensional left atrium model were obtained using a

10-F SoundStar ICE catheter (Biosense Webster). Briefly, the right femoral access was first constructed, and an 11-F sheath for advancing the ICE catheter was inserted into the middle of the right atrium. The catheter was rotated until the atrial septal was fully visible. Finally, the posterior and inferior areas of the fossa ovalis were punctured. The delivery device to the sheath was advanced to the left atrium through the punctured hole. In addition, during the LAAC procedure, the ICE probe was advanced into the left atrium through the same atrial septal puncture hole. The WATCHMAN device (Boston Scientific) was used for the procedure. If the LAA morphology was unsuitable for the WATCHMAN device implantation, the LACbes device (PushMed, Shanghai, China) was instead implanted. Both sheaths have a diameter of 12-F. The diagrammatic flow of these steps is shown in Figure 2.

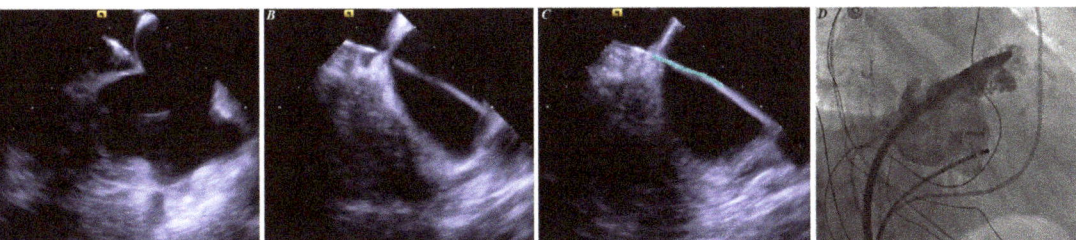

Figure 2. Steps of ICE-guided TP procedure. Panel (**A**) shows ICE image of tenting sign. Panel (**B**) shows ICE image of SL1 sheath positioned in the left atrium. Panel (**C**) shows delivered guide wire (green line) into the left atrium along the SL1 sheath. Panel (**D**) shows that SL1 sheath and guide wire were replaced, and device delivery sheath and ICE catheter were positioned in the left atrium through the same puncture hole. ICE = intracardiac echocardiography; TP = transseptal puncture.

2.2.2. TEE- or DSA-Guided TP Procedure

The TEE- or DSA-guided TP procedure was performed as previously described [5–8]. Briefly, a single femoral vein access was first constructed. A posterior and inferior TP was attempted under TEE or DSA guidance. Throughout the LAAC procedure, only the device delivery sheath was advanced to the left atrium through the punctured hole. During the TEE-guided TP procedure, the patients were given general anesthesia and intubated when the TEE probe was introduced. The principle of the closure device use was the same as that for the ICE-guided TP procedure.

2.3. Outpatient Follow-Up

Postimplant FU was scheduled at 2, 6, and 12 months post-procedure. The iASD results were collected at months 2 and 12. The presence and size of the iASDs were detected and measured using three-dimensional TEE, and the blood flow direction through the iASD was detected by color Doppler ultrasonography. The hemodynamic parameters, especially the pulmonary artery pressure, were also assessed by echocardiography. TTE was used as an alternative to TEE for the iASD examination.

In addition to the echocardiography data, the incidence of clinical adverse events, including cardiovascular death, ischemic stroke, migraine, and readmission for acute heart failure, was also captured during each FU.

2.4. Statistical Analysis

Continuous normally distributed variables were presented as mean ± SD. Differences between the groups were analyzed by one-way ANOVA. Non-normally distributed data were expressed as the median and interquartile range (IQR), and corresponding groups were compared by the Mann–Whitney U test. Categorical variables were expressed as count (percentage) and compared by Fisher's exact test.

The unadjusted risk ratio of each variable was estimated by univariable logistic regression analysis. The relationship between ICE-guided LAAC and the risk of iASD was analyzed by multivariable logistic regression analysis after adjustment for several covariates: the CHA$_2$DS$_2$-VASc score and the HASBLED score (model 1); age, sex, body mass index (BMI), non-paroxysmal AF, AF duration, heart failure, hypertension, diabetes mellitus, prior ischemic stroke, coronary heart disease, left atrial diameter (LAD), left ventricular ejection fraction (LVEF), pathological mitral regurgitation and tricuspid regurgitation, patent foramen ovale (PFO) occlusion, and the use of different closure devices (model 2). Statistical significance was set at $p \leq 0.05$. Statistical analysis was performed using IBM SPSS software, version 26.0 (IBM SPSS Inc., Chicago, IL, USA), and R software, version 4.2.0 (Ross Ihaka and Robert Gentleman, Auckland, New Zealand).

3. Results

3.1. Patient Characteristics at Baseline

A total of 177 patients were enrolled in this study (Figure 1). Among them, 112 were classified in group 1, and 65 patients were classified in group 2. The baseline characteristics of the study patients are summarized in Table 1. The mean age, CHA$_2$DS$_2$-VASc score, and HASBLED score were 64.5 ± 9.1 years, 3.4 ± 1.8, and 1.8 ± 1.1, respectively. Moreover, 65.5% of the study participants were males. Except for non-paroxysmal AF and pulmonary hypertension, which were significantly higher in the patients in group 2 (non-paroxysmal AF: 61.6% vs. 83.1%, $p = 0.004$ and pulmonary hypertension: 6.3% vs. 24.6%, $p = 0.001$), there was no significant difference in patient characteristics at the baseline between the two groups.

Table 1. Baseline characteristics.

	Group 1 (n = 112)	Group 2 (n = 65)	p-Value
Demographics			
Age, years	n = 112, 64.6 ± 8.8	n = 65, 64.4 ± 9.6	0.844
Male sex	n = 112, 72 (64.3)	n = 65, 44 (67.7)	0.743
BMI, kg/m^2	n = 112, 25.1 ± 3.2	n = 65, 25.0 ± 3.5	0.783
AF overview			
Paroxysmal AF	n = 112, 43 (38.4)	n = 65, 11 (16.9)	0.004
Non-paroxysmal AF	n = 112, 69 (61.6)	n = 65, 54 (83.1)	0.004
AF duration, months	n = 112, 12.0 (4.0, 48.0)	n = 65, 24.0 (6.0, 90.0)	0.041
Risk factors			
CHA$_2$DS$_2$-VASc score	n = 112, 3.3 ± 1.7	n = 65, 3.5 ± 1.9	0.551
Heart failure	n = 112, 34 (30.4)	n = 65, 22 (33.8)	0.738
Hypertension	n = 112, 58 (51.8)	n = 65, 41 (63.1)	0.160
Age ≥ 75 years	n = 112, 11 (9.8)	n = 65, 9 (13.8)	0.464
Stroke/TIA/SE	n = 112, 39 (34.8)	n = 65, 19 (29.2)	0.508
Coronary artery disease	n = 112, 32 (28.6)	n = 65, 19 (29.2)	1.000
Age 65–74 years	n = 112, 50 (44.6)	n = 65, 25 (38.5)	0.435
HASBLED score	n = 112, 1.8 ± 1.1	n = 65, 1.8 ± 1.2	0.812
Echocardiographic index			
LAD, mm	n = 112, 44.6 ± 5.6	n = 65, 46.1 ± 6.7	0.120
LVEF, %	n = 112, 55.4 ± 6.0	n = 65, 55.3 ± 5.8	0.886
Pathological mitral regurgitation	n = 112, 28 (25.0)	n = 65, 17 (26.2)	0.860
Pathological tricuspid regurgitation	n = 112, 37 (33.0)	n = 65, 26 (40.0)	0.416
Pulmonary hypertension	n = 112, 7 (6.3)	n = 65, 16 (24.6)	0.001
Mean pressure, mmHg	n = 7, 45.0 ± 3.5	n = 16, 43.6 ± 8.6	0.678

BMI = body mass index; AF = atrial fibrillation; TIA = transient ischemic attack; SE = systemic embolism; LAD = left atrial diameter; LVEF = left ventricular ejection fraction.

3.2. Procedure Characteristics

All the patients underwent successful TP. For group 2, 37 (56.9%) patients underwent TEE-guided LAAC, and 28 (43.1%) patients underwent DSA-guided LAAC. The successful

LAAC rate in group 1 was 99.1%, and it was 98.5% for the group 2 patients. Significantly more patients in group 1 underwent radiofrequency catheter ablation (RFCA) at the time of LAAC (90.2% vs. 40.0%, $p = 0.000$). All nine patients who underwent PFO occlusion were in group 2. After discharge, all the patients received OAC or antiplatelet therapy (Table 2).

Table 2. Procedure characteristics.

	Group 1 (n = 112)	Group 2 (n = 65)	p-Value
Device			0.414
WATCHMAN	n = 112, 90 (80.4)	n = 65, 55 (84.6)	
LACbes	n = 112, 22 (19.6)	n = 65, 9 (13.8)	
Intra-procedure details			
LAAC success	n = 112, 111 (99.1)	n = 65, 64 (98.5)	1.000
Combined with RFCA	n = 112, 101 (90.2)	n = 65, 26 (40.0)	0.000
PFO occlusion	n = 112, 0 (0.0)	n = 65, 9 (13.8)	0.000
Discharge medication			0.011
OAC monotherapy	n = 112, 107 (95.5)	n = 65, 57 (87.7)	
OAC plus single antiplatelet therapy	n = 112, 5 (4.5)	n = 65, 3 (4.6)	
Dual antiplatelet therapy	n = 112, 0 (0.0)	n = 65, 5 (7.7)	

LAAC = left atrial appendage closure; RFCA = radiofrequency catheter ablation; PFO = patent foramen ovale; OAC = oral anticoagulant.

3.3. Two Months FU

At a median of 57 (IQR: 47, 74) days of FU, 24 (21.4%) patients in group 1 had iASD (Table 3). Among them, 9 were detected by TEE and 15 by TTE. The total incidence of iASD was comparable between the two groups (21.4% vs. 15.4%, $p = 0.429$). All the patients with a patent iASD had LR shunts. The mean size of the patent iASD in the group 1 patients was 2.8 ± 0.9 [range: 1.5–5.1] mm, which was numerically larger than the 2.2 ± 0.8 [range: 1.4–3.5] mm for the patients in group 2 ($p = 0.065$). A total of two (1.8%) patients in group 1 developed two patent iASDs: the sizes of the iASDs were 4.5 + 2.0 mm and 2.3 + 1.7 mm. New-onset pulmonary hypertension was detected in three patients; all of them were in group 1, and none of them had a patent iASD. Two patients died, one (ICE-guided, with iASD in the first month) from device-related thrombus and the other (ICE-guided, without iASD in the second month) from catastrophic heart failure with delayed cardiac tamponade. No other adverse events occurred.

3.4. Twelve Months FU

There were 25 patients with patent iASD who received repeat TTE checks on day 243, on average (IQR: 186–382), after LAAC (Table 3). iASD was still present in five patients in group 1. The closure rate of patent iASD was comparable between the groups (70.6% vs. 71.4%, $p = 1.000$). No RL shunts were detected. The size of the residual iASD for the patients in group 1 was 2, 2, 3, 3, and 4 mm, and it was 1.5 and 2 mm for the patients in group 2 ($p = 0.190$). One patient in group 1 had two 4.0- and 1.0-mm shunts. The iASD occlusion of the patent is shown in Figure 3. None of the patients developed new-onset pulmonary hypertension. The data for all the patients who were alive after the first FU were available, and none of the patients died or developed adverse events.

3.5. Relationship between Patent iASD and ICE-Guided LAAC

Univariable logistic regression showed that ICE-guided LAAC did not increase the risk of iASD (Figure 4). However, both the history of ischemic stroke (OR = 2.488; 95% CI, 1.159–5.340; $p = 0.019$) and the use of the LACbes device (OR = 2.401; 95% CI, 1.005–5.737; $p = 0.049$) significantly increased the risk of iASD.

Table 3. Follow-up.

	Group 1 (*n* = 112)	Group 2 (*n* = 65)	*p*-Value
First FU (month 2)			
Time to review, days	*n* = 112, 57.5 (44.0, 75.0)	*n* = 65, 57.0 (50.0, 71.0)	0.236
Examination			0.001
TEE	*n* = 112, 33 (29.5)	*n* = 65, 35 (53.8)	
TTE	*n* = 112, 79 (70.5)	*n* = 65, 30 (46.2)	
Patent iASD	*n* = 112, 24 (21.4)	*n* = 65, 10 (15.4)	0.429
TEE-detected	*n* = 33, 9 (27.3)	*n* = 35, 4 (11.4)	0.128
TTE-detected	*n* = 79, 15 (19.0)	*n* = 30, 6 (20.0)	1.000
Shunt			1.000
LR shunt	*n* = 24, 24 (100.0)	*n* = 10, 10 (100.0)	
RL shunt	*n* = 24, 0 (0.0)	*n* = 10, 0 (0.0)	
Size, mm	*n* = 24, 2.8 ± 0.9	*n* = 10, 2.2 ± 0.8	0.065
New-onset pulmonary hypertension	*n* = 112, 3 (2.68)	*n* = 65, 0 (0.0)	0.299
Final FU (month 12)			
Time to review, days	*n* = 17, 221.0 (161.0, 392.0)	*n* = 7, 260.0 (204.0, 364.0)	0.619
Residual iASD	*n* = 17, 5 (29.4)	*n* = 7, 2 (28.6)	1.000
Shunt			1.000
LR shunt	*n* = 5, 5 (100.0)	*n* = 2, 2 (100.0)	
RL shunt	*n* = 5, 0 (0.0)	*n* = 2, 0 (0.0)	

FU = follow-up; TEE = transesophageal echocardiography; TTE = transthoracic echocardiography; iASD = iatrogenic atrial septal defect; LR = left-to-right; RL = right-to-left.

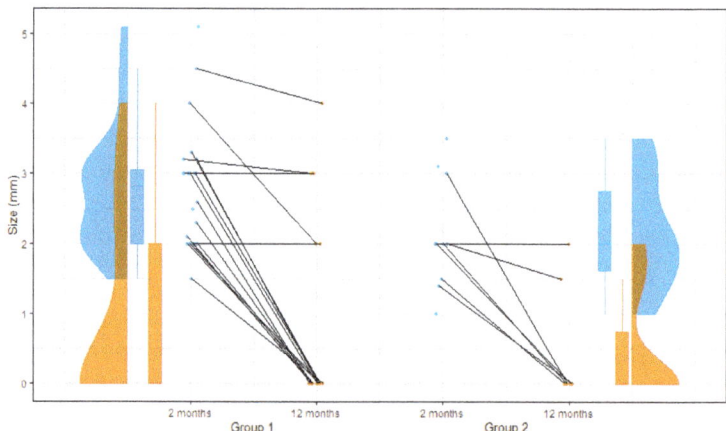

Figure 3. Occlusion of patent iASD. iASD = iatrogenic atrial septal defect.

Even after adjustment for the CHA_2DS_2-VASc and HASBLED scores, we found no relationship between ICE-guided LAAC and the development of iASD (adjusted OR: 1.588 (95%CI, 0.696–3.623; *p* = 0.272)). We also found no relationship between ICE-guided LAAC and the development of iASD after adjustment for demographic characteristics (age, sex, and BMI); certain underlying diseases (non-paroxysmal AF, AF duration, heart failure, hypertension, diabetes mellitus, prior ischemic stroke, and coronary heart disease); the echocardiographic index (LAD, LVEF, pulmonary hypertension, pathological mitral, and tricuspid regurgitation); and peri-procedure characteristics (PFO closure and the use of different devices) (adjusted OR: 1.681 (95% CI, 0.634–4.455; *p* = 0.296)).

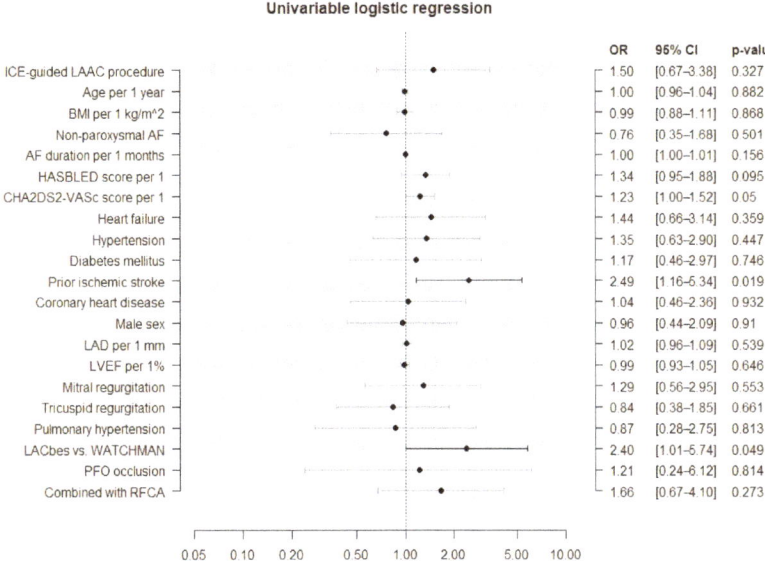

Figure 4. Predictors of patent iatrogenic atrial septal defect. ICE = intracardiac echocardiography; LAAC = left atrial appendage closure; BMI = body mass index; AF = atrial fibrillation; LAD = left atrial diameter; LVEF = left ventricular ejection fraction; PFO = patent foramen ovale; RFCA = radiofrequency catheter ablation.

4. Discussion

The present study revealed the incidence, size, and clinical outcomes of iASDs after the ICE-guided LAAC procedure. The incidence of iASDs at month 2 after the ICE-guided LAAC procedure was 21.4%. The occlusion rate of iASDs at month 12 after the ICE-guided LAAC was 70.6%. There was no difference in the incidence of iASDs between the ICE-guided LAAC group and the TEE- or DSA-guided LAAC group at month 2 and 12. However, the size of iASD was numerically larger in the ICE-guided LAAC group than in the TEE- or ICE-guided LAAC group. Univariate and multivariable logistic regression analyses showed that the ICE-guided LAAC did not increase the risk of iASD. All the iASDs were LR shunt and did not cause pulmonary hypertension. The residual iASD was not associated with the development of adverse events. We found that both the history of ischemic stroke and the use of the LACbes device increased the risk of patent iASD, which, to the best of our knowledge, was never reported in the previous studies. To our knowledge, this is the first report on the dynamic incidence of patent iASD after ICE-guided LAAC.

4.1. Incidence and Size of Patent iASD after LAAC

The incidence of iASD shortly after LAAC has been reported in several studies. For instance, Korsholm et al. compared the efficacy and safety of ICE-guided LAAC and the traditional TEE-guided LAAC of the left upper chamber, with the iASD being one of the secondary efficacy parameters. The incidence and size of the residual iASD in the ICE group at day 55 of FU were 35% and 3.5 (IQR: 1–8) mm, respectively. For the TEE group, the incidence and size of the residual iASD were 26% and 3.5 (2–6) mm, respectively, which were not significantly different between the groups ($p = 0.21$ for the incidence of iASD and $p = 0.58$ for the iASD size) [8]. Puga et al. conducted single-center research on the risk of developing iASD. Thirty patients underwent ICE-guided LAAC on the left atrium, and 36 underwent TEE-guided LAAC. The results showed that the iASD incidence was higher in the ICE group (65.4% in the ICE group vs. 40.9% in the TEE group, $p = 0.048$), but there was no significant difference in the size of the iASD between the two groups

(5 mm (IQR 4–5.5 mm) vs. 5 mm (2–5 mm), p = 0.712) at the first FU. Multivariable analysis showed that ICE alone was associated with a higher iASD (OR = 3.745, 95%CI: 1.197–11.715 incidence [9]. In the present study, we determined the incidence of iASD at month 2 of FU after LAAC. The results showed that the ICE-guided LAAC did not increase the risk of iASD. However, the size of the iASD was numerically larger in the ICE-guided LAAC group. Compared to the above reports, the incidence of iASD in our study was relatively low, and the size of the iASD was small. The mean iASD in the ICE group in this study was only 2.8 mm. For the long-term occlusion rate, Chen et al. reported that the incidence of iASD after the ICE-guided LAAC procedure dropped from 57.9% at month 2 of FU to 4.2% at month 12 of FU [12]. In our study, the incidence of iASD in the ICE-guided LAAC group was 21.4% at month 2 of FU, and the occlusion rate of iASD at month 12 of FU was 70.6%. Nelles et al. reported that the incidence of iASD under TEE-guided LAAC dropped from 34.7% at month 3 of FU to 18.1% at month 12 [13]. Singh et al. reported that the incidence of iASD in 253 patients in a "PROTECT AF" cohort at month 12 of FU was 6.8% [14]. The occlusion of iASD over time is a common phenomenon. To sum up, the short-term and long-term incidence and size of iASD following ICE-guided LAAC in our study are within the acceptable range.

4.2. Predictive Indicators of iASD

It is necessary to discuss the lack of difference between the ICE-guided group and the TEE- or DSA-guided group. The occurrence of iASD is related to many factors, such as sheath diameter, excessive operations, and FU duration. A sheath diameter $\geq$ 14-F increased the risk of iASD [15]. It was worth noting that the device delivery sheath was 12 F, and the sheath of the ICE catheter was 11-F, which meant that that the largest diameter of the puncture hole was almost 9 mm. However, our results showed that ICE-guided LAAC did not increase the risk of developing iASD, and the mean size of the patent iASD was 2.8 mm. During the procedure, the device delivery sheath and ICE catheter were advanced into the left atrium through the same puncture hole. Because the posterior and inferior area of the fossa ovalis was thick and elastic, we hypothesized that a further additional TP operation could not substantially damage the atrial septum. Two patients in group 1 had two patent iASDs at month 2 of FU, which might be related to extra damage caused by the poor operation. In addition, empirically speaking, ICE was more accurate in finding the device delivery pathway best suited to the LAAC procedure. Operators could look for an ideal puncture site using ICE images and the left atrial model. However, for the TEE-guided LAAC procedure, the primary use of the TEE images in TP was for safety purposes. The significant deviation between the axial direction of the device delivery catheter and the LAA inevitably increases the number of catheter operations, or there could even be a need re-perform the TP operation. Thirdly, iASD had a high spontaneous closure rate. The earlier the FU, the easier it was to observe the patent iASD. Puga et al. also reported that the ICE-guided approach was associated with a higher incidence of iASD. Their scheduled FU was quite early, even before the LAAC review, and the long-term occlusion rate was not reported [9]. To sum up, the ICE-guided approach did not increase the incidence of patent iASD.

We found that a history of ischemic stroke and the use of the LACbes device increased the risk of patent iASD. A relative observational study revealed that the cauliflower-shaped LAA was complex and was associated with cardiac embolism [16]. This kind of LAA would increase the difficulty of the operation, resulting in a higher number of LAAC attempts. In theory, because of the same sheath size, the use of the LACbes device does not increase the risk of iASD. In our study, the LACbes device was implanted if the LAA morphology was unsuitable for the WATCHMAN device implantation. Once the patient received the LACbes device implantation, he or she experienced a higher number of LAAC attempts compared to the patients who received the WATCHMAN device implantation. Excessive operations could increase the risk of iASD. A long-term observation study revealed that a higher number of cryoballoon (CBA) applications was an independent predictor of patent iASD

(OR = 1.207, 95%CI, 1.033–1.411, p = 0.018) [17]. To minimize iASD development, a more precise evaluation before and during LAAC is necessary to improve the first successful deployment rate and minimize the TP attempts.

4.3. Clinical Outcomes of Patent iASD

The clinical relevance of patent iASD is still controversial. The previous studies show that blood flows through the LAAC-related iASD from the left to the right shunt, and the iASD resolves itself over time. In the present concept, the iASD was seen as a phenomenon rather than a complication, and the subsequent exclusive closure operation was rarely performed. Reports on the outcomes of iASDs after LAAC are scanty, but several studies have reported immediate or long-term iASDs after MitraClip. Schueler et al. reviewed 66 patients who underwent the MitraClip procedure and found that the iASD was the only indicator associated with death in 6 months [18]. Morikawa et al. investigated the outcomes of RL shunt through iASD and found that although RL shunt was only observed in 5% of the patients, it significantly increased the risk of acute deoxygenation. Moreover, the composite of major adverse cardiac events was significantly higher in the patients with RL shunt than those with LR shunt. By comparison, the patients with severe tricuspid regurgitation, higher serum B-type natriuretic peptide, higher pulmonary artery pressure, and right atrial pressure increased the risk of RL shunt [10]. For our cohort, cardiac function impairment was only mild; 39.7% of the patients presented with left heart failure; the mean LVEF was 55.4 ± 6.2%; the rate of pathological valve regurgitation at the baseline was less than 40%; none of the patients was in New York Heart Association functional class IV; and none of the patients had RL shunt through iASD over the FU period. It is worth noting that LAAC is appropriate for patients who have intolerance to anticoagulants or have a high risk of thromboembolism rather than those with severe hemodynamic disturbance. In addition, lifelong antithrombotic medications are recommended for patients who have undergone LAAC. In addition, the sheath diameter of the MitraClip catheter is 22-F, significantly larger than the 12-F LAAC catheter; a larger catheter can cause larger defects when punctured. Most studies have shown that LAAC-related iASD is not life-threatening and is not associated with adverse clinical events [9,11–13]. We believe that it is unnecessary to focus too much on LAAC-related iASD, whether TEE-, DSA-, or ICE-guided. Rather, there is a need to focus on better heart failure management to prevent iASD-associated complications.

4.4. Study Limitations

There were several limitations in our study. The rate of patent iASD was numerically higher in the ICE-guided LAAC group than in the TEE- or DSA-guided LAAC group. Considering that significantly more patients in the ICE-guided LAAC group than in the TEE- or DSA-guided LAAC group underwent RFCA in the same period of LAAC, we could not determine whether this difference was related to the insufficient sample size or was caused by the additional RFCA procedure. The sensitivity of TTE in detecting iASD is lower than that of TEE, which may lead to an underestimation of iASD. Given that this was a retrospective study, the accuracy of some data, such as the prevalence of migraine, might be inaccurate.

5. Conclusions

In the present study, the incidence of iASD following ICE-guided LAAC at month 2 of FU was 21.4%, and the 12-month closure rate of iASD was 70.6%. No patient had RL shunt. ICE-guided LAAC did not increase the risk of patent iASD. Despite the size of the iASD being numerically larger for the patient who underwent ICE-guided LAAC than the patient who underwent TEE- or DSA-guided LAAC, this did not increase the risk of developing pulmonary hypertension and other adverse clinical complications.

Author Contributions: Conceptualization, F.Y. and H.L. (Haitao Liu); methodology, Y.M. and J.X.; software, Y.M. and H.D.; validation, J.L.; formal analysis, Y.M. and Y.W.; investigation, J.L., Y.W. and H.L. (Huihui Li); resources, F.Y.; data curation, H.D., Y.W. and H.L. (Huihui Li); writing—original draft preparation, Y.M.; writing—review and editing, L.G. and H.L. (Haitao Liu). All authors have read and agreed to the published version of the manuscript.

Funding: This research was funded by the General program of National Natural Science Foundation of China, grant number 81970274.

Institutional Review Board Statement: The study was conducted according to the guidelines of the Declaration of Helsinki and approved by the Institutional Review Board of the First Affiliated Hospital of Air Force Military Medical University.

Informed Consent Statement: Informed consent was obtained from all subjects involved in the study.

Data Availability Statement: The datasets used and/or analyzed during the current study are be available from the corresponding author on reasonable request.

Conflicts of Interest: The authors declare no conflict of interest.

References

1. Reddy, V.Y.; Möbius-Winkler, S.; Miller, M.A.; Neuzil, P.; Schuler, G.; Wiebe, J.; Sick, P.; Sievert, H. Left atrial appendage closure with the Watchman device in patients with a contraindication for oral anticoagulation: The ASAP study (ASA Plavix Feasibility Study with Watchman Left Atrial Appendage Closure Technology). *J. Am. Coll. Cardiol.* **2013**, *61*, 2551–2556. [CrossRef] [PubMed]
2. Osmancik, P.; Herman, D.; Neuzil, P.; Hala, P.; Taborsky, M.; Kala, P.; Poloczek, M.; Stasek, J.; Haman, L.; Branny, M.; et al. Left Atrial Appendage Closure Versus Direct Oral Anticoagulants in High-Risk Patients with Atrial Fibrillation. *J. Am. Coll. Cardiol.* **2020**, *75*, 3122–3135. [CrossRef] [PubMed]
3. Hindricks, G.; Potpara, T.; Dagres, N.; Arbelo, E.; Bax, J.J.; Blomström-Lundqvist, C.; Boriani, G.; Castella, M.; Dan, G.A.; Dilaveris, P.E.; et al. 2020 ESC Guidelines for the diagnosis and management of atrial fibrillation developed in collaboration with the European Association for Cardio-Thoracic Surgery (EACTS). *Eur. Heart J.* **2021**, *42*, 373–498. [CrossRef]
4. Rich, M.E.; Tseng, A.; Lim, H.W.; Wang, P.J.; Su, W.W. Reduction of Iatrogenic Atrial Septal Defects with an Anterior and Inferior Transseptal Puncture Site when Operating the Cryoballoon Ablation Catheter. *J. Vis. Exp.* **2015**, *100*, e52811. [CrossRef] [PubMed]
5. Meier, B.; Blaauw, Y.; Khattab, A.A.; Lewalter, T.; Sievert, H.; Tondo, C.; Glikson, M.; ESC Scientific Document Group. EHRA/EAPCI expert consensus statement on catheter-based left atrial appendage occlusion. *Europace* **2014**, *16*, 1397–1416. [CrossRef] [PubMed]
6. Berti, S.; Paradossi, U.; Meucci, F.; Trianni, G.; Tzikas, A.; Rezzaghi, M.; Stolkova, M.; Palmieri, C.; Mori, F.; Santoro, G. Periprocedural intracardiac echocardiography for left atrial appendage closure: A dual-center experience. *JACC Cardiovasc. Interv.* **2014**, *7*, 1036–1044. [CrossRef] [PubMed]
7. Yuniadi, Y.; Hanafy, D.A.; Raharjo, S.B.; Yugo, D. Left atrial appendage closure device implantation guided with fluoroscopy only: Long-term results. *J. Arrhythm.* **2019**, *35*, 262–266. [CrossRef] [PubMed]
8. Korsholm, K.; Jensen, J.M.; Nielsen-Kudsk, J.E. Intracardiac Echocardiography from the Left Atrium for Procedural Guidance of Transcatheter Left Atrial Appendage Occlusion. *JACC Cardiovasc. Interv.* **2017**, *10*, 2198–2206. [CrossRef] [PubMed]
9. Puga, L.; Teixeira, R.; Paiva, L.; Ribeiro, J.M.; Gameiro, J.; Sousa, J.P.; Costa, M.; Gonçalves, L. Iatrogenic atrial septal defect after percutaneous left atrial appendage closure: A single-center study. *Int. J. Cardiovasc. Imaging* **2021**, *37*, 2359–2368. [CrossRef] [PubMed]
10. Morikawa, T.; Miyasaka, M.; Flint, N.; Manabe, O.; Dawkins, S.; Cheng, R.; Hussaini, A.; Makar, M.; Kar, S.; Nakamura, M. Right-to-Left Shunt Through Iatrogenic Atrial Septal Defect After MitraClip Procedure. *JACC Cardiovasc. Interv.* **2020**, *13*, 1544–1553. [CrossRef] [PubMed]
11. Rosu, R.; Cismaru, G.; Muresan, L.; Puiu, M.; Gusetu, G.; Istratoaie, S.; Pop, D.; Zdrenghea, D. Intracardiac echocardiography for transseptal puncture. A guide for cardiac electrophysiologists. *Med. Ultrason.* **2019**, *21*, 183–190. [CrossRef] [PubMed]
12. Chen, Y.H.; Wang, L.G.; Zhou, X.D.; Fang, Y.; Su, L.; Wu, S.J.; Huang, W.J.; Xiao, F.Y. Outcome and safety of intracardiac echocardiography guided left atrial appendage closure within zero-fluoroscopy atrial fibrillation ablation procedures. *J. Cardiovasc. Electrophysiol.* **2022**, *33*, 667–676. [CrossRef] [PubMed]
13. Nelles, D.; Vij, V.; Al-Kassou, B.; Weber, M.; Vogelhuber, J.; Beiert, T.; Nickenig, G.; Schrickel, J.W.; Sedaghat, A. Incidence, persistence, and clinical relevance of iatrogenic atrial septal defects after percutaneous left atrial appendage occlusion. *Echocardiography* **2022**, *39*, 65–73. [CrossRef] [PubMed]
14. Singh, S.M.; Douglas, P.S.; Reddy, V.Y. The incidence and long-term clinical outcome of iatrogenic atrial septal defects secondary to transseptal catheterization with a 12F transseptal sheath. *Circ. Arrhythm. Electrophysiol.* **2011**, *4*, 166–171. [CrossRef] [PubMed]
15. Alkhouli, M.; Sarraf, M.; Holmes, D.R. Iatrogenic Atrial Septal Defect. *Circ. Cardiovasc. Interv.* **2016**, *9*, e003545. [CrossRef] [PubMed]

6. Kimura, T.; Takatsuki, S.; Inagawa, K.; Katsumata, Y.; Nishiyama, T.; Nishiyama, N.; Fukumoto, K.; Aizawa, Y.; Tanimoto, Y.; Tanimoto, K.; et al. Anatomical characteristics of the left atrial appendage in cardiogenic stroke with low CHADS2 scores. *Heart. Rhythm.* **2013**, *10*, 921–925. [CrossRef] [PubMed]
7. Chan, N.Y.; Choy, C.C.; Yuen, H.C.; Chow, H.F.; Fong, H.F. A Very Long-term Longitudinal Study on the Evolution and Clinical Outcomes of Persistent Iatrogenic Atrial Septal Defect After Cryoballoon Ablation. *Can. J. Cardiol.* **2019**, *35*, 396–404. [CrossRef] [PubMed]
8. Schueler, R.; Öztürk, C.; Wedekind, J.A.; Werner, N.; Stöckigt, F.; Mellert, F.; Nickenig, G.; Hammerstingl, C. Persistence of iatrogenic atrial septal defect after interventional mitral valve repair with the MitraClip system: A note of caution. *JACC Cardiovasc. Interv.* **2015**, *8*, 450–459. [CrossRef] [PubMed]

Disclaimer/Publisher's Note: The statements, opinions and data contained in all publications are solely those of the individual author(s) and contributor(s) and not of MDPI and/or the editor(s). MDPI and/or the editor(s) disclaim responsibility for any injury to people or property resulting from any ideas, methods, instructions or products referred to in the content.

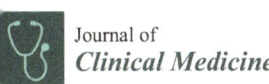

Article

Impact of Amiodarone Therapy on the Ablation Outcome of Ventricular Tachycardia in Arrhythmogenic Right Ventricular Cardiomyopathy

Chin-Yu Lin [1,2], Fa-Po Chung [1,2,*], Nwe Nwe [3], Yu-Cheng Hsieh [2,4], Cheng-Hung Li [2,4], Yenn-Jiang Lin [1,2], Shih-Lin Chang [1,2], Li-Wei Lo [1,2], Yu-Feng Hu [1,2], Ta-Chuan Tuan [1,2], Tze-Fan Chao [1,2], Jo-Nan Liao [1,2], Ting-Yung Chang [1,2], Ling Kuo [1,2], Cheng-I Wu [1,2], Chih-Min Liu [1,2], Shin-Huei Liu [1,2], Wen-Han Cheng [1,2] and Shih-Ann Chen [2,4]

[1] Heart Rhythm Center, Division of Cardiology, Department of Medicine, Taipei Veterans General Hospital, No. 201, Sec. 2, Shih-Pai Road, Taipei 112, Taiwan
[2] Department of Medicine, National Yang-Ming Chiao-Tung University, No. 155, Sec. 2, Linong St., Taipei 112, Taiwan
[3] Department of Cardiology, Yangon General Hospital, Yangon Q4HX+MH5, Myanmar
[4] Cardiovascular Center, Taichung Veterans General Hospital, No. 1650, Taiwan Boulevard Sect. 4, Taichung City 40705, Taiwan
* Correspondence: marxtaiji@gmail.com

Abstract: (1) Background: Catheter ablation (CA) is an accepted treatment option for drug-refractory ventricular tachycardia (VT) in patients with arrhythmogenic right ventricular cardiomyopathy (ARVC). This study investigates the effect of amiodarone on ablation outcomes in ARVC. (2) Methods: The study enrolled patients with ARVC undergoing CA of sustained VT. In all patients, substrate modification was performed to achieve non-inducible VT. The patients were categorized into two groups according to whether they had used amiodarone before CA. Baseline and electrophysiological characteristics, substrate, and outcomes were compared. (3) Results: A total of 72 ARVC patients were studied, including 29 (40.3%) "off" amiodarone and 43 (56.7%) "on" amiodarone. The scar area was similar between the two groups. Patients "off" amiodarone had smaller endocardial and epicardial areas with abnormal electrograms. Twenty of 43 patients (47.5%) "on" amiodarone discontinued it within 3 months after CA. During a mean follow-up period of 43.2 ± 29.5 months, higher VT recurrence was observed in patients "on" amiodarone. Patients "on" amiodarone who discontinued amiodarone after CA had a lower recurrence than those without. (4) Conclusions: Patients with ARVC "on" amiodarone before CA had distinct substrate characteristics and worse ablation outcomes than patients "off" amiodarone, especially in those who had used amiodarone continuously.

Keywords: amiodarone; arrhythmogenic right ventricular cardiomyopathy; abnormal electrograms; ventricular tachycardia; ablation

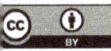

1. Introduction

Arrhythmogenic right ventricular cardiomyopathy (ARVC) is an inherited cardiomyopathy, characterized by fibro-fatty infiltration of the right ventricle owing to mutations in the desmosomal proteins [1]. Consequently, the heterogeneous substrates in the right ventricle are predisposed to delayed wavefront propagation and inhomogeneity of electrical conduction [2], which could contribute to ventricular tachycardia/fibrillation (VT/VF). Current guidelines recommend implanting an implantable cardioverter-defibrillator (ICD) in high-risk patients to prevent sudden cardiac death (SCD) or recurrence of fatal VT/VF in survivors [3]. Anti-arrhythmic drugs (AADs) are commonly used to prevent VT recurrences despite the implantation of an ICD. Amiodarone is the most common AAD used for the prevention of VT recurrences in patients with ARVC [4]. Amiodarone is, however, frequently limited by its ineffective reduction of recurrences of VT or well-known side effects [5]. Catheter ablation (CA) has therefore been used as an alternative procedure for patients who are intolerant to AADs or who have drug-refractory VT/VF in the ARVC [3] However, the impact of amiodarone on substrate mapping and the subsequent effect on preventing VT recurrence after CA were not known.

Furthermore, a recent study demonstrated that concomitant amiodarone therapy may affect outcomes in patients with ischemic VT who are undergoing CA [6]. The above findings may be explained by changes in substrate characteristics and electrogram properties. It is unknown whether concomitant amiodarone therapy affects procedural outcomes in patients with ARVC. Accordingly, the aim of this study was to investigate the substrate characteristics and ablation outcomes between ARVC patients receiving CA with and without concomitant amiodarone therapy.

2. Materials and Methods

2.1. Study Population

From 2013 to 2020, we retrospectively screened patients with ARVC who had undergone successful CA of drug-refractory VT in three medical centers (Taipei Veterans General Hospital, Yangon General Hospital, and Taichung Veterans General Hospital). Based on the 2010 modified Task Force criteria, all patients met the diagnosis of definite ARVC [7] The indications for catheter ablation included the following: (1) individuals with recurrent, sustained monomorphic VT refractory to antiarrhythmic drugs; and (2) symptomatic individuals with a high burden of ventricular ectopy and documented non-sustained VT refractory to antiarrhythmic drugs. Patients without documented sustained VT or successful CA were excluded. Patients had a minimum follow-up period of six months after CA. Written informed consent was obtained in all cases. The institutional review boards of each participating center approved the collection of data. From the electronic medical records, clinical data, such as baseline characteristics, 12 lead ECGs, 24 h Holter monitoring, transthoracic echocardiography, coronary angiography, and electrophysiological (EP)/ablation parameters, were collected for comparison. In the study, patients were divided into two groups based on their use of amiodarone before CA ("Off" amiodarone for at least 8 weeks before ablation and "On" amiodarone within 8 weeks). The use of amiodarone depends on physicians' discretion or intolerable side effects.

2.2. Electrophysiological Study, Mapping, and Ablation

In previous publications, we described details of an electrophysiological study, substrate mapping, and ablation strategies [8]. After obtaining informed consent, we performed a standardized electrophysiological study on all patients under fasting and sedated conditions. Except for amiodarone, all anti-arrhythmic drugs (AADs) have been discontinued for at least five half-lives prior to CA [8]. The induction protocol and mapping strategy were described in the previous article [9]. Epicardial mapping/ablation is conducted in patients with failed endocardial ablation or in those who may have extensive epicardial involvement and limited abnormal substrates within the endocardium [8]. The RV endocardial bipolar scar and low voltage zone (LVZ) were defined as areas with peak-to-peak bipolar voltage < 0.5 mV and 0.5–1.5 mV, respectively, whereas the RV endocardial unipolar LVZ area was defined as an area with peak-to-peak unipolar voltage < 5.5 mV [10].

The RV epicardial bipolar scar and LVZ were defined as areas with a peak-to-peak bipolar voltage of <0.5 mV and 0.5–1 mV, respectively. The voltage maps were manually edited to avoid intracavitary points. An average bipolar or unipolar voltage was calculated. The scar, LVZ, and areas with abnormal electrograms (defined as either continuous, late, or fragmented potentials during sinus or paced rhythm) were assessed by using the standard surface area measurement tool on the navigation system [11]. When multiple areas of confluent low voltage were present, the aggregate area of the individual regions of interest was calculated. All patients received complete endocardial and/or epicardial substrate modification targeting the areas with abnormal electrograms. Successful ablation was defined as the non-inducibility of any VTs with or without isoproterenol [8].

2.3. Follow-Up and Recurrences of Ventricular Arrhythmia (VA)

Patients were followed up at the first, third, and sixth months after CA, as well as every three–six months thereafter. ICD interrogation, ECG, and Holter monitoring were performed. Recurrent VA, defined as sustained VT or VT/VF, requires ICD interventions [12].

2.4. Statistical Analysis

The continuous and categorical variables were expressed as mean ± standard deviation and percentage, respectively. The Student's *t*-test was used to compare continuous variables, while chi-square tests with or without Yate's correction for continuity or Fisher's exact tests were used for categorical variables, as indicated. A multivariate Cox proportional hazards regression analysis was performed with variables with a *p*-value of less than 0.2 in the univariate analysis for a hazard ratio to predict the VT/VF recurrence. We considered a *p*-value of 0.05 to be statistically significant. The statistical analyses were conducted using the Statistical Package for the Social Sciences, Version 22.0 (IBM Corporation, Armonk, NY, USA).

3. Results

3.1. Study Population

3.1.1. Patient Selection and Baseline Characteristics of ARVC Patients

In total, we screened 106 patients who were diagnosed with definite ARVC and had received successful CA of VA (Figure 1). The analysis included 72 patients (67.9%) (age 45.3 ± 14.5 years, 61.1% male) who received CA for clinically documented sustained VT with successful ablation. (Figure 1). Of these, 29 (40.3%) and 43 (59.7%) patients were classified as "off" and "on" amiodarone groups, respectively (Figure 1). The median (25–75%) duration of amiodarone use in patients "on" amiodarone was 11 (4–18) months before CA. The characteristics of these two groups are shown in Table 1. There were fewer men in patients "off" amiodarone (13 (44.8%) vs. 31 (72.1%); *p* = 0.027). Patients "off" amiodarone received more class Ic AAD medications (10 (34.5%) vs. 3 (7.0%); *p* = 0.004). In terms of the other parameters and Task Force criteria, there were no significant differences between the two groups.

Table 1. Comparison of baseline characteristics between patients with ARVC "On" and "Off" amiodarone before CA.

	"Off" Amiodarone (N = 29)	"On" Amiodarone (N = 43)	*p*-Value
Baseline characteristics			
Age	43.0 ± 13.1	46.9 ± 15.4	0.260
Sex (Men, %)	13 (44.8%)	31 (72.1%)	0.027
Hypertension	7 (24.1%)	14 (32.6%)	0.598
Diabetes mellitus	2 (6.9%)	2 (4.7%)	0.999
LVEF (%)	57.2 ± 8.1	53.5 ± 8.7	0.081
RVEF (%)	41.0 ± 9.7	38.0 ± 11.5	0.240
Medication			
Amiodarone dose before CA (mg)	0	232.6 ± 97.9	
Beta blocker before CA	21 (72.4%)	29 (67.4%)	0.795
Class Ic AAD before CA	10 (34.5%)	3 (7.0%)	0.004
Class Ib AAD before CA	7 (24.1%)	4 (9.3%)	0.105

Table 1. Cont.

	"Off" Amiodarone (N = 29)	"On" Amiodarone (N = 43)	p-Value
"Continued" amiodarone before discharge	0	38 (88.4%)	
"Continued" amiodarone 3 months after CA	0 (0.0%)	23 (53.5%)	
Amiodarone dose after CA (mg)	0	223.9 ± 106.5	
Task Force criteria *			
Structural abnormalities			
Major	9 (31.0%)	25 (58.1%)	0.076
Minor	15 (51.7%)	14 (32.6%)	
Fibrofatty replacement			
Major	7 (24.1%)	9 (20.9%)	0.483
Minor	2 (6.9%)	13 (30.2%)	
Depolarization abnormalities			
Major	2 (6.9%)	9 (20.9%)	0.138
Minor	26 (89.7%)	30 (69.8%)	
Repolarization abnormalities			
Major	9 (27.3%)	7 (15.2%)	0.421
Minor	13 (39.4%)	21 (45.7%)	
Ventricular arrhythmias			
Major	10 (34.5%)	19 (44.2%)	0.469
Minor	19 (65.5%)	24 (55.8%)	
Family history			
Major	5 (17.2%)	10 (23.3%)	0.568
Minor	0 (0.0%)	1 (2.3%)	

* According to the 2010 revised Task Force criteria (9). AAD, anti-arrhythmic drug; ARVC, arrhythmogenic right ventricular cardiomyopathy; CA, catheter ablation; LVEF, left ventricular ejection fraction; RVEF, right ventricular ejection fraction.

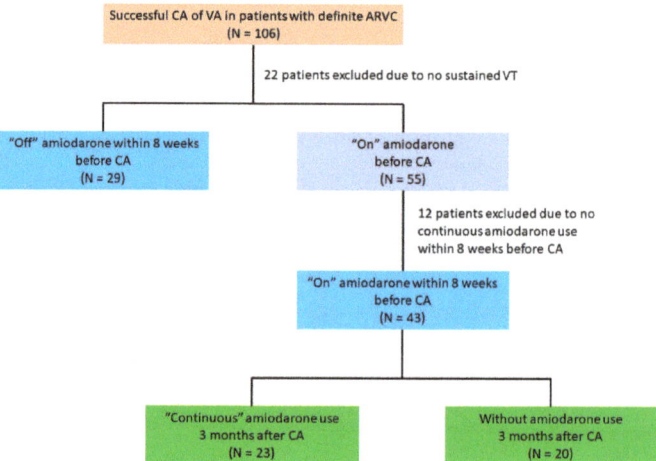

Figure 1. Patient selection in the present study. Patients with ARVC receiving successful CA for ventricular arrhythmia were screened. We enrolled ARVC patients with clinically documented sustained VT, and patients were further categorized into two groups based on their use of amiodarone within the 8 weeks before CA. ARVC = arrhythmogenic right ventricular cardiomyopathy; CA = catheter ablation; VT = ventricular tachycardia.

3.1.2. Endocardial and Epicardial Substrate Characteristics

Epicardial approach was performed in 47 (65.3%) patients, including 12 (41.4%) and 35 (81.4%) patients "off" and "on" amiodarone, respectively ($p = 0.001$). The characteristics of the RV substrate are shown in Table 2. There were no significant differences between the two groups regarding endocardial and epicardial bipolar voltage, unipolar voltage, and LVZ/scar area. The total activation time of the endocardium and epicardium was longer in patients "on" amiodarone than those in patients "off" amiodarone (158.2 ± 31.8 ms vs. 144.0 ± 32.7 ms, $p < 0.001$; 211.2 ± 26.0 ms vs. 183.6 ± 24.2 ms, $p = 0.002$). In addition, the areas of abnormal electrograms within the endocardium and epicardium were significantly larger in patients "on" amiodarone (Figure 2) than those in patients "off" amiodarone (Figure 3). (Endo: 16.8 ± 15.4 cm^2 vs. 6.8 ± 5.0 cm^2, $p = 0.001$; Epi: 28.2 ± 29.0 cm^2 vs. 13.7 ± 21.4 cm^2, $p = 0.024$). In the patients with amiodarone before CA, there was no significant difference in the substrate characteristics between patients with amiodarone durations of more than 6 months or not (Supplemental Table S1).

Table 2. Comparison of baseline characteristics between patients with ARVC "On" and "Off" amiodarone before ablation.

	"Off" Amiodarone (N = 29)	"On" Amiodarone (N = 43)	p-Value
VT morphologies	1.3 ± 0.6	1.7 ± 0.9	0.014
VT cycle length	309.2 ± 54.7	304.5 ± 72.5	0.774
Procedure time (minutes)	184.5 ± 51.1	220.3 ± 43.9	0.019
Ablation time (minutes)	28.2 ± 24.4	55.4 ± 37.7	0.001
RV endocardium			
Mapping points	600.7 ± 528.5	850.0 ± 666.8	0.096
Bipolar voltage *	2.1 ± 0.6	1.9 ± 0.7	0.142
Unipolar voltage *	5.3 ± 0.7	4.9 ± 1.4	0.253
Total activation time (ms)	144.0 ± 32.7	158.2 ± 31.8	<0.001
Bipolar low voltage zone (cm^2)	28.4 ±17.1	34.7± 27.4	0.275
Bipolar low voltage zone, %	13.5 ± 7.6	15.4 ± 10.7	0.415
Bipolar scar (cm^2)	14.2 ± 12.5	17.4 ± 13.6	0.317
Bipolar scar, %	6.8 ± 5.3	8.0 ± 5.5	0.341
Unipolar low voltage zone (cm^2)	55.1 ± 36.3	65.3 ± 27.9	0.183
Unipolar low voltage zone, %	22.6 ± 11.7	25.8 ±10.2	0.215
Area with abnormal electrograms	6.8 ± 5.0	16.8 ± 15.4	0.001
RV epicardium	(N = 12)	(N = 35)	
Mapping points	1495.8 ± 950.9	2076.8 ± 1776.9	0.270
Averaged bipolar voltage (mV) *	1.3 ± 0.5	1.3 ± 0.8	0.919
Total activation time (ms)	183.6 ± 24.2	211.2 ± 26.0	0.002
Bipolar low voltage zone (cm^2)	95.0 ± 54.8	111.5 ± 55.8	0.378
Bipolar low voltage zone, %	36.0 ± 22.2	36.3 ± 20.4	0.968
Bipolar scar (cm^2)	53.4 ± 43.7	56.6 ± 34.2	0.797
Bipolar scar, %	19.0 ± 14.9	19.1 ± 11.4	0.842
Area with abnormal electrograms	13.7 ± 21.4	28.2 ± 29.0	0.024

* The average of bipolar or unipolar median voltage. ARVC, arrhythmogenic right ventricular cardiomyopathy; RV, right ventricular; VT, ventricular tachycardia.

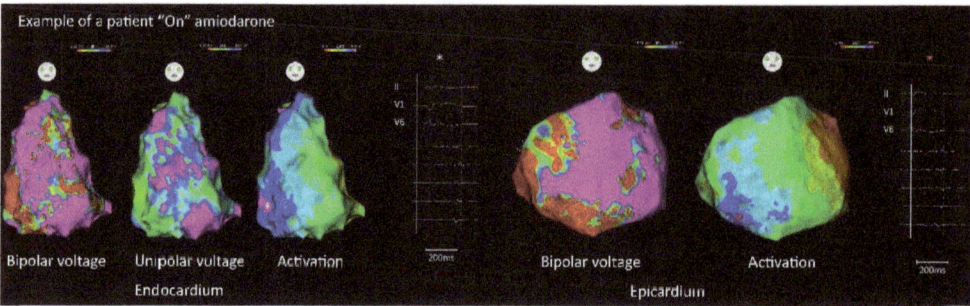

Figure 2. An example of electrophysiological and substrate characteristics in a patient "on" amiodarone before CA. Patients with ARVC "on" amiodarone had a longer total activation time and larger areas with abnormal electrograms. The (**left panel**) showed an endocardial voltage map and activation map with local abnormal electrograms. The (**right panel**) showed an epicardial voltage map and activation map with local abnormal electrograms (* indicated the location of corresponding signal). "See text for details".

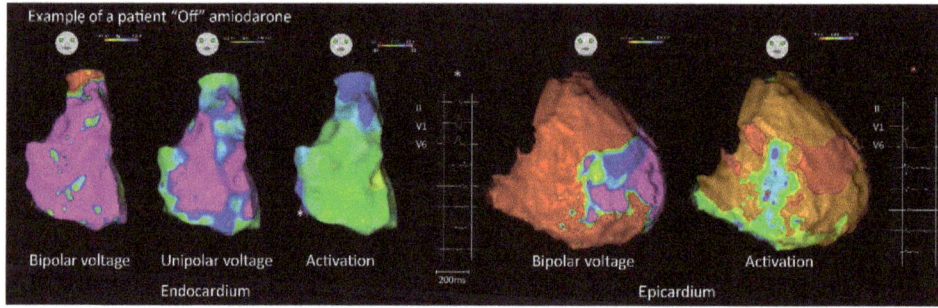

Figure 3. An example of electrophysiological and substrate characteristics in a patient "off" amiodarone before CA. The (**left panel**) showed an endocardial voltage map and activation map with local abnormal electrograms. The (**right panel**) showed an epicardial voltage map and activation map with local abnormal electrograms (* indicated the location of corresponding signal). "See text for details".

3.1.3. Mapping of Ventricular Tachycardia and Catheter Ablation

During the electrophysiological study, 112 VTs (1.6 ± 0.8/patient) were induced, including 37 and 75 VTs in patients "off" and "on" amiodarone, respectively ($p = 0.008$). The mean cycle length of inducible VTs was 306.3 ± 66.1 ms. Of 112 inducible VTs, 61 VTs were mappable (14 in the "off" amiodarone group and 47 in the "on" amiodarone group, $p = 0.007$). Nine of the 61 mappable VT circuits were considered intramural because they lacked identifiable diastolic paths despite simultaneous epicardial and endocardial mapping. Three in the "off" amiodarone and six in the "on" amiodarone, ($p = 0.731$), all identified VT isthmuses and were correlated with areas with abnormal electrograms and abnormal substrates.

Each patient underwent ablation of the isthmus if mappable, and complete elimination of the endocardial and/or epicardial abnormal substrates. In patients "on" amiodarone, the total procedure duration and ablation time were significantly longer than in those "off" amiodarone (220.3 ± 43.9 min vs. 184.5 ± 51.1 min, $p = 0.019$, and 55.4 ± 37.7 min vs. 28.2 ± 24.4 min, $p = 0.001$, respectively). In all patients, non-inducibility of VT was achieved following CA. There were no procedural complications.

3.1.4. Follow-Up

After a follow-up period of 43.2 ± 29.5 months, two patients (2.5%) died of non-cardiovascular causes (pneumonia: 2), and 24 (33.3%) experienced VT/VF recurrences. The incidence of VT/VF recurrence was significantly higher in patients "on" amiodarone than those "off" amiodarone (19/43 (44.2%) vs. 5/29 (17.2%), log-rank p-value = 0.011, Figure 4A). Among patients "on" amiodarone, the use of amiodarone was continued in 23 cases (53.5%) 3 months after CA. The incidence of VT/VF recurrence among patients on amiodarone before CA was still higher for those with continuous amiodarone use than for those without (14/23 (60.9%) vs. 5/20 (25.0%), log-rank p-value = 0.002, Figure 4B). Univariate and multivariate analyses (Table 3) showed that the use of amiodarone before CA (hazard ratio (HR): 3.04, 95% confidence interval (CI): 1.07–8.66, p = 0.038) is the only independent predictor of VT/VF recurrence.

Table 3. Univariate and multivariate analyses of VT/VF recurrence after catheter ablation.

	Univariate Analysis		Multivariate Analysis	
	p-Value	HR (95% CI)	p-Value	HR (95% CI)
Age (year)	0.995	1.00 (0.97–1.03)	-	-
Sex (male)	0.051	2.56 (0.99–6.56)	0.605	1.38 (0.41–4.68)
Hypertension	0.062	2.21 (0.96–5.10)	0.665	1.24 (0.47–3.22)
Diabetes mellitus	0.758	1.38 (0.18–10.46)	-	-
LVEF (%)	0.642	0.99 (0.95–1.04)	-	-
RVEF (%)	0.049	0.96 (0.93–1.00)	0.494	0.98 (0.94–1.03)
Amiodarone before CA	0.013	3.54 (1.31–9.60)	0.038	3.04 (1.07–8.66)
Amiodarone > 6 months	0.283	1.56 (0.69–3.54)	-	-
Task Force score	0.550	1.08 (0.84–1.38)	-	-
Total activation time (RV endo)	0.009	1.02 (1.00–1.03)	0.385	1.03 (0.96–1.12)
Bipolar scar (%, RV endo)	0.283	1.04 (0.97–1.12)	-	-
Epicardial approach	0.413	1.44 (0.60–3.46)	-	-

CA = catheter ablation; CI = confidence interval; HR = hazard ratio; LVEF = left ventricular ejection fraction; RV = right ventricle; RVEF = RV ejection fraction.

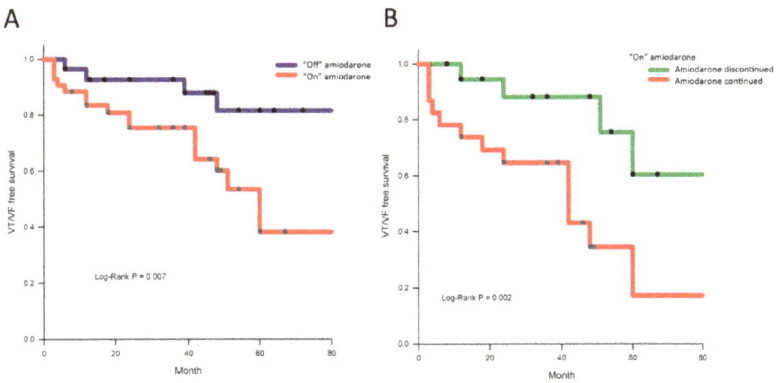

Figure 4. Kaplan–Meier curve for ablation outcomes during follow-up. (**A**) The Kaplan–Meier curve showed the recurrence-free survival in patients "on" and "off" amiodarone. Higher VT/VF recurrences were observed in patients "on" amiodarone than in those "off" amiodarone. (**B**) The Kaplan–Meier curve demonstrated the VT/VF recurrence-free survival in the patients with or without continuous amiodarone use after the successful ablation in patients "on" amiodarone before CA.

4. Discussion

4.1. Main Findings

According to our study, amiodarone use before CA in patients with ARVC is associated with a longer activation time and a greater area of abnormal electrograms within the RV endocardium and epicardium. Despite the similar ablation strategy and endpoints (complete elimination of arrhythmogenic potential and non-inducible VT), VT recurrence was higher in patients "on" amiodarone before CA. Regardless of acute success, patients whose amiodarone use was discontinued 3 months after CA experienced fewer VT recurrences during subsequent follow-up.

4.2. Amiodarone and the Abnormal Substrate

Amiodarone has been shown to prolong the total QRS duration and result in low amplitude signals in previous studies [13], which is consistent with the present findings that a longer activation time was observed in patients "on" amiodarone compared with those without. One of the main effects of chronic amiodarone therapy is the inhibition of potassium outward currents, which may prolong the action potential duration of the ventricular myocytes and delay conduction velocity [14]. Amiodarone may also increase the refractory periods of ischemic scar tissue and organize fractionated electrograms [15]. Luigi et al. reported that patients with ischemic VT "on" amiodarone had a smaller area of abnormal electrogram compared to those without [6]. These findings suggest that the use of amiodarone may mask "abnormal" electrical activity within the scar tissue in patients with ischemic VT. However, the impact of amiodarone on abnormal electrograms in patients with ARVC or other non-ischemic cardiomyopathies remains to be determined.

In contrast to the above-mentioned study regarding ischemic cardiomyopathy, we found that patients "on" amiodarone had larger areas of abnormal electrograms than those "off" amiodarone. Inconsistent findings as compared to ischemic substrates can be attributed to the following plausible explanations: (1) amiodarone prolongs conduction velocity heterogeneously in fatty-infiltrated myocytes and creates more abnormal electrograms in patients with ARVC; and (2) there is a diversity of disease progression and scarring in ARVCs, which could also contribute to nonuniform ablation outcomes. However, as a result of the study design, we cannot determine the cause-and-effect relationship between amiodarone use and the extent of abnormal electrogram extension in the present study. Further studies focusing on the effects of amiodarone on the diseased substrate in ARVC will be warranted.

4.3. Amiodarone Use and Ablation Outcomes

In this study, we found that patients who were "on" amiodarone had higher recurrences of VT than those who were "off" amiodarone before CA. These findings may be explained by the following reasons: First, a greater extent of diseased substrates has been observed in amiodarone users, suggesting a worse disease status and/or faster disease progression in these individuals. Previously, we found that the progression of the disease could also cause the expansion of abnormal substrates, which was linked to VT recurrences [8]. The second issue is that, despite the larger area with abnormal electrograms, there were still some arrhythmogenic substrates that were hidden after amiodarone use as seen in ischemic substrates. As a result, substrate modification could not be performed completely. Moreover, amiodarone could possess good antiarrhythmic properties and prevent ventricular arrhythmias from being induced after CA [16]. Nonetheless, the possibility of this is negated by the findings that these patients were refractory to amiodarone before CA. Furthermore, the pro-arrhythmic effect was reported with a relatively low incidence but was not negligible [4,17]. Amiodarone might prolong the QT interval and cause polymorphic ventricular tachycardia (i.e., torsade de pointes), especially in patients with drug-drug interactions [18]. The above hypothesis might be indirectly supported by the observation that patients with continuous use of amiodarone after ablation experience VT recurrences at higher rates. Amiodarone, however, causes proarrhythmia at a rate of less than one percent per year [19]. A previous study demonstrated that long-term amiodarone use did not increase mortality or hospitalization [20]. Further investigation is needed to determine the exact reason for the higher incidence of VT recurrence in ARVC patients with amiodarone use before CA.

4.4. Clinical Implications

To the best of our knowledge, this is the first study to investigate the impact of amiodarone use before CA in patients with ARVC. Amiodarone use before CA can result in distinct substrate characteristics, such as longer activation times and larger areas with abnormal electrograms and was associated with worse ablation outcomes. According to the above findings, we suggest the physician withdraw amiodarone before CA if the patient can tolerate it. Despite the standard ablation strategies and endpoints, VT recurrences were still higher in patients without discontinuation, reflecting the importance of alternative strategies to assess the ablation endpoints in these patients who could not withdraw the amiodarone. Future studies are warranted to address this aspect.

4.5. Limitations

There were some limitations in the present study. This is a retrospective study in which only patients who had successfully undergone ablation were included. The prescription of amiodarone was based on the clinical physician's discretion. In patients with ARVC before CA, it is difficult to standardize the use of AADs. Furthermore, the use of amiodarone after CA was also at the discretion of the physicians, which may have affected the present findings. In this retrospective study, it is difficult to determine whether the amiodarone or the need for amiodarone affects substrate characteristics and recurrence. Nevertheless, the bias can be minimized by multivariate analysis and collaboration between referral centers. Additionally, epicardial approaches were not performed in all patients. However, even with the above-mentioned differences, there are more patients "on" amiodarone who are undergoing epicardial ablation to achieve the same outcome. In this regard, we concluded that epicardial ablation was not the cause of the differences between the two groups. A prospective study is warranted to validate the impact of amiodarone on the ablation outcome in patients with definite ARVC.

5. Conclusions

Despite similar ablation strategies and endpoints, amiodarone use before CA may be associated with a higher rate of VT recurrence in patients with ARVC. Higher VT recurrences were observed in ARVC patients who continued to take amiodarone despite the acute success.

Supplementary Materials: The following supporting information can be downloaded at: https://www.mdpi.com/article/10.3390/jcm11247265/s1. Supplemental Table S1. Comparison of substrate characteristics between patients with different periods on amiodarone before ablation.

Author Contributions: Conceptualization, C.-Y.L. and F.-P.C.; methodology, C.-Y.L. and F.-P.C.; formal analysis, C.-Y.L. and F.-P.C.; investigation, Y.-J.L., L.-W.L., Y.-F.H., S.-L.C., S.-A.C., C.-H.L., N.N., Y.-C.H., T.-C.T., F.-P.C. and C.-Y.L.; resources, Y.-J.L., L.-W.L., Y.-F.H., S.-L.C., S.-A.C., C.-H.L., N.N., Y.-C.H., T.-C.T., F.-P.C. and C.-Y.L.; data curation, C.-Y.L.; writing—original draft preparation, C.-Y.L. and F.-P.C.; writing—review and editing, C.-Y.L., F.-P.C., N.N., Y.-C.H., C.-H.L., Y.-J.L., S.-L.C., L.-W.L., Y.-F.H., T.-C.T., T.-F.C., J.-N.L., T.-Y.C., L.K., C.-I.W., C.-M.L., S.-H.L., W.-H.C. and S.-A.C.; funding acquisition, C.-Y.L. and F.-P.C. All authors have read and agreed to the published version of the manuscript.

Funding: This work was supported by the Ministry of Science and Technology (111-2314-B-075-007-MY3, 109-2314-B-075-076-MY3, 109-2314-B-010-058-MY2, 109-2314-B-075-074-MY3, 109-2314-B-075-076 -MY3, grant nos. 107-2314-B-010-061-MY2, 106-2314-B-075-006-MY3, 106-2314-B-010-046-MY3 and 106-2314-B-075-073-MY3), Research Foundation of Cardiovascular Medicine, Szu-Yuan Research Foundation of Internal Medicine, and Taipei Veterans General Hospital (grant no. V106C-158, V106C-104, V107B-014, V107C-060, V107C-054, V108C-107, and V109C-113).

Institutional Review Board Statement: The study was conducted in accordance with the Declaration of Helsinki and approved by the Institutional Review Board of Taipei Veterans General Hospital (2018-07-006B).

Informed Consent Statement: Patient consent was waived due to the anonymized nature of the information and the fact that the submission did not include images that might identify the person.

Data Availability Statement: The authors confirm that the data supporting the findings of this study are available within the article.

Conflicts of Interest: The authors declare no conflict of interest.

References

1. Corrado, D.; Link, M.S.; Calkins, H. Arrhythmogenic Right Ventricular Cardiomyopathy. *N. Engl. J. Med.* **2017**, *376*, 61–72. [CrossRef] [PubMed]
2. Dalal, D.; Nasir, K.; Bomma, C.; Prakasa, K.; Tandri, H.; Piccini, J.; Roguin, A.; Tichnell, C.; James, C.; Russell, S.D.; et al Arrhythmogenic right ventricular dysplasia: A United States experience. *Circulation* **2005**, *112*, 3823–3832. [CrossRef] [PubMed]
3. Towbin, J.A.; McKenna, W.J.; Abrams, D.J.; Ackerman, M.J.; Calkins, H.; Darrieux, F.C.C.; Daubert, J.P.; de Chillou, C.; DePasquale, E.C.; Desai, M.Y.; et al. 2019 HRS expert consensus statement on evaluation, risk stratification, and management of arrhythmogenic cardiomyopathy. *Heart Rhythm* **2019**, *16*, e301–e372. [CrossRef] [PubMed]
4. Vassallo, P.; Trohman, R.G. Prescribing amiodarone: An evidence-based review of clinical indications. *JAMA* **2007**, *298*, 1312–1322. [CrossRef] [PubMed]
5. Colunga Biancatelli, R.M.; Congedo, V.; Calvosa, L.; Ciacciarelli, M.; Polidoro, A.; Iuliano, L. Adverse reactions of Amiodarone. *J. Geriatr. Cardiol.* **2019**, *16*, 552–566. [CrossRef]
6. Di Biase, L.; Romero, J.; Du, X.; Mohanty, S.; Trivedi, C.; Della Rocca, D.G.; Patel, K.; Sanchez, J.; Yang, R.; Alviz, I.; et al. Catheter ablation of ventricular tachycardia in ischemic cardiomyopathy: Impact of concomitant amiodarone therapy on short- and long-term clinical outcomes. *Heart Rhythm* **2021**, *18*, 885–893. [CrossRef] [PubMed]
7. Marcus, F.I.; McKenna, W.J.; Sherrill, D.; Basso, C.; Bauce, B.; Bluemke, D.A.; Calkins, H.; Corrado, D.; Cox, M.G.; Daubert, J.P.; et al. Diagnosis of arrhythmogenic right ventricular cardiomyopathy/dysplasia: Proposed modification of the Task Force Criteria. *Eur. Heart J.* **2010**, *31*, 806–814. [CrossRef] [PubMed]
8. Lin, C.Y.; Chung, F.P.; Kuo, L.; Lin, Y.J.; Chang, S.L.; Lo, L.W.; Hu, Y.F.; Tuan, T.C.; Chao, T.F.; Liao, J.N.; et al. Characteristics of recurrent ventricular tachyarrhythmia after catheter ablation in patients with arrhythmogenic right ventricular cardiomyopathy. *J. Cardiovasc. Electrophysiol.* **2019**, *30*, 582–592. [CrossRef] [PubMed]
9. Lin, C.Y.; Chung, F.P.; Lin, Y.J.; Chang, S.L.; Lo, L.W.; Hu, Y.F.; Tuan, T.C.; Chao, T.F.; Liao, J.N.; Chang, T.Y.; et al. Clinical significance of J waves with respect to substrate characteristics and ablation outcomes in patients with arrhythmogenic right ventricular cardiomyopathy. *Europace* **2021**, *23*, 1418–1427. [CrossRef]
10. Marchlinski, F.E.; Callans, D.J.; Gottlieb, C.D.; Zado, E. Linear ablation lesions for control of unmappable ventricular tachycardia in patients with ischemic and nonischemic cardiomyopathy. *Circulation* **2000**, *101*, 1288–1296. [CrossRef] [PubMed]
11. Aliot, E.M.; Stevenson, W.G.; Almendral-Garrote, J.M.; Bogun, F.; Calkins, C.H.; Delacretaz, E.; Della Bella, P.; Hindricks, G.; Jais, P.; Josephson, M.E.; et al. EHRA/HRS Expert Consensus on Catheter Ablation of Ventricular Arrhythmias: Developed in a partnership with the European Heart Rhythm Association (EHRA), a Registered Branch of the European Society of Cardiology (ESC), and the Heart Rhythm Society (HRS); in collaboration with the American College of Cardiology (ACC) and the American Heart Association (AHA). *Heart Rhythm* **2009**, *6*, 886–933. [CrossRef] [PubMed]
12. Chung, F.P.; Li, H.R.; Chong, E.; Pan, C.H.; Lin, Y.J.; Chang, S.L.; Lo, L.W.; Hu, Y.F.; Tuan, T.C.; Chao, T.F.; et al. Seasonal variation in the frequency of sudden cardiac death and ventricular tachyarrhythmia in patients with arrhythmogenic right ventricular dysplasia/cardiomyopathy: The effect of meteorological factors. *Heart Rhythm* **2013**, *10*, 1859–1866. [CrossRef] [PubMed]
13. Brembilla-Perrot, B.; Claudon, O.; Houriez, P.; Beurrier, D.; Suty-Selton, C. Absence of change of signal-averaged electrocardiogram identifies patients with ventricular arrhythmias who are non-responders to amiodarone. *Int. J. Cardiol.* **2002**, *83*, 47–55. [CrossRef] [PubMed]
14. Van Herendael, H.; Dorian, P. Amiodarone for the treatment and prevention of ventricular fibrillation and ventricular tachycardia. *Vasc. Health Risk Manag.* **2010**, *6*, 465–472. [CrossRef] [PubMed]
15. Kawase, A.; Ikeda, T.; Nakazawa, K.; Ashihara, T.; Namba, T.; Kubota, T.; Sugi, K.; Hirai, H. Widening of the excitable gap and enlargement of the core of reentry during atrial fibrillation with a pure sodium channel blocker in canine atria. *Circulation* **2003**, *107*, 905–910. [CrossRef] [PubMed]

Kirchhof, P.; Degen, H.; Franz, M.R.; Eckardt, L.; Fabritz, L.; Milberg, P.; Laer, S.; Neumann, J.; Breithardt, G.; Haverkamp, W. Amiodarone-induced postrepolarization refractoriness suppresses induction of ventricular fibrillation. *J. Pharmacol. Exp. Ther.* **2003**, *305*, 257–263. [CrossRef] [PubMed]

Corrado, D.; Wichter, T.; Link, M.S.; Hauer, R.N.; Marchlinski, F.E.; Anastasakis, A.; Bauce, B.; Basso, C.; Brunckhorst, C.; Tsatsopoulou, A.; et al. Treatment of Arrhythmogenic Right Ventricular Cardiomyopathy/Dysplasia: An International Task Force Consensus Statement. *Circulation* **2015**, *132*, 441–453. [CrossRef] [PubMed]

Siddoway, L.A. Amiodarone: Guidelines for use and monitoring. *Am. Fam. Physician* **2003**, *68*, 2189–2196. [PubMed]

Connolly, S.J. Evidence-based analysis of amiodarone efficacy and safety. *Circulation* **1999**, *100*, 2025–2034. [CrossRef] [PubMed]

Doyle, J.F.; Ho, K.M. Benefits and risks of long-term amiodarone therapy for persistent atrial fibrillation: A meta-analysis. *Mayo Clin. Proc.* **2009**, *84*, 234–242. [CrossRef] [PubMed]

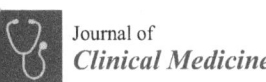

Article

The Impact of COVID-19 Pandemic on the Clinical Practice Patterns in Atrial Fibrillation: A Multicenter Clinician Survey in China

Feng Hu [1], Minhua Zang [1], Lihui Zheng [2], Wensheng Chen [3], Jinrui Guo [4], Zhongpeng Du [5], Erpeng Liang [6], Lishui Shen [7], Xiaofeng Hu [8], Xuelian Xu [9], Gaifeng Hu [10], Aihua Li [11], Jianfeng Huang [1], Yan Yao [2,*] and Jun Pu [1,*]

[1] Department of Cardiology, Renji Hospital, School of Medicine, Shanghai Jiaotong University, Shanghai 200127, China
[2] Department of Cardiology, Fuwai Hospital, National Center for Cardiovascular Diseases, Chinese Academy of Medical Sciences and Peking Union Medical College, Beijing 100037, China
[3] Department of Cardiology, Guangdong Provincial Hospital of Chinese Medicine, Guangzhou 510120, China
[4] Department of Cardiology, Fuwai Yunnan Cardiovascular Hospital, Kunming 650102, China
[5] Department of Cardiology, Zhu Jiang Hospital of Southern Medical University, Guangzhou 510280, China
[6] Heart Center of Henan Provincial People's Hospital, Central China Fuwai Hospital, Zhengzhou University, Zhengzhou 451460, China
[7] Department of Cardiology, Affiliated Hangzhou First People's Hospital, Zhejiang University School of Medicine, Hangzhou 310003, China
[8] Department of Cardiology, Shanghai Chest Hospital, Shanghai Jiao Tong University, Shanghai 200030, China
[9] Department of Cardiology, University-Town Hospital of Chongqing Medical University, Chongqing 400042, China
[10] Department of Cardiology, The First Affiliated Hospital of Wenzhou Medical University, Wenzhou 325035, China
[11] Department of Cardiology, The Affiliated Hospital of Yangzhou University, Yangzhou 225007, China
* Correspondence: ianyao@263.net.cn (Y.Y.); pujun310@hotmail.com (J.P.)

Abstract: The COVID-19 pandemic has severely impacted healthcare systems worldwide. This study investigated cardiologists' opinions on how the COVID-19 pandemic impacted clinical practice patterns in atrial fibrillation (AF). A multicenter clinician survey, including demographic and clinical questions, was administered to 300 cardiologists from 22 provinces in China, in April 2022. The survey solicited information about their treatment recommendations for AF and their perceptions of how the COVID-19 pandemic has impacted their clinical practice patterns for AF. The survey was completed by 213 cardiologists (71.0%) and included employees in tertiary hospitals (82.6%) and specialists with over 10 years of clinical cardiology practice (53.5%). Most respondents stated that there were reductions in the number of inpatients and outpatients with AF in their hospital during the pandemic. A majority of participants stated that the pandemic had impacted the treatment strategies for all types of AF, although to different extents. Compared with that during the assumed non-pandemic period in the hypothetical clinical questions, the selection of invasive interventional therapies (catheter ablation, percutaneous left atrial appendage occlusion) was significantly decreased (all $p < 0.05$) during the pandemic. There was no significant difference in the selection of non-invasive therapeutic strategies (the management of cardiovascular risk factors and concomitant diseases, pharmacotherapy for stroke prevention, heart rate control, and rhythm control) between the pandemic and non-pandemic periods (all $p > 0.05$). The COVID-19 pandemic has had a profound impact on the clinical practice patterns of AF. The selection of catheter ablation and percutaneous left atrial appendage occlusion was significantly reduced, whereas pharmacotherapy was often stated as the preferred option by participating cardiologists.

Keywords: COVID-19 pandemic; atrial fibrillation; interventional therapy; catheter ablation; percutaneous left atrial appendage occlusion; pharmacotherapy

1. Introduction

The coronavirus disease 2019 (COVID-19) pandemic has severely disrupted medical care systems worldwide [1–5]. The adverse influence of the pandemic on the healthcare system has impacted the prevention and treatment of COVID-19 itself, and has destabilized the relationship between clinicians and patients. In particular, the highly contagious and widespread Omicron variant has made the epidemic difficult to control and has presented challenges for the diagnosis and treatment of other common diseases [6,7].

Atrial fibrillation (AF) treatment is a comprehensive and multifaceted strategy involving heart rhythm control, heart rate control, stroke prevention therapy, interventional or surgical therapy, and the management of cardiovascular risk factors and concomitant diseases [8,9]. Several previous studies have found increased morbidity in AF patients who also have COVID-19, which affects their prognosis [10–14]. Zoubi M et al. demonstrated that new-onset AF is a poor prognostic sign in patients with severe COVID-19 [15]. Alkhameys S et al. performed an interrupted time series analysis of anticoagulant prescription between January 2019 and February 2021 using the English Prescribing Dataset. Although the prescription of direct-acting oral anticoagulants during the COVID-19 pandemic increased by 19%, the overall prescription of oral anticoagulants during this period was lower than expected, possibly owing to medication adherence [16]. A recently published questionnaire analysis also revealed that the COVID-19 pandemic significantly impaired the quality of life of patients awaiting AF ablation procedures [17]. Thus, COVID-19 continues to impact the management of AF and brings increasing challenges for clinicians.

However, no relevant studies have extensively investigated the impact of the COVID-19 pandemic on the clinical practice patterns of AF. In the present study, we invited 300 cardiologists from 22 provinces in China, in April 2022, to fill out a questionnaire survey investigating their perspectives on how the COVID-19 pandemic has impacted their treatment strategies for AF patients.

2. Methods

2.1. Study Design and Participants

To better understand the impact of the COVID-19 pandemic on AF treatment practices, we conducted a multicenter physician survey of 300 cardiologists in China. Research team members at the Renji Hospital, School of Medicine, Shanghai Jiaotong University, developed and distributed the survey. This survey was implemented using an online questionnaire as the primary source of data collection. The intended target population was physicians in cardiovascular departments who treated patients with AF in their routine clinical work. An initial questionnaire draft informed by the study aims was developed, pilot-tested, and revised from 1 April 2022 to 10 April 2022. A detailed questionnaire including demographic questions and clinical questions was distributed via the WeChat software to 300 cardiologists from 22 provinces in China, in April 2022. The clinician survey was administered anonymously, and all responses were submitted by 30 April 2022. This study was approved by the Institutional Ethics Committee of Renji Hospital Affiliated to Medical College of Shanghai Jiaotong University.

2.2. Questionnaire Design

The questionnaire, entitled "Clinician Perspectives on the Impact of the COVID-19 Pandemic on the Clinical Practice Patterns in Atrial Fibrillation", consisted of single-choice, multiple-choice, and open-ended free-text response questions (Supplement S1). Questions 1 to 5 collected the participant's demographic information, including years of practice, subspecialty, hospital grade, and province. Questions 6 and 7 aimed to investigate the severity of the COVID-19 pandemic at the participant's location. Questions 8 to 24 were designed to obtain the participant's perspectives on how the COVID-19 pandemic has impacted the clinical practice patterns of AF and their treatment strategy decisions for AF patients during the pandemic. On the basis of the standard recommendations for treating AF in the latest guidelines [8,9], we explored the participant's AF treatment practices via various clinical scenarios in questions 11 to 19. Because there is an overlap in the treatment strategies for the first diagnosed AF and other types of AF, we did not design separate questions about the first diagnosed AF. In addition, the difference between long-standing persistent AF and permanent AF mainly lies in the therapeutic attitudes of the patient and physician about the rhythm control strategy, and there is no notable difference in the clinical characteristics of these patient groups. Therefore, we combined these two types of AF when designing the questionnaire in accordance with the point of view of physicians. Clinical decisions for emergencies such as hemodynamic instability induced by AF were excluded from the clinical survey. Some rarely used AF treatments, such as AF surgery, hybrid surgical/catheter ablation procedures, atrioventricular node ablation and pacing, and surgical left atrial appendage exclusion were also not included in the questionnaire. This questionnaire defines the "previous non-pandemic period" as the year 2019 before the COVID-19 pandemic outbreak.

2.3. Statistical Analysis

All statistical analyses were performed using the SPSS 24.0 software (IBM Corp, Armonk, NY, USA). Continuous measures were described as mean ± standard deviation. Categorical measures were described as counts or as the number (percentage) of participants and compared by a Pearson chi-squared test. Standard $p < 0.05$ was considered statistically significant.

3. Results

3.1. Characteristics of Survey Respondents

In this multicenter survey, 300 questionnaires were distributed via WeChat. A total of 213 questionnaires were returned with a response rate of 71.0%. The characteristics of the respondents are summarized in Table 1. Among the respondents, 82.6% were employed in tertiary hospitals, 53.5% reported more than 10 years of clinical cardiology practice, 59.6% had cardiac arrhythmia as a subspecialty, and 40.8% were electrophysiologists who performed catheter ablation for arrhythmias. The locations of all participated cardiologists are summarized in Table S1.

3.2. Severity of COVID-19 Pandemic at the Locations of the Participants

The participating cardiologists were from 22 provinces in China with different levels of severity of the COVID-19 pandemic. The characteristics of the pandemic are summarized in Table 2. Overall, 20.7% of participants reported more than 1000 new COVID-19 cases per day in their province during the week before responding to the survey, and 16.4% worked in a city where there were more than 1000 new COVID-19 cases per day in the week before the survey.

3.3. Impact of COVID-19 Pandemic on the Clinical Practice Patterns in AF

3.3.1. Impact of COVID-19 Pandemic on the Numbers of AF Inpatients and Outpatients

The vast majority of respondents stated that there was an obvious reduction in the number of inpatients and outpatients with a chief complaint of AF-related symptoms, although in different proportions. Only sporadic respondents reported an increase in such patients, and a small proportion of respondents reported that there was only a slight increase or decrease (Figure 1). Similar results were seen for the number of AF patients who underwent catheter ablation therapy.

3.3.2. Perception of Participating Cardiologists on the Impact of COVID-19 Pandemic on the Clinical Practice Patterns in AF

In questions 20 to 24, participants were asked: "Regarding the treatment of first diagnosed/paroxysmal/persistent/long-standing persistent/permanent AF, at what level do you think the COVID-19 pandemic has impacted you?". The response statistics are shown in Figure 2. Less than one in five participating cardiologists stated that the pandemic had almost no impact on their treatment of first diagnosed, paroxysmal, persistent, and long-standing persistent AF. At the same time, 22.07% thought that the COVID-19 pandemic had almost no influence on their treatment of permanent AF. By contrast, the vast majority of the other participants believed that the COVID-19 pandemic had varying degrees of impact on their AF treatment practices.

Table 1. Characteristics of survey respondents ($n = 213$).

Characteristic	n (%)
Years in practice (years)	
≤5	50 (23.5)
6–10	49 (23.0)
11–20	89 (41.8)
>20	25 (11.7)
Classification of employed hospital	
Primary general hospital	4 (1.9)
Secondary general hospital	16 (7.5)
Tertiary general hospital	176 (82.6)
Cardiovascular hospital	17 (8.0)
Subspecialty (multiple choice)	
Arrhythmias	127 (59.6)
Coronary heart disease	103 (48.4)
Congenital heart disease/structural heart disease	19 (9.0)
Heart failure	64 (30.0)
Hypertension	68 (31.9)
Dyslipidemia	47 (22.1)
Critical cardiovascular diseases	36 (16.9)
Cardiovascular diseases without detailed subspecialty	50 (23.5)
Other subspecialty	10 (4.7)
Subspecialty in interventional therapy (multiple choice)	
Electrophysiology	87 (40.8)
Coronary artery intervention therapy	91 (42.7)
Cardiac device implantation	75 (35.2)
Interventional therapy for congenital heart disease	16 (7.5)
Interventional therapy for peripheral vascular diseases	3 (1.4)
Other interventional therapy	2 (0.9)
Not interventional physicians	53 (24.9)

Table 2. The severity of COVID-19 pandemic at the locations of the participants ($n = 213$).

Characteristic	n (%)
Newly reported COVID-19 cases per day in the province of the respondents	
>1000 cases per day	44 (20.66)
501–1000 cases per day	0 (0.00)
101–500 cases per day	7 (3.29)
11–100 cases per day	50 (23.47)
≤10 cases per day	112 (52.58)
Newly reported COVID-19 cases per day in the city of the respondents	
>1000 cases per day	35 (16.43)
501–1000 cases per day	3 (1.41)
101–500 cases per day	5 (2.35)
11–100 cases per day	21 (9.86)
≤10 cases per day	149 (69.95)

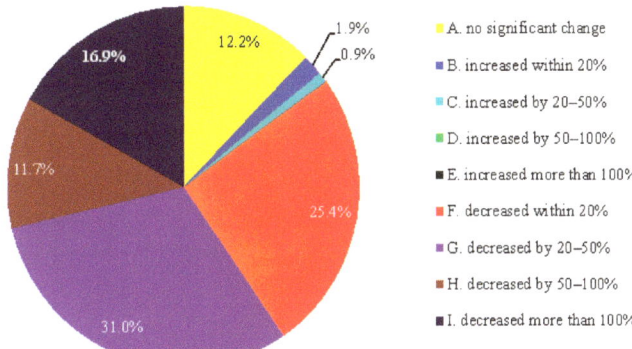

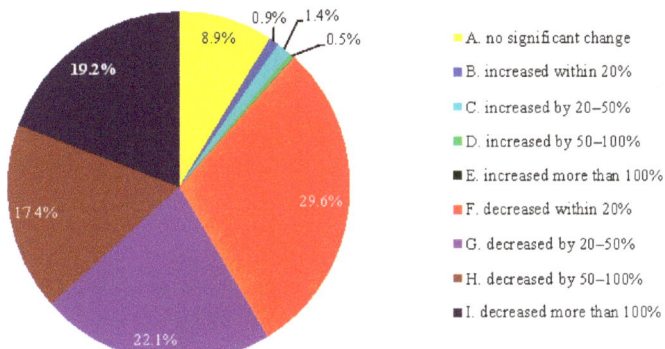

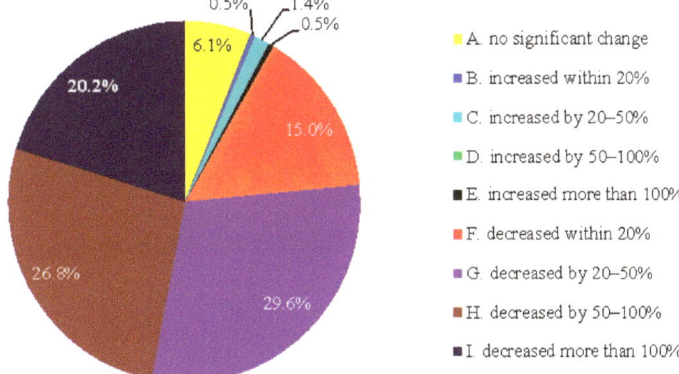

Figure 1. Impact of the COVID-19 pandemic on the numbers of outpatients and inpatients with AF. (**A**) Impact of the COVID-19 pandemic on the number of outpatients with AF. (**B**) Impact of the COVID-19 pandemic on the number of inpatients with AF. (**C**) Impact of the COVID-19 pandemic on the number of AF patients who underwent catheter ablation therapy.

(A) Perception of participated cardiologists on the impact of COVID-19 pandemic on the clinical practice patterns in first diagnosed AF

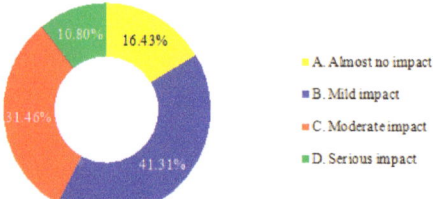

- A. Almost no impact
- B. Mild impact
- C. Moderate impact
- D. Serious impact

(B) Perception of participated cardiologists on the impact of COVID-19 pandemic on the clinical practice patterns in paroxysmal AF

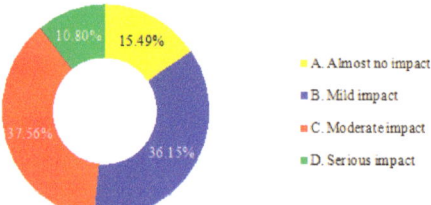

- A. Almost no impact
- B. Mild impact
- C. Moderate impact
- D. Serious impact

(C) Perception of participated cardiologists on the impact of COVID-19 pandemic on the clinical practice patterns in persistent AF

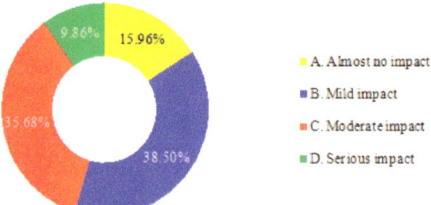

- A. Almost no impact
- B. Mild impact
- C. Moderate impact
- D. Serious impact

(D) Perception of participated cardiologists on the impact of COVID-19 pandemic on the clinical practice patterns in long-standing persistent AF

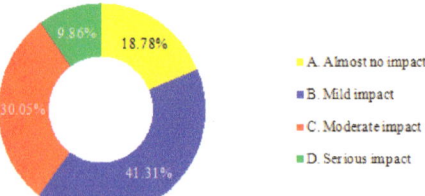

- A. Almost no impact
- B. Mild impact
- C. Moderate impact
- D. Serious impact

(E) Perception of participated cardiologists on the impact of COVID-19 pandemic on the clinical practice patterns in permanent AF

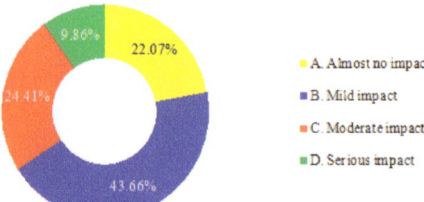

- A. Almost no impact
- B. Mild impact
- C. Moderate impact
- D. Serious impact

Figure 2. Cardiologists' perceptions of how the COVID-19 pandemic affected AF clinical practice patterns.

(**A**) Cardiologists' perceptions on how the COVID-19 pandemic impacted the clinical practice patterns for first diagnosed AF. (**B**) Cardiologists' perceptions on how the COVID-19 pandemic impacted the clinical practice patterns for paroxysmal AF. (**C**) Cardiologists' perceptions on how the COVID-19 pandemic impacted the clinical practice patterns for persistent AF. (**D**) Cardiologists' perceptions on how the COVID-19 pandemic impacted the clinical practice patterns for long-standing persistent AF. (**E**) Cardiologists' perceptions on how the COVID-19 pandemic impacted the clinical practice patterns for permanent AF.

3.3.3. Impact of COVID-19 Pandemic on the Clinical Practice Patterns in the Paroxysmal AF

Regarding the therapeutic recommendations for patients with paroxysmal AF (Figure 3A), there were no significant differences in the management of cardiovascular risk factors and concomitant diseases or in the use of pharmacotherapy for stroke prevention, heart rate control, and rhythm control among COVID-19-positive patients, COVID-19-negative patients during the pandemic period, and patients in the non-pandemic period. However, only 13.6%, 7.5%, and 4.2% of respondents chose electrical cardioversion, catheter ablation, and percutaneous left atrial appendage occlusion, respectively, for treating COVID-19-positive patients, which were significantly lower responses than for treating COVID-19-negative patients in the pandemic period and patients in the non-pandemic period (all $p < 0.05$). Intergroup analyses revealed that the percentage of respondents recommending catheter ablation for COVID-19-negative patients with paroxysmal AF during the pandemic period was also significantly lower than in the non-pandemic period (all $p < 0.05$).

3.3.4. Impact of COVID-19 Pandemic on the Clinical Practice Patterns in the Persistent AF

For patients with persistent AF, significantly fewer respondents recommended catheter ablation and percutaneous left atrial appendage occlusion for COVID-19-positive patients than for COVID-19-negative patients during the pandemic and patients in the non-pandemic period (all $p < 0.05$) (Figure 3B). Furthermore, compared with respondents who chose either of the two invasive interventional strategies for COVID-19-negative patients during the non-pandemic period, significantly fewer respondents chose either of the strategies for such patients during the pandemic period (all $p < 0.05$).

3.3.5. Impact of COVID-19 Pandemic on the Clinical Practice Patterns in the Long-Standing Persistent or Permanent AF

Regarding the therapeutic recommendations for long-standing persistent or permanent AF (Figure 3C), only 4.2%, 4.2%, and 7.5% of participants chose electrical cardioversion, catheter ablation, and percutaneous left appendage occlusion, respectively, for treating COVID-19-positive patients during the pandemic period. These percentages were significantly lower than for COVID-19-negative patients during the pandemic period and patients in the non-pandemic period (all $p < 0.05$). There was no significant difference in the recommendation of electrical cardioversion, catheter ablation, and percutaneous left atrial appendage occlusion between COVID-19-negative patients during the pandemic period and non-pandemic period (all $p > 0.05$).

3.3.6. Impact of COVID-19 Pandemic on the Invasive Interventional Therapies Recommended by the Participating Cardiologists for AF Patients

As shown in Figure 4, during the COVID-19 pandemic, the recommendations of invasive interventional therapies (catheter ablation and percutaneous left atrial appendage occlusion) were inversely related to the number of new COVID-19 cases in the cities of participating cardiologists (all $p < 0.05$).

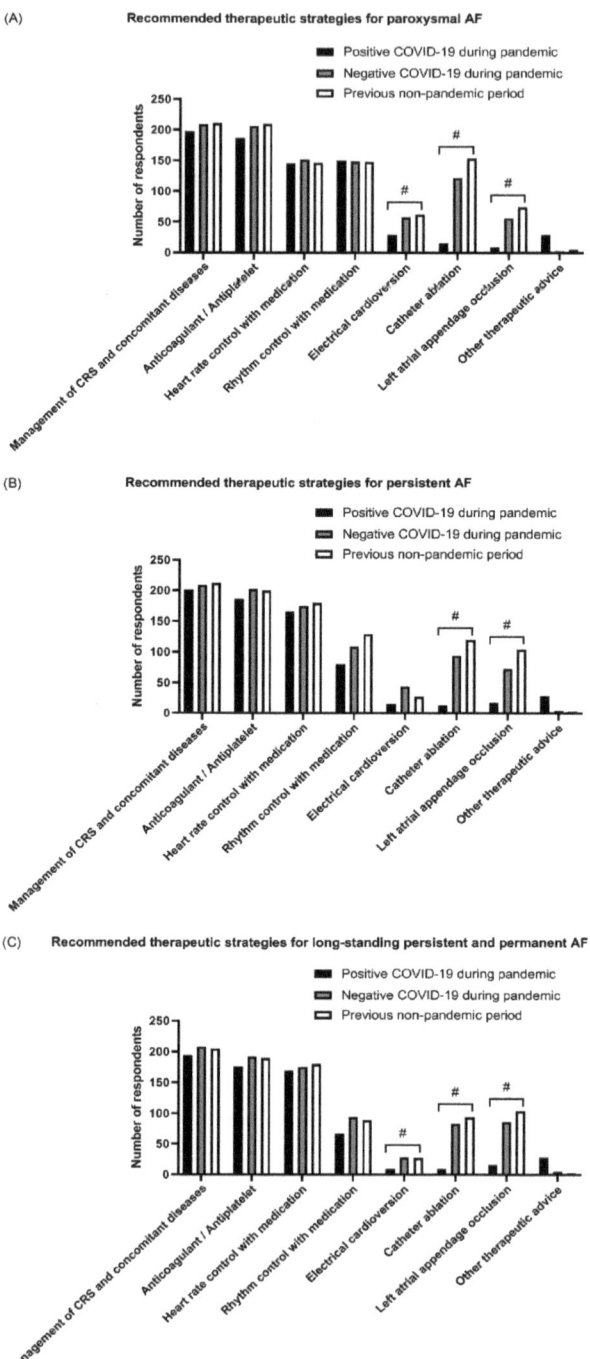

Figure 3. Therapeutic strategies recommended by the participating cardiologists. (**A**) Recommended therapeutic strategies for paroxysmal AF. (**B**) Recommended therapeutic strategies for persistent AF. (**C**) Recommended therapeutic strategies for long-standing persistent and permanent AF. #, $p < 0.05$.

(A) Recommendation of catheter ablation for AF patients during COVID-19 pandemic

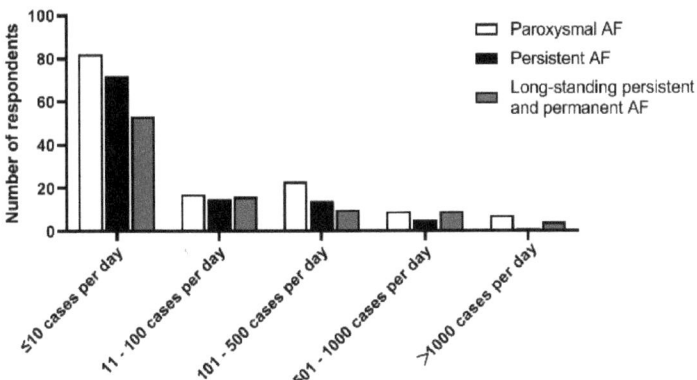

(B) Recommendation of left atrial appendage occlusion for AF patients during COVID-19 pandemic

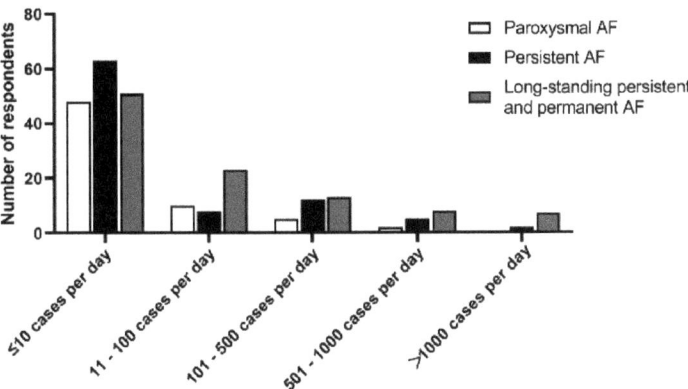

Figure 4. Invasive interventional therapies recommended by the participating cardiologists for AF patients during the COVID-19 pandemic. (**A**) Recommendation of catheter ablation for AF patients during COVID-19 pandemic. (**B**) Recommendation of left atrial appendage occlusion for AF patients during COVID-19 pandemic.

4. Discussion

The COVID-19 pandemic has had a severe impact on healthcare systems around the world. In this multicenter physician survey, we found that the number of inpatients and outpatients with a chief complaint of AF-related symptoms and the number of AF patients who received catheter ablation therapy decreased during the pandemic period. The overwhelming majority of participating cardiologists stated that the COVID-19 pandemic had markedly affected the treatment strategies for AF patients to varying degrees. Compared with respondents who chose to use treatments for all types of AF in the period before the COVID-19 pandemic, fewer respondents chose to use invasive interventional therapies such as catheter ablation and percutaneous left atrial appendage occlusion during the pandemic period. Meanwhile, physicians were more likely to recommend pharmacotherapy for AF patients.

AF is the most common cardiac arrhythmia in adults and is associated with an increased risk of ischemic stroke, cognitive impairment, and heart failure, and it can be a considerable burden to the patient, their family, and society [18–20]. This study found a significant decrease in the number of inpatients and outpatients with AF treated at a hospital during the pandemic. The main reason for this phenomenon is that AF is a chronic disease and these patients were likely worried about the potential risk of contracting COVID-19 during their hospital visit. Except for those with severe symptoms, many patients with AF chose at-home oral medication treatment. Meanwhile, some patients were also limited in traveling between regions during the pandemic, limiting their ability to attend hospital visits. Besides, COVID-19 infections among medical staff would dramatically reduce the number of available staff to provide medical services [21,22]. Although some studies identified an improvement in the physician-patient relationship during the COVID-19 pandemic preventive strategies such as wearing face masks, face shields, and protective clothing create barriers to effective physician-patient communication and has led to decline in trust in doctors during this challenging period [23,24]. Under such circumstances, the communication and interaction between doctors and patients are vital to ensure the comprehensive clinical management of AF. Because the COVID-19 pandemic led to a reduction in hospital visits by AF patients, it is conceivable that the ongoing pandemic could be accompanied by increases in AF-related complications and disability. In China, there are some measures to devote medical resources to the prevention and control of the COVID-19 pandemic, such as the widespread use of vaccines, nationwide free tests for COVID-19, continuous reshaping of the health emergency system, quick and effective cooperation in the joint prevention and the control of various departments, etc. [25]. The pandemic has harmed China and the global economy. That will pose a severe challenge to the health resources of countries, thereby increasing the medical burden of patients [26]. AF interventional therapies, such as catheter ablation and percutaneous left atrial appendage occlusion, are regularly carried out in general tertiary hospitals and have a unique value in the comprehensive treatment of AF. Compared with other types of medical treatment, catheter ablation can significantly prevent the recurrent of atrial arrhythmias and reduce the AF burden in any type of AF, as revealed by the recently published CABANA (Catheter Ablation versus Antiarrhythmic Drug Therapy for Atrial Fibrillation) trial [27,28]. In the AF patients enrolled in the CABANA trial who also had clinically diagnosed heart failure, catheter ablation also showed superiority for improvements in survival and quality of life when compared with medical therapy [27]. Previous studies have verified that early rhythm control therapy leads to a lower risk of cardiovascular complications in AF patients [29–31]. Emerging clinical evidence has also indicated that percutaneous left atrial appendage occlusion is a safe and effective therapeutic strategy for cardioembolic stroke prevention in non-valvular AF patients [32–35]. With the development of many cities in China, Shanghai has the highest rate of elderly, and the AF burden in the aging population has become substantial. Based on the data from medical insurance in the Shanghai municipal health commission database, the left atrial appendage occlusion, as an effective alternative option for AF-related stroke prevention, showed a significant increment from 0.16% in 2015 to 1.23% in 2020 [36]. Compared to other uncommon therapeutic strategies (AF surgery, hybrid surgical/catheter ablation procedures, atrioventricular node ablation and pacing, and surgical left atrial appendage exclusion), the proportion of left atrial appendage occlusion increased 7.68 times from 2015 to 2020 in Shanghai [36]. The application of left atrial appendage occlusion in AF patients who meet the indications may vary among different provinces in China. However, the present study found that the COVID-19 pandemic decreased the proportion of cardiologists who recommended catheter ablation and percutaneous left atrial appendage occlusion for AF patients (who were either positive or negative for COVID-19) during the pandemic period compared with the proportion during the non-pandemic period. According to data from the Hellenic Cardiology Society Ablation Registry, the number of ablation procedures conducted in 2019 (before the COVID-19 pandemic) and 2020 (during the COVID-19 pandemic) was reduced from 3182 cases to 2759 cases, and the number of atrial fibrillation ablation procedures was reduced by 13.8% [37]. The Spanish Catheter Ablation Registry data showed that the number of ablation procedures conducted and the success rate were both affected by the COVID-19 pandemic [38]. The quality of life of patients awaiting AF ablation has also been significantly impaired by the COVID-19 pandemic [17]. Moreover, interventional treatment during the pandemic may involve arranging a dedicated catheter room and specialized medical staff, which is a possible reason why fewer physicians chose interventional therapeutics during the pandemic than in the pre-pandemic period.

Non-invasive therapeutic strategies, such as pharmacotherapy for stroke prevention, heart rate control, rhythm control, and the management of risk factors and comorbidities, are essential cornerstones for improving long-term outcomes in patients with AF [8,9]. Handy A et al. evaluated the use of antithrombotic therapy and COVID-19 outcomes in England's nationwide atrial fibrillation cohort. The authors found that pre-existing antithrombotic therapy was associated with lower odds of COVID-19 death in AF patients during the pandemic [39]. At the peak of COVID-19 lockdown, patients with AF-related symptoms faced various medical problems. An effective antiarrhythmic medication may be used carefully in selected AF outpatients to address these problems [40]. In the present study, there was no significant difference in the recommendations of these non-invasive strategies between the pandemic and non-pandemic periods. Although the proportion of participating physicians who recommended basic non-invasive strategies was not small, the reduction in hospital visits by AF patients during the pandemic had a potentially negative impact on the effectiveness of these treatments. Recently, the concept of Internet hospitals has become more common. Depending on the attributes of such a platform, increasing the communication between doctors and patients may be a promising approach to improve the comprehensive treatment of AF patients during the COVID-19 pandemic. Telemedicine is an important complementary strategy for the management and follow-up of some chronic diseases during the pandemic [41–46]. Previous studies have demonstrated that telemedicine could be of great value for the management of many chronic diseases during the epidemic, especially the long-term management of hypertension, chronic heart failure, and atrial fibrillation in the cardiology department during such a challenging period [41–43].

The current study has several limitations. Firstly, this study is a multicenter clinician survey analysis and all participated cardiologists from 22 provinces in China. Given the severity of the COVID-19 pandemic and the distribution of healthcare resources in different countries or regions, the results of this study may be biased in different regions. Secondly, the treatment of AF is complex and requires individual solutions according to guidelines' recommendations. Thus, the hypothetical clinical scenarios based on the questionnaires may not reflect actual practice management accurately. Besides, the conclusions of this clinician survey still need to be confirmed by further clinical studies. Meanwhile, this survey mainly recruited cardiologists in hospitals that can carry out the common interventional therapeutic strategies for AF. Therefore, the higher proportions of respondents specializing in arrhythmia and working in tertiary hospitals also have potential bias.

5. Conclusions

In summary, the ongoing COVID-19 pandemic has had a profound impact on the clinical practice patterns of AF. During the pandemic period, the selections of catheter ablation and percutaneous left atrial appendage occlusion decreased significantly, whereas pharmacotherapy was often stated as the preferred option by participating cardiologists.

Supplementary Materials: The following are available online at https://www.mdpi.com/article/10.3390/jcm11216469/s1, Supplement S1: Clinician Perspectives on the Impact of the COVID-19 Pandemic on the Clinical Practice Patterns in Atrial Fibrillation; Table S1: Locations of participated cardiologists (n = 213).

Author Contributions: Conceptualization, F.H. and J.P.; methodology, F.H.; software, F.H. and M.Z. validation, J.P. and Y.Y.; formal analysis, A.L.; investigation, J.H.; data curation, W.C., J.G., Z.D., E.L. L.S., X.H., X.X., Z.D. and G.H.; writing—original draft preparation, F.H.; writing—review and editing M.Z. and L.Z.; supervision, J.P.; project administration, F.H. and J.P. All authors have read and agreed to the published version of the manuscript.

Funding: This research received no external funding.

Institutional Review Board Statement: The study was conducted according to the guidelines of the Declaration of Helsinki, and approved by the Institutional Ethics Committee of Renji Hospital Affiliated to Medical College of Shanghai Jiaotong University (No.2022096, 15 March 2022).

Informed Consent Statement: Informed consent was obtained from all subjects involved in the study.

Data Availability Statement: The data used to support the findings of this study are available from the corresponding author upon reasonable request.

Conflicts of Interest: The authors declare no conflict of interest.

References

1. Coronaviridae Study Group of the International Committee on Taxonomy of Viruses. The species Severe acute respiratory syndrome-related coronavirus: Classifying 2019-nCoV and naming it SARS-CoV-2. *Nat. Microbiol.* **2020**, *5*, 536–544. [CrossRef] [PubMed]
2. Girum, T.; Lentiro, K.; Geremew, M.; Migora, B.; Shewamare, S. Global strategies and effectiveness for COVID-19 prevention through contact tracing, screening, quarantine, and isolation: A systematic review. *Trop. Med. Health* **2020**, *48*, 91. [CrossRef]
3. He, X.; Lau, E.H.Y.; Wu, P.; Deng, X.; Wang, J.; Hao, X.; Lau, Y.C.; Wong, J.Y.; Guan, Y.; Tan, X.; et al. Temporal dynamics in viral shedding and transmissibility of COVID-19. *Nat. Med.* **2020**, *26*, 672–675. [CrossRef]
4. Rothan, H.A.; Byrareddy, S.N. The epidemiology and pathogenesis of coronavirus disease (COVID-19) outbreak. *J. Autoimmun.* **2020**, *109*, 102433. [CrossRef] [PubMed]
5. Wang, D.; Hu, B.; Hu, C.; Zhu, F.; Liu, X.; Zhang, J.; Wang, B.; Xiang, H.; Cheng, Z.; Xiong, Y.; et al. Clinical Characteristics of 138 Hospitalized Patients With 2019 Novel Coronavirus—Infected Pneumonia in Wuhan, China. *JAMA* **2020**, *323*, 1061–1069. [CrossRef] [PubMed]
6. Araf, Y.; Akter, F.; Tang, Y.; Fatemi, R.; Alam Parvez, S.; Zheng, C.; Hossain, G. Omicron variant of SARS-CoV-2: Genomics, transmissibility, and responses to current COVID-19 vaccines. *J. Med. Virol.* **2022**, *94*, 1825–1832. [CrossRef] [PubMed]
7. Mohiuddin, M.; Kasahara, K. Investigating the aggressiveness of the COVID-19 Omicron variant and suggestions for possible treatment options. *Respir. Med.* **2021**, *191*, 106716. [CrossRef]
8. January, C.T.; Wann, L.S.; Calkins, H.; Chen, L.Y.; Cigarroa, J.E.; Cleveland, J.C., Jr.; Ellinor, P.T., Jr.; Ezekowitz, M.D.; Field, M.E.; Furie, K.L.; et al. 2019 AHA/ACC/HRS Focused Update of the 2014 AHA/ACC/HRS Guideline for the Management of Patients With Atrial Fibrillation: A Report of the American College of Cardiology/American Heart Association Task Force on Clinical Practice Guidelines and the Heart Rhythm Society in Collaboration With the Society of Thoracic Surgeons. *Circulation* **2019**, *140*, e125–e151. [CrossRef]
9. Hindricks, G.; Potpara, T.; Dagres, N.; Arbelo, E.; Bax, J.J.; Blomström-Lundqvist, C.; Boriani, G.; Castella, M.; Dan, G.-A.; Dilaveris, P.E.; et al. 2020 ESC Guidelines for the diagnosis and management of atrial fibrillation developed in collaboration with the European Association for Cardio-Thoracic Surgery (EACTS): The Task Force for the diagnosis and management of atrial fibrillation of the European Society of Cardiology (ESC) Developed with the special contribution of the European Heart Rhythm Association (EHRA) of the ESC. *Eur. Heart J.* **2021**, *42*, 373–498. [CrossRef]
10. Gawałko, M.; Kapłon-Cieślicka, A.; Hohl, M.; Dobrev, D.; Linz, D. COVID-19 associated atrial fibrillation: Incidence, putative mechanisms and potential clinical implications. *IJC Heart Vasc.* **2020**, *30*, 100631. [CrossRef]
11. Bhatla, A.; Mayer, M.M.; Adusumalli, S.; Hyman, M.C.; Oh, E.; Tierney, A.; Moss, J.; Chahal, A.A.; Anesi, G.; Denduluri, S.; et al. COVID-19 and cardiac arrhythmias. *Heart Rhythm* **2020**, *17*, 1439–1444. [CrossRef] [PubMed]
12. Romiti, G.; Corica, B.; Lip, G.; Proietti, M. Prevalence and Impact of Atrial Fibrillation in Hospitalized Patients with COVID-19: A Systematic Review and Meta-Analysis. *J. Clin. Med.* **2021**, *10*, 2490. [CrossRef] [PubMed]
13. Kelesoglu, S.; Yilmaz, Y.; Ozkan, E.; Calapkorur, B.; Gok, M.; Dursun, Z.B.; Kilic, A.U.; Demirelli, S.; Simsek, Z.; Elcık, D. New onset atrial fibrillation and risk faktors in COVID-19. *J. Electrocardiol.* **2021**, *65*, 76–81. [CrossRef] [PubMed]
14. Li, Z.; Shao, W.; Zhang, J.; Ma, J.; Huang, S.; Yu, P.; Zhu, W.; Liu, X. Prevalence of Atrial Fibrillation and Associated Mortality Among Hospitalized Patients With COVID-19: A Systematic Review and Meta-Analysis. *Front. Cardiovasc. Med.* **2021**, *8*, 720129. [CrossRef] [PubMed]
15. Zoubi, M.; Hejly, A.; Amital, H.; Mahroum, N. New-onset Atrial Fibrillation as Poor Outcome Predictor in Patients with Severe COVID-19. *Isr. Med. Assoc. J.* **2022**, *24*, 445–447.

6. Alkhameys, S.; Barrett, R. Impact of the COVID-19 pandemic on England's national prescriptions of oral vitamin K antagonist (VKA) and direct-acting oral anticoagulants (DOACs): An interrupted time series analysis (January 2019–February 2021). *Curr. Med. Res. Opin.* **2022**, *38*, 1081–1092. [CrossRef]
7. Pius, C.; Ahmad, H.; Snowdon, R.; Ashrafi, R.; Waktare, J.E.; Borbas, Z.; Luther, V.; Mahida, S.; Modi, S.; Hall, M.; et al. Impact of COVID-19 on patients awaiting ablation for atrial fibrillation. *Open Heart* **2022**, *9*, e001969. [CrossRef]
8. Alkhouli, M.; Friedman, P.A. Ischemic Stroke Risk in Patients With Nonvalvular Atrial Fibrillation: JACC Review Topic of the Week. *J. Am. Coll. Cardiol.* **2019**, *74*, 3050–3065. [CrossRef]
9. Andrade, J.; Khairy, P.; Dobrev, D.; Nattel, S. The Clinical Profile and Pathophysiology of Atrial Fibrillation: Relationships among clinical features, epidemiology, and mechanisms. *Circ. Res.* **2014**, *114*, 1453–1468. [CrossRef]
10. Morin, D.P.; Bernard, M.L.; Madias, C.; Rogers, P.A.; Thihalolipavan, S.; Estes, N.A., 3rd. The State of the Art: Atrial Fibrillation Epidemiology, Prevention, and Treatment. *Mayo Clin. Proc.* **2016**, *91*, 1778–1810. [CrossRef]
11. Wosik, J.; Clowse, M.E.; Overton, R.; Adagarla, B.; Economou-Zavlanos, N.; Cavalier, J.; Henao, R.; Piccini, J.P.; Thomas, L.; Pencina, M.J.; et al. Impact of the COVID-19 pandemic on patterns of outpatient cardiovascular care. *Am. Heart J.* **2020**, *231*, 1–5. [CrossRef] [PubMed]
12. Borrelli, E.; Grosso, D.; Vella, G.; Sacconi, R.; Querques, L.; Zucchiatti, I.; Prascina, F.; Bandello, F.; Querques, G. Impact of COVID-19 on outpatient visits and intravitreal treatments in a referral retina unit: Let's be ready for a plausible "rebound effect". *Graefes Arch. Clin. Exp. Ophthalmol.* **2020**, *258*, 2655–2660. [CrossRef] [PubMed]
13. Zhou, Y.; Ma, Y.; Yang, W.F.Z.; Wu, Q.; Wang, Q.; Wang, D.; Ren, H.; Luo, Y.; Yang, D.; Liu, T.; et al. Doctor-patient relationship improved during COVID-19 pandemic, but weakness remains. *BMC Fam. Pr.* **2021**, *22*, 255. [CrossRef]
14. Gopichandran, V.; Sakthivel, K. Doctor-patient communication and trust in doctors during COVID 19 times—A cross sectional study in Chennai, India. *PLoS ONE* **2021**, *16*, e0253497. [CrossRef] [PubMed]
15. Wang, J.; Wang, Z. Strengths, Weaknesses, Opportunities and Threats (SWOT) Analysis of China's Prevention and Control Strategy for the COVID-19 Epidemic. *Int. J. Environ. Res. Public Health* **2020**, *17*, 2235. [CrossRef]
16. Shen, J.; Shum, W.Y.; Cheong, T.S.; Wang, L. COVID-19 and Regional Income Inequality in China. *Front. Public Health* **2021**, *9*, 687152. [CrossRef]
17. Packer, D.L.; Piccini, J.P.; Monahan, K.H.; Al-Khalidi, H.R.; Silverstein, A.P.; Noseworthy, P.A.; Poole, J.E.; Bahnson, T.D.; Lee, K.L.; Mark, D.B.; et al. Ablation Versus Drug Therapy for Atrial Fibrillation in Heart Failure: Results From the CABANA Trial. *Circulation* **2021**, *143*, 1377–1390. [CrossRef]
18. Poole, J.E.; Bahnson, T.D.; Monahan, K.H.; Johnson, G.; Rostami, H.; Silverstein, A.P.; Al-Khalidi, H.R.; Rosenberg, Y.; Mark, D.B.; Lee, K.L.; et al. Recurrence of Atrial Fibrillation After Catheter Ablation or Antiarrhythmic Drug Therapy in the CABANA Trial. *J. Am. Coll. Cardiol.* **2020**, *75*, 3105–3118. [CrossRef]
19. Solimene, F.; Santoro, M.G.; Stabile, G.; Msc, M.M.; De Simone, A.; Pandozi, C.; Pelargonio, G.; Rossi, P.; Battaglia, A.; Pecora, D.; et al. Early rhythm-control ablation therapy to prevent atrial fibrillation recurrences: Insights from the CHARISMA Registry. *Pacing Clin. Electrophysiol.* **2021**, *44*, 2031–2040. [CrossRef]
20. Kirchhof, P.; Camm, A.J.; Goette, A.; Brandes, A.; Eckardt, L.; Elvan, A.; Fetsch, T.; van Gelder, I.C.; Haase, D.; Haegeli, L.M.; et al. Early Rhythm-Control Therapy in Patients with Atrial Fibrillation. *N. Engl. J. Med.* **2020**, *383*, 1305–1316. [CrossRef]
21. Kim, D.; Yang, P.-S.; You, S.C.; Sung, J.-H.; Jang, E.; Yu, H.T.; Kim, T.-H.; Pak, H.-N.; Lee, M.-H.; Lip, G.Y.H.; et al. Treatment timing and the effects of rhythm control strategy in patients with atrial fibrillation: Nationwide cohort study. *BMJ* **2021**, *373*, n991. [CrossRef] [PubMed]
22. Holmes, D.R.; Kar, S.; Price, M.J.; Whisenant, B.; Sievert, H.; Doshi, S.K.; Huber, K.; Reddy, V.Y. Prospective Randomized Evaluation of the Watchman Left Atrial Appendage Closure Device in Patients With Atrial Fibrillation Versus Long-Term Warfarin Therapy: The PREVAIL trial. *J. Am. Coll. Cardiol.* **2014**, *64*, 1–12. [CrossRef] [PubMed]
23. Sievert, H.; Lesh, M.D.; Trepels, T.; Omran, H.; Bartorelli, A.; Della Bella, P.; Nakai, T.; Reisman, M.; DiMario, C.; Block, P.; et al. Percutaneous Left Atrial Appendage Transcatheter Occlusion to Prevent Stroke in High-Risk Patients With Atrial Fibrillation: Early clinical experience. *Circulation* **2002**, *105*, 1887–1889. [CrossRef]
24. Reddy, V.Y.; Sievert, H.; Halperin, J.; Doshi, S.K.; Buchbinder, M.; Neuzil, P.; Huber, K.; Whisenant, B.; Kar, S.; Swarup, V.; et al. Percutaneous Left Atrial Appendage Closure vs Warfarin for Atrial Fibrillation: A randomized clinical trial. *JAMA* **2014**, *312*, 1988–1998. [CrossRef]
25. Osmancik, P.; Herman, D.; Neuzil, P.; Hala, P.; Taborsky, M.; Kala, P.; Poloczek, M.; Stasek, J.; Haman, L.; Branny, M.; et al. Left Atrial Appendage Closure Versus Direct Oral Anticoagulants in High-Risk Patients With Atrial Fibrillation. *J. Am. Coll. Cardiol.* **2020**, *75*, 3122–3135. [CrossRef] [PubMed]
26. Chen, M.; Li, C.; Liao, P.; Cui, X.; Tian, W.; Wang, Q.; Sun, J.; Yang, M.; Luo, L.; Wu, H.; et al. Epidemiology, management, and outcomes of atrial fibrillation among 30 million citizens in Shanghai, China from 2015 to 2020: A medical insurance database study. *Lancet Reg. Health West. Pac.* **2022**, *23*, 100470. [CrossRef]
27. Vassilikos, V.P.; Giannopoulos, G.; Billis, A.; Efremidis, M.; Andrikopoulos, G.; Katsivas, A.; Kossyvakis, C.; Kallergis, E.; Letsas, K.; Kanoupakis, E.; et al. Effect of the COVID-19 pandemic on cardiac electrophysiological ablation procedures in Greece—Data from the Hellenic Society of Cardiology Ablation Registry. *Hell. J. Cardiol.* **2022**, *67*, 76–78. [CrossRef]

38. Cózar León, R.; Anguera Camós, I.; Cano Pérez, Ó.; en Representación de los Colaboradores del Registro Español de Ablación con Catéter. Spanish Catheter Ablation Registry. 20th Official Report of the Heart Rhythm Association of the Spanish Society of Cardiology. *Rev. Esp. Cardiol.* **2021**, *74*, 1073–1084. [CrossRef]
39. Handy, A.; Banerjee, A.; Wood, A.M.; Dale, C.; Sudlow, C.L.M.; Tomlinson, C.; Bean, D.; Thygesen, J.H.; A Mizani, M.; Katsoulis M.; et al. Evaluation of antithrombotic use and COVID-19 outcomes in a nationwide atrial fibrillation cohort. *Heart* **2022**, *108*, 923–931. [CrossRef]
40. Mascarenhas, D.A.N.; Mudumbi, P.C.; Kantharia, B.K. Outpatient initiation of dofetilide: Insights from the complexities of atrial fibrillation management during the COVID-19 lockdown. *J. Interv. Card. Electrophysiol.* **2021**, *63*, 21–28. [CrossRef]
41. Severino, P.; D'Amato, A.; Prosperi, S.; Magnocavallo, M.; Maraone, A.; Notari, C.; Papisca, I.; Mancone, M.; Fedele, F. Clinical Support through Telemedicine in Heart Failure Outpatients during the COVID-19 Pandemic Period: Results of a 12-Months Follow Up. *J. Clin. Med.* **2022**, *11*, 2790. [CrossRef] [PubMed]
42. Hu, Y.-F.; Cheng, W.-H.; Hung, Y.; Lin, W.-Y.; Chao, T.-F.; Liao, J.-N.; Lin, Y.-J.; Lin, W.-S.; Chen, Y.-J.; Chen, S.-A. Management of Atrial Fibrillation in COVID-19 Pandemic. *Circ. J.* **2020**, *84*, 1679–1685. [CrossRef] [PubMed]
43. Colbert, G.B.; Venegas-Vera, A.V.; Lerma, E.V. Utility of telemedicine in the COVID-19 era. *Rev. Cardiovasc. Med.* **2020**, *21*, 583–587 [CrossRef] [PubMed]
44. Gareev, I.; Gallyametdinov, A.; Beylerli, O.; Valitov, E.; Alyshov, A.; Pavlov, V.; Izmailov, A.; Zhao, S. The opportunities and challenges of telemedicine during COVID-19 pandemic. *Front. Biosci. Biosci.-Elite* **2021**, *13*, 291–298. [CrossRef]
45. Bokolo, A.J. Exploring the adoption of telemedicine and virtual software for care of outpatients during and after COVID-19 pandemic. *Ir. J. Med. Sci.* **2020**, *190*, 1–10. [CrossRef]
46. Ohannessian, R.; Duong, T.A.; Odone, A. Global Telemedicine Implementation and Integration Within Health Systems to Fight the COVID-19 Pandemic: A Call to Action. *JMIR Public Health Surveill.* **2020**, *6*, e18810. [CrossRef]

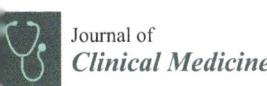

A Four-Stepwise Electrocardiographic Algorithm for Differentiation of Ventricular Arrhythmias Originated from Left Ventricular Outflow Tract

Hong-Wei Tan [1,†], Wei-Dong Gao [2,†], Xin-Hua Wang [3], Zhi-Song Chen [1] and Xue-Bo Liu [1,*]

1. Department of Cardiology, Tongji Hospital, Tongji University School of Medicine, No. 389 Xincun Road, Shanghai 200065, China
2. Department of Cardiology, Jiangmen Central Hospital, Jiangmen 529030, China
3. Department of Cardiology, Ren Ji Hospital, School of Medicine, Shanghai Jiao Tong University, 1630 Dongfang Rd., Shanghai 200127, China
* Correspondence: lxb70@hotmail.com
† These authors contributed equally to this work.

Abstract: Several electrocardiographic algorithms have been proposed to identify the site of origin for the ventricular arrhythmias (VAs) from the left ventricular outflow tract (LVOT) versus right ventricular outflow tract. However, the electrocardiographic criteria for distinguishing VAs originated from the different sites of LVOT is lacking. We aimed to develop a simple and efficient ECG algorithm to differentiate LVOT VAs originated from the aortic root, AMC and LV summit. We analyzed 12-lead ECG characteristics of 68 consecutive patients who underwent successful radiofrequency catheter ablation of symptomatic VAs from LVOT. Patients were divided into RCC (right coronary cusp) group ($n = 8$), the L-RCC (the junction between the LCC and RCC) group ($n = 21$), the LCC (left coronary cusp) group ($n = 24$), the aortomitral continuity (AMC) group ($n = 9$) and the LV summit group ($n = 6$) according to the final ablation sites. Measurements with the highest diagnostic performance were modeled into a 4-stepwise algorithm to discriminate LVOT VAs. The performance of this novel algorithm was prospectively tested in a validation cohort of 43 consecutive patients undergoing LVOT VAs ablation. Based on the accuracy of AUC, a 4-stepwise ECG algorithm was developed. First, the QS duration in aVL > 134 ms was used to distinguish VAs from AMC, LV summit and VAs from aortic root (80% sensitivity and 76% specificity). Second, the R duration in II > 155 ms was used to differentiate VAs from LV summit and VAs from AMC (67% sensitivity and 56% specificity). Third, the ratio of III/II < 0.9 was used to discriminate VAs from RCC and VAs from LCC, L-RCC (82% sensitivity and 63% specificity). Fourth, the QS duration of aVR > 130 ms was used to discern VAs from LCC and VAs from L-RCC (75% sensitivity and 62% specificity). In the prospective evaluation, our 4-stepwise ECG algorithm exhibited a good predictive value. We have developed a novel and simple 4-stepwise ECG algorithm with good predictive value to discriminate the AVs from different sites of LVOT.

Keywords: ventricular arrhythmias; catheter ablation; electrocardiogram; algorithm; left ventricular outflow tract

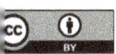

1. Introduction

Idiopathic ventricular arrhythmias (VAs) often originate from the left ventricular outflow tract (LVOT) [1–4], and up to one third of all VAs are thought to arise from the LVOT region [5]. Anatomically, LVOT lies in the center of the heart and includes the aortic root, aortomitral continuity (AMC), the superior basal septum and LV summit [3]. LVOT VAs can be successfully treated by endocardial radiofrequency catheter ablation (RFCA) from the aortic root, AMC or from the LV summit via cardiac venous system [3,4]. The surface electrocardiogram (ECG) is a simple and relatively accurate evaluation tool for localization of VAs before ablation. The electrocardiographic characteristics of VAs originating from the aortic root, AMC and LV summit have been studied [3–5], and several ECG criteria have been proposed to identify the site of origin for the VAs from the LVOT versus right ventricular outflow tract [6–10]. However, the electrocardiographic criterion for distinguishing VAs originating from the different sites of LVOT is still lacking. The aim of our study was to develop a simple and efficient ECG algorithm to differentiate LVOT VAs that originated from the aortic root, AMC and LV summit.

2. Methods

2.1. Study Design

This study was designed in 2 phases: (1) a retrospective analysis of successful LVOT VAs ablation cases in order to develop an ECG algorithm; and (2) a prospective cohort study to verify the accuracy and effectiveness of our ECG algorithm.

2.2. Study Populations

Consecutive patients with symptomatic LVOT VAs who were successfully ablated from January 2019 to December 2020 were included in this study. LVOT VAs were defined as VAs with inferior axis, a R/S transition in lead V3 or earlier and a site of the earliest ventricular activation in the aortic root, AMC and LV summit [11]. Physical examination, 12-lead ECG, 24-h Holter monitor, and echocardiography demonstrated no evidence of structural heart disease in any patients. Baseline characteristics, including age, gender, nature of the clinical arrhythmia, and 12-lead ECG during the VAs, were recorded. All antiarrhythmic drugs were discontinued for at least five-lives before the study. The Institutional Review Board approved the study protocol, and informed consent for the procedure was obtained from all the patients.

2.3. Electrophysiological Study

All patients underwent electrophysiological examination in the postabsorptive, nonsedated state. A catheter was placed in the right ventricle, or within the distal coronary sinus via femoral veins if necessary. Surface ECG leads were applied in the standard manner. ECG and intracardiac electrograms were recorded simultaneously by digital multichannel system (EPMed, St Jude Medical or Pruca Cardiolab, GE Healthcare), filtered at 30 to 500 Hz for bipolar electrograms and at 0.05 to 400 Hz for unipolar electrograms. If VAs were not inducible at baseline, intravenous isoproterenol infusion (2–5 ug/min) was administrated to induce the clinical VAs. If clinical arrhythmia failed to occur spontaneously, programmed stimulation was performed. The standard protocol consisted of ventricular stimulation at 2 basic drive cycle length with ≤2 extrastimuli to a minimum coupling interval of 230 ms as described previously [12]. Mapping and pacing were performed using a 7.5Fr, 3.5-mm-tip irrigated ablation catheter (Navistar ThermoCool; Biosense Webster, Diamond Bar, CA, USA) introduced from the right femoral vein for sites in the right ventricular outflow tract and LV summit or right femoral artery for the endocardial LVOT and AMC. Intravenous heparin was administered to maintain an activated clot time > 250 s when mapping at the aortic root and left ventricle.

2.4. Mapping and Radiofrequency Catheter Ablation

The procedure was performed under the guidance of fluoroscopy and the 3-dimensional electroanatomic mapping system (CARTO 3, Biosense Webster, Diamond Bar, CA). In patients with frequent premature ventricular contractions (PVC), activation mapping was performed in the right ventricular outflow tract, the aortic root, AMC and great cardiac veins. In some cases, the area underneath aortic sinus cusps was reached by an antegrade trans-septal approach as described previously [12]. When PVC was infrequent, pace mapping was performed during sinus rhythm at a pacing cycle length of 500 ms at an output just greater than a diastolic threshold, as previously described [8,13]. The ablation target was defined as the earliest bipolar electrogram preceding the QRS onset during the PVC and/or an excellent pace map (>11/12 leads) [8]. When the earliest ventricular activation at the intended local site preceded QRS onset by >20 ms [14] and/or excellent pace mapping was achieved, RFCA was performed in temperature-controlled mode with a maximum power of 35 W, temperature limit of 43 °C, and flush rate of 20 mL/min in aortic root, AMC and with a maximum power of 30 W, temperature limit of 43 °C, and flush rate of 30 mL/min in great cardiac veins. If the impedance was too high (more than 200 Ω, even more), we usually flush the catheter first and wait for the impedance to decrease to less than 180 Ω, then we begin ablation. If the earliest ventricular activation site was identified in RVOT or ablation was performed in RVOT, the patients were excluded from the study. If the VAs require multiple sites (≥2) ablation, the cases were also excluded.

Coronary angiography was performed to assess the course of left and right coronary artery and catheter ablation from the aortic root/coronary cusp; this was only performed if the distance from the electrode tip to the ostium of each left and right coronary ostium was >8 mm as detected by simultaneous coronary angiography [4]. Radiofrequency energy application from the great cardiac veins was performed at sites where the distance to the adjacent coronary artery was >5 mm, as determined by simultaneous coronary angiography [4]. During radiofrequency energy delivery, if a decreased frequency/ elimination of VAs occurred within the initial 15 s, the radiofrequency delivery was continued for 30 to 60 s. Otherwise, the energy delivery was terminated, and the ventricular arrhythmias were re-mapped. Successful ablation was defined as the absence of spontaneous or inducible VAs with isoproterenol infusion (2–5 ug/min) and burst pacing from the RV or LV 30 min after the final radiofrequency application.

2.5. ECG Analysis

The surface 12-lead ECG were recorded during sinus rhythm and during the VAs at a sweep speed of 100 mm/s for all patients. The electrodes of leads V1 and V2 were placed at the fourth intercostal space with careful attention to minimize the effect of incorrect electrode placement on the QRS morphology [15].The following parameters were measured during clinical VAs: (1) total QRS duration; (2) R wave duration and amplitude of inferior leads (II, III, aVF) and the R wave amplitude ratio of lead III/II; (3) QS wave duration and amplitude in leads aVL and aVR and the QS wave amplitude ratio of aVL/aVR; (4) R and S wave amplitude in leads V1-V6; and (5) the site of R wave transition in the precordial leads. The T-P segment was considered the isoelectric baseline for measurement of R wave and S wave amplitudes. The total QRS duration was measured from the site of earliest initial deflection from the isoelectric line in any lead to the time of latest activation in any lead. The R-wave duration was measured from the site of the earliest initial deflection from the isoelectric line to the time at which the R-wave intersected the isoelectric line [16]. For all cases, QRS measurements were performed before mapping and ablation. The ECG analysis was performed by two experienced investigators blinded to the site of the origin with electronic calipers.

2.6. Procedure Success and Follow-Up

Acute success was defined as absence of spontaneous or provoked clinical VAs at 30 min after the last radiofrequency energy application. Follow-up was performed by referring physicians or outpatient clinics.

2.7. Statistical Analysis

Continuous variables are expressed as mean ± SD. Analysis of variance (ANOVA) followed by the Tukey test was used to compare the difference among groups. Categorical variables were compared by a chi-squared test analysis or Fisher's exact test. For those ECG measurements that were significantly different between the anatomical sites, a receiver operating characteristic (ROC) curve was performed to determine cut-offs with optimal performance. These were then subjected to stepwise mechanistic analysis in varying order and combination to derive an algorithm with optimal statistical accuracy and the sensitivity, specificity, positive predictive value (PPV), and negative predictive value (NPV) for predicting the origins of VAs were assessed using the standard formula. All statistical analyses were performed using SPSS 15.0 software (SPSS Inc., Chicago, IL, USA), and the differences were considered significant at $p < 0.05$.

3. Results

3.1. Patient Characteristics

The study population consisted of 68 patients (28 men, mean age 54 ± 17 years [range 17–85]) with symptomatic idiopathic sustained ventricular tachycardia (VT; $n = 2$, non-sustained VT ($n = 5$), or premature ventricular contractions (PVCs; $n = 61$). The VAs origin was identified in the LVOT by 3-dimensional mapping and a successful catheter ablation. The patients were further divided into five groups according to the final ablation site which includes the RCC (right coronary cusp) group ($n = 8$), the L-RCC (the junction between the LCC and RCC) group ($n = 21$), the LCC (left coronary cusp) group ($n = 24$), the AMC group ($n = 9$) and the LV summit group ($n = 6$). No structural heart disease was found on physical examination, 12-lead ECG or echocardiography. All patients were refractory to ≥1 antiarrhythmic drug before ablation. The demographic and clinical data are shown in Table 1. There was no significant difference in terms of age, gender, diameter of LV, burdens of VAs and comorbidity. Patients in LV summit groups showed significant longer VAs history than patients in RCC and L-RCC groups.

Table 1. Patients and clinical characteristics.

Characteristic	RCC Group ($n = 8$)	L-RCC Group ($n = 21$)	LCC Group ($n = 24$)	AMC Group ($n = 9$)	LV Summit Group ($n = 6$)
Age (year)	45 ± 19	50 ± 16	56 ± 16	66 ± 15	54 ± 20
Gender (male)	1 (13%)	7 (33%)	11 (46%)	5 (56%)	4 (67%)
BMI (kg/m^2)	24.9 ± 4.8	26.3 ± 6.2	25.2 ± 5.3	27.0 ± 7.1	25.3 ± 4.8
Hypertension (n,%)	3 (37%)	7 (33%)	9 (37%)	4 (44%)	2 (33%)
Diabetes	1 (14%)	2 (9%)	3 (14%)	1 (11%)	0
LVd (mm)	45 ± 5	48 ± 4	50 ± 5	51 ± 3	49 ± 3
LVEF (%)	59 ± 3	65 ± 6	61 ± 5	61 ± 6	61 ± 7
History (month)	17 ± 13	21 ± 28	30 ± 31	30 ± 26	65 ± 58 *#
PVC burden (n/24 h)	20,653 ± 13,707	23,279 ± 12,299	22,302 ± 8208	23,751 ± 11,356	34,843 ± 13,899
VT (%)	1 (13%)	2 (9%)	2 (8%)	0	2 (33%)
Antiarrhythmics (n)	2.1 ± 1.1	1.9 ± 1.3	2.0 ± 1.2	2.2 ± 1.2	1.8 ± 1.3

Values are presented as mean ± SD or as n (%). BMI, body mass index; LVd, left ventricular diameter; LVEF, left ventricular ejection fraction; PVC, premature ventricular contraction; VT, ventricular tachycardia. * $p < 0.05$ compared with RCC group; # $p < 0.05$ compared with L-RCC group.

3.2. Mapping and Ablation

All patients underwent electrophysiological study and 3-dimensional mapping. The successful ablation site was located in the RCC in 8 patients, L-RCC in 21, LCC in 24, AMC in 9 and LV summit in 6 patients. There were no significant differences in local ventricular activation time relative to QRS onset at the successful ablation sites, or duration of radiofrequency application among groups. Compared to other groups, all patients in the LV summit group demonstrated larger A wave at the ablation site.

3.3. ECG Analysis

All patients showed R morphology in inferior leads and QS morphology in aVR and aVL. As for the precordial leads, all the patients demonstrated a R/S transition in lead V3 or earlier. Patients in AMC and LV summit groups demonstrated Rs morphology in lead V1 while patients with VAs from aortic root showed rs or rS morphology in lead V1.

The results of the electrocardiographic parameters of the VAs are showed in Tables 2 and 3 and Figure 1. The total QRS duration was significantly increased in the LV summit group than in other groups ($p < 0.05$ or $p < 0.01$) and was significantly increased in the LV summit group than in the AMC group ($p < 0.05$). The R wave duration in lead II, III and aVF was significantly increased in the LV summit group than in RCC, L-RCC, and LCC groups (all $p < 0.01$), and was significantly increased in the AMC group than in the RCC and L-RCC groups (all $p < 0.01$). The R wave duration in lead II showed significant difference between LV summit group and AMC group ($p < 0.05$). The QS duration in lead aVL and aVR was significantly increased in the LV summit group than in VAs from aortic root (all $p < 0.01$), and was significantly increased in the AMC group than in VAs from RCC and L-RCC groups (all $p < 0.01$). The QS duration in lead aVL was significantly increased in the AMC group compared to VAs from LCC ($p < 0.01$).

Table 2. Comparison of ECG characteristics of limb leads.

Characteristic	RCC Group (n = 8)	L-RCC Group (n = 21)	LCC Group (n = 24)	AMC Group (n = 9)	LV Summit Group (n = 6)
Total QRS duration (ms)	150 ± 28	142 ± 15	147 ± 13	158 ± 13 #	178 ± 26 *#&$
R wave duration (ms)					
Lead I	100 ± 35	88 ± 33	83 ± 35	73 ± 26	103 ± 41
Lead II	132 ± 13	134 ± 16	142 ± 14	152 ± 11 *#	171 ± 30 *#&$
Lead III	131 ± 11	129 ± 19	139 ± 16	152 ± 11 *#	169 ± 34 *#&
Lead aVF	130 ± 10	133 ± 17	141 ± 16	151 ± 11 *#	168 ± 30 *#&
QS wave duration (ms)					
Lead I (S wave)	35 ± 7	59 ± 23	64 ± 27	81 ± 29	71 ± 46
Lead aVL	113 ± 19	124 ± 18	130 ± 17 *	147 ± 13 *#&	153 ± 24 *#&
Lead aVR	125 ± 14	128 ± 14	139 ± 15 *#	146 ± 14 *#	155 ± 15 *#&
R wave amplitude (mV)					
Lead I	0.46 ± 0.27	0.43 ± 0.30	0.32 ± 0.22	0,20 ± 0.11	0.29 ± 0.21
Lead II	1.75 ± 0.33	2.07 ± 0.81	2.11 ± 0.57	1.71 ± 0.28	1.84 ± 0.53
Lead III	1.40 ± 0.45	1.95 ± 0.86	2.18 ± 0.69 *	1.89 ± 0.39	1.93 ± 0.55
Lead aVF	1.60 ± 0.42	2.05 ± 0.89	2.14 ± 0.59 *	1.79 ± 0.34	1.86 ± 0.53
The ratio of III/II	0.78 ± 0.15	0.94 ± 0.16*	1.03 ± 0.13 *	1.10 ± 0.16 *#	1.06 ± 0.10 *
QS wave amplitude (mV)					
Lead I (S wave)	0.07 ± 0.03	0.22 ± 0.13	0.31 ± 0.17	0.39 ± 0.11	0.24 ± 0.16
Lead aVL	0.58 ± 0.29	1.14 ± 0.53 *	1.24 ± 0.35 *	1.12 ± 0.21 *	1.12 ± 0.30 *
Lead aVR	1.02 ± 0.18	1.09 ± 0.42	1.09 ± 0.21	0.79 ± 0.15 #&	0.96 ± 0.25
The ratio of aVL/aVR	0.58 ± 0.28	1.12 ± 0.36 *	1.20 ± 0.36 *	1.45 ± 0.38 *#	1.18 ± 0.18 *

Values are presented as mean ± SD or as n (%). * $p < 0.01$ compared with RCC group; # $p < 0.01$ compared with L-RCC group; & $p < 0.01$ compared with LCC group; $ $p < 0.05$ compared with AMC group.

Table 3. Comparison of ECG characteristics of precordial leads.

Characteristic	RCC Group (n = 8)	L-RCC Group (n = 21)	LCC Group (n = 24)	AMC Group (n = 9)	LV Summit Group (n = 6)
R wave duration (ms)					
Lead V1	46 ± 10	52 ± 24	72 ± 32 *	101 ± 52 *#&	134 ± 17 *#&
Lead V2	54 ± 14	72 ± 33	88 ± 27	113 ± 35 *#&	127 ± 12 *#&
Lead V3	92 ± 25	108 ± 24	112 ± 23 *	124 ± 31 *	132 ± 18 *
Lead V4	129 ± 15	127 ± 16	131 ± 14	137 ± 23	148 ± 22 *#&
Lead V5	134 ± 14	130 ± 14	135 ± 14	139 ± 22	150 ± 23
Lead V6	113 ± 41	130 ± 13	134 ± 12 *	142 ± 16 *	147 ± 28 *
S wave duration (ms)					
Lead V1	79 ± 23	69 ± 23	60 ± 23	30 ± 1 *#&	44 ± 7 *
Lead V2	73 ± 18	62 ± 29	56 ± 23	44 ± 13 *	43 ± 6 *
Lead V3	45 ± 15	47 ± 21	40 ± 21	37 ± 12	42 ± 15
R wave amplitude (mV)					
Lead V1	0.22 ± 0.07	0.34 ± 0.24	0.53 ± 0.42 *	0.68 ± 0.57 *#	0.83 ± 0.26 *#
Lead V2	0.45 ± 0.17	0.98 ± 0.65	1.07 ± 0.58	1.22 ± 0.76	1.47 ± 0.58
Lead V3	0.93 ± 0.32	1.57 ± 0.97	1.85 ± 0.83 *	1.77 ± 0.71 *	2.42 ± 0.94 *#
Lead V4	1.79 ± 0.53	2.06 ± 1.11	2.25 ± 0.68	1.84 ± 0.52	2.68 ± 0.88
Lead V5	1.92 ± 0.30	2.10 ± 0.88	2.18 ± 0.68	1.33 ± 0.43 #&	2.28 ± 0.89 $
Lead V6	1.75 ± 0.33	1.84 ± 0.67	1.77 ± 0.56	0.91 ± 0.34 *#&	1.22 ± 0.37 #&
S wave amplitude (mV)					
Lead V1	1.28 ± 0.67	1.00 ± 0.58	0.61 ± 0.48 *#	0.16 ± 0.11 *#	0.37 ± 0.28 *
Lead V2	1.36 ± 0.61	1.25 ± 0.86	1.12 ± 0.66	0.48 ± 0.35 *#&	0.50 ± 0.16 *
Lead V3	0.55 ± 0.43	0.69 ± 0.49	0.81 ± 0.52	0.58 ± 0.51	0.45 ± 0.17

Values are presented as mean ± SD or as n (%). * $p < 0.01$ compared with RCC group; # $p < 0.01$ compared with L-RCCgroup; & $p < 0.01$ compared with LCC group; $ $p < 0.05$ compared with AMC group.

The R wave amplitude in Lead III and aVF was significantly higher in VAs localized in LCC compared to VAs originated from RCC ($p < 0.01$). Compared to other groups, the QS wave amplitude in lead aVL was significantly decreased in the RCC group (all $p < 0.01$). The QS wave amplitude in lead aVR was significantly decreased in the AMC group than in the L-RCC and LCC groups (all $p < 0.01$).

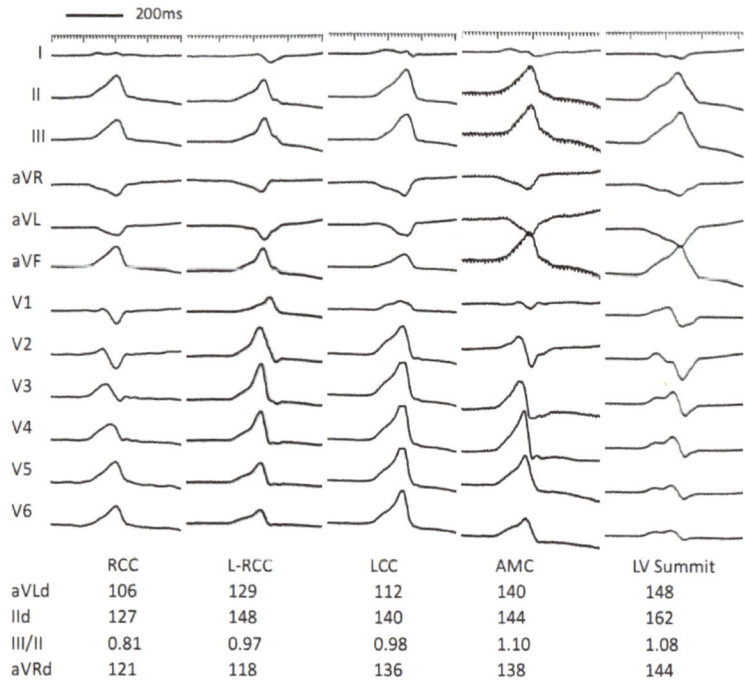

Figure 1. Examples of the electrocardiographic morphology of ventricular arrhythmias originating from different sites of LVOT. aVLd, The QS duration in aVL; IId, The R duration in II; III/II, The ratio of III/II; aVRd, The QS duration in aVR.

The R wave amplitude ratio of lead III/II was significantly decreased in the RCC group compared to VAs from other groups (all $p < 0.01$). The R wave amplitude ratio of lead III/II was significantly decreased in the L-RCC group than in the AMC group ($p < 0.01$). The QS wave amplitude ratio of aVL/aVR was significantly decreased in the RCC group compared to VAs from other groups (all $p < 0.01$). The QS wave amplitude ratio of aVL/aVR was significantly decreased in the L-RCC group than in the AMC group ($p < 0.01$).

In the precordial leads, the R wave duration and amplitude in Lead V1 and V2 demonstrated a progressive increment with significant difference between VAs from AMC, LV summit and VAs from aortic root, while the S wave duration and amplitude showed a tendency to decrease from aortic root to AMC and LV summit groups.

3.4. Develop a Stepwise ECG Algorithm to Differentiate LVOT VAs

The ability of ECG parameters to distinguish LVOT VAs was assessed by using an ROC curve. The area under the curve for the ROC curve of the QS duration in aVL was 0.846 [95% confidential interval 0.735–0.956]. The QS duration in aVL >134 ms had 80% sensitivity and 76% specificity for differentiating VAs from AMC, LV summit and VAs from aortic root. The area under the curve for the ROC curve of the R duration in II was 0.667 [95% confidential interval 0.369–0.965]. The R duration in II > 155 ms had 67% sensitivity and 56% specificity for differentiating VAs from AMC and VAs from LV summit. The area under the curve for the ROC curve of the ratio of III/II was 0.833 [95% confidential interval 0.711–0.955]. The ratio of III/II < 0.9 had 82% sensitivity and 63% specificity for differentiating VAs from RCC and VAs from L-RCC, LCC. The area under the curve for the ROC curve of the QS duration in aVR was 0.724 [95% confidential interval 0.573–0.876]. The QS duration in aVR > 130 ms had 75% sensitivity and 62% specificity for differentiating VAs from LCC and VAs from L-RCC (Figure 2).

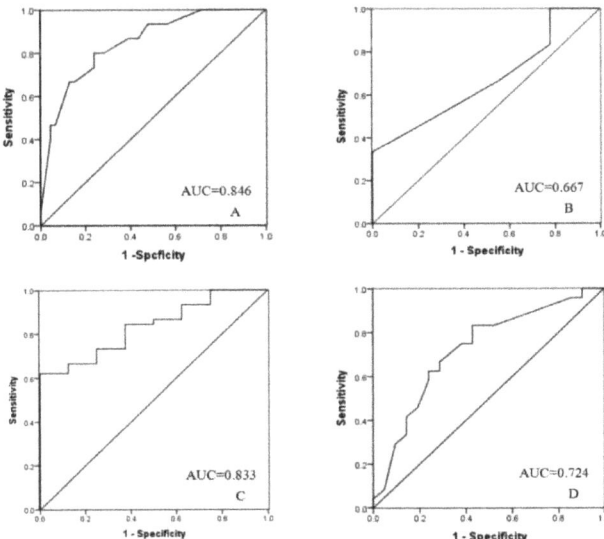

Figure 2. Receiver operating characteristic (ROC) curve of the QS duration in aVL (**A**), the R duration in II (**B**), the ratio of III/II (**C**) and the QS duration in aVR (**D**) to distinguish LVOT VAs.

According to the accuracy of AUC, a stepwise ECG algorithm was developed (Figure 3). First, QS duration in aVL > 134 ms was used to distinguish VAs from AMC, LV summit and VAs from aortic root. Second, R duration in II > 155 ms was used to differentiate VAs from LV summit and VAs from AMC. Third, the ratio of III/II < 0.9 was used to discriminate VAs from RCC and VAs from LCC, L-RCC. Fourth, the QS duration of aVR > 130 ms was used to discern VAs from LCC and VAs from L-RCC.

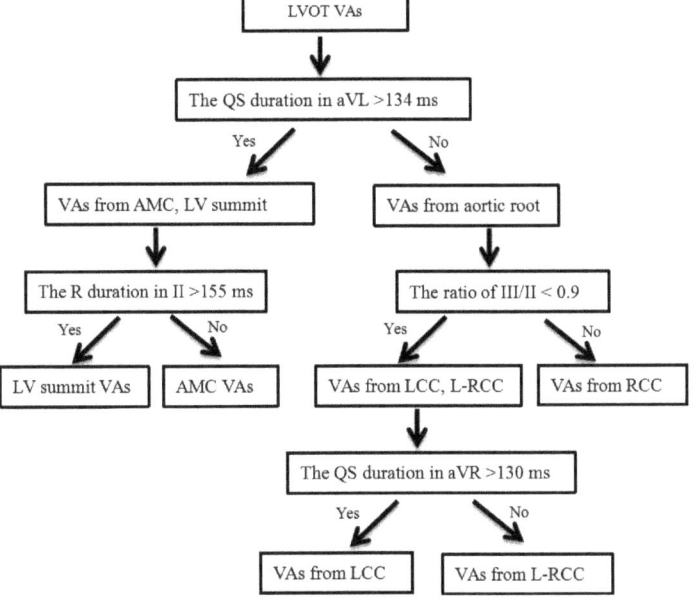

Figure 3. Flowchart of 4-stepwise electrocardiographic algorithm.

3.5. Validation of Four-Stepwise ECG Algorithm in the Prospective Study

A total of 43 consecutive patients (22 males and 21 females) with a left branch block pattern and inferior axis QRS morphology, and with precordial transition before lead V3 that indicate VAs from LVOT, were selected to verify the effectiveness of our four-stepwise algorithms. All these patients underwent successful RFCA for VAs between January 2021 and December 2021 at the sites of LVOT. The successful ablation site was located in the RCC in 6 patients, L-RCC in 8, LCC in 16, AMC in 5 and LV summit in 8 patients. The QS duration in aVL > 134 ms exhibited 100% sensitivity, 86.7% specificity, 76.5% positive predictive value and 100% negative predictive value for differentiating VAs from AMC, LV summit and VAs from aortic root. The R duration in II > 155 ms had 75.0% sensitivity, 80.0% specificity, 85.7% positive predictive value and 66.7% negative predictive value for differentiating VAs from AMC and VAs from LV summit. The ratio of III/II < 0.9 showed 100% sensitivity, 95.0% specificity, 85.7% positive predictive value and 100% negative predictive value for distinguishing VAs from RCC and VAs from LCC, L-RCC. The QS duration in aVR > 130 ms showed 66.7% sensitivity, 62.5% specificity, 72.7% positive predictive value and 55.6% negative predictive value for differentiating VAs from LCC and VAs from L-RCC (Table 4, Figure 4).

Table 4. The accuracy of ECG algorithm for predicting the origins of VAs from LVOT in prospective cohort.

	Sensitivity, %	Specificity, %	PPV, %	NPV, %
The QS duration in aVL > 134 ms for differentiating VAs from AMC, LV summit and VAs from aortic root	100.0	86.7	76.5	100.0
The R duration in II > 155 ms for differentiating VAs from AMC and VAs from LV summit	75.0	80.0	85.7	66.7
The ratio of III/II < 0.9 for differentiating VAs from RCC and VAs from L-RCC, LCC	100.0	95.0	85.7	100.0
The QS duration in aVR > 130 ms for differentiating VAs from LCC and VAs from L-RCC	66.7	62.5	72.7	55.6

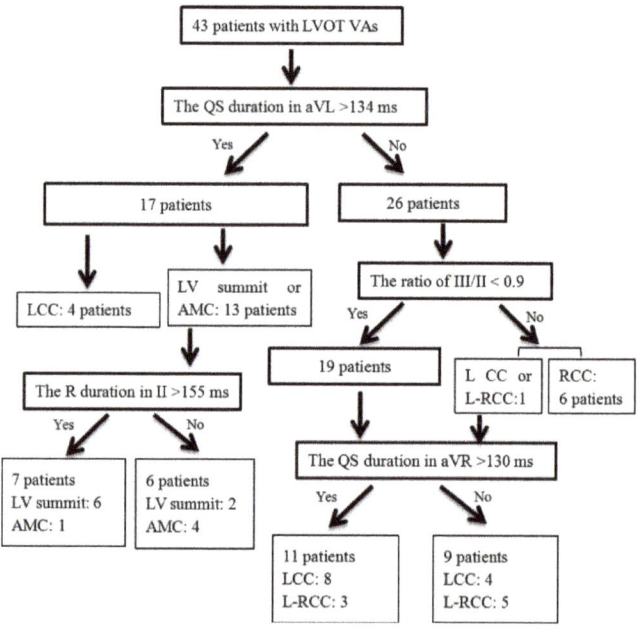

Figure 4. Process of validation in the prospective cohort patients.

4. Discussion

This study explored the surface ECG characteristics of VAs originating from LVOT and we present a simple four-stepwise ECG algorithm to differentiate VAs from different sites of LVOT. We have demonstrated that in patients with VAs when ECG strongly favors an LVOT origin, our four-stepwise ECG algorithm can help localize the likely sites of origin during planning for VAs ablation. First, AMC and LV summit VAs can be differentiated from aortic root VAs by measuring the QS duration in aVL. Then, differentiation between AMC and LV summit VAs can be made by the R duration in II. Third, the ratio of III/II was used to distinguish VAs from RCC and VAs from LCC, L-RCC. Last, LCC VAs could be differentiated from L-RCC VAs by using the QS duration in aVR. For patients referred for catheter ablation of LVOT VAs, this simple ECG measurement might be performed to help plan an ablation strategy and to enhance patient counseling with regard to potential outcome, procedure risk associated with mapping and ablation.

Anatomically, the aortic root occupies a central location within the heart, and the RVOT is located anteriorly and leftward to the aortic root, with the AMC and LV summit anterosuperior to the aortic root. The AMC and the LV summit face each other at the basal portion of the LV muscle between them [5,12]. The aortic root consists of three sinuses of Valsalva. The RCC and LCC are connected with the ventricular musculature at their bases, and the NCC is located between the right and the left atria, immediately anterior to the interatrial septum [13,14]. It has been proven that ventricular myocardial extensions into the aorta beyond ventriculo-arterial junction and these myocardial extensions are the target of ablation [17]. AMC consists of the aortic annulus and the anterior side around the mitral annulus. Although this is a fibrous structure, it is known to be an arrhythmogenic site for ventricular tachyarrhythmias in both normal and diseased heart [18,19]. The LV summit constitutes the superior-most aspect of the LV ostium. It is defined as a triangular region, the apex of which is formed by the bifurcation of the left anterior descending and left circumflex arteries, with its base formed by the arc between the first septal perforator of the left anterior descending artery and the left circumflex artery [5]. The VAs originating from the LV summit can be ablated through the great cardiac vein [5,20].

The ECG characteristics of LVOT VAs are very similar and may even overlap because they all originate from adjacent cardiac structures [21]. It is important to differentiate the ECG characteristics of LVOT VAs in order to safely perform radiofrequency catheter ablation. Ouyang et al. [22] found that a great R wave duration and R/S wave amplitude ratio in lead V1 or V2 reliably predicted an aortic sinus cusp compared with right ventricular outflow tract origin. Lin et al. [23] found that the LCC VAs typically produce a precordial transition by V2, whereas RCC VAs demonstrated a precordial transition by lead V3 and precordial transition is a simple criterion for distinguishing VAs from LCC to RCC. Chen et al. [18] found that AMC VAs showed an early R/S transition pattern in the precordial leads, and VAs from anterior AMC demonstrated equal R and S amplitudes in V2, rS in V1, and R in V3, while VAs from the middle part of the AMC demonstrated a special ('rebound') transition pattern, with which equal R and S amplitudes occurred in V2, and high R waves in V1 and V3. However, one shortcoming of the R wave transition in the precordial leads is the QRS morphology that could alter markedly with an incorrect electrode placement [15]. Komatsu et al. [24] found that The R-wave amplitude ratio in lead III/II, Q-wave amplitude ratio in leads aVL/aVR, and ratio of R wave/S wave in lead V1 were higher in LV summit VAs than in the RVOT and the RCC VAs, the ECG characteristics of LV summit VAs were similar to those in LCC VAs, except for the presence of an initial Q wave in lead I, an initial R wave in lead V1.

In the present study, we have demonstrated that the QS duration in aVL was significantly increased in VAs from AMC and LV summit than in VAs from aortic root, and the QS duration in aVL > 134 ms could be used to distinguish VAs from AMC, LV summit and VAs from aortic root. The R duration in II increased more in the LV summit group than in the AMC group. Anatomically, the aortic root, AMC and LV summit area lie in a continuum from the medial to the lateral, and the QRS duration of VAs from aortic root,

AMC and LV summit would be increased gradually as demonstrated in our study because of synchronous rather than sequential ventricular activation [11]. For differentiating VAs from aortic root, we have found that the ratio of III/II was significantly decreased in VAs from RCC compared to VAs from L-RCC and LCC. The LCC typically sits slightly superior to the RCC. As a result, the VAs from LCC have more of an inferior axis relative to the VAs from RCC [23]. We also found that the QS duration of aVR increased in VAs from LCC than in VAs from L-RCC, and the QS duration of aVR > 130 ms can be used to distinguishing VAs from these two sites.

To the best of our knowledge, this study is the first to investigate the surface ECG characteristics of VAs from different sites of LVOT. We found that patients with VAs from different sites of LVOT demonstrated distinct ECG characteristics, and we also presented a simple four-stepwise ECG algorithm with satisfactory sensitivity and specificity to distinguish VAs from different sites of LVOT. The utility of this ECG algorithm to predict the precise origin of LVOT VAs was validated in a prospective cohort, and the algorithm also exhibited a good predictive value in discriminating LVOT VAs. The last step of the algorithm showed relatively low sensitivity and specificity; this would be explained as the population of our study was small, LCC and L-RCC are closely related, and it is difficult for ECG to distinguish VAs from these areas. Our algorithm uses limb leads, which are less influenced by lead position. Moreover, based upon the duration and amplitude of the QRS wave, the algorithm is simple and practicable in routine clinical practice to help plan an ablation strategy and to enhance patient counseling.

Study Limitations

There were several limitations in the present study. First, the study population was relatively small, which might result in statistical bias, and the results of our study should be validated further in larger populations. Second, the origins of LOVT VAs were defined by the successful ablation sites, which might not be the real origin but anatomically in close proximity to it. Furthermore, the patients requiring multiple sites ablation were excluded from this study, and these may lead to subjective bias. Third, cases with structural heart disease that affect cardiac anatomy were excluded, and the stepwise ECG algorithm would not be suitable for patients with structural heart disease. Fourth, intracardiac echocardiography was not used, only coronary angiography and 3-dimensional electroanatomic mapping were used to determine the final ablation sites; sometimes it is difficult for us to distinguish LCC-RCC VAs from LCC VAs. Finally, the long-term success was not confirmed in this study, as there might be late recurrence cases in these subjects.

5. Conclusions

We have developed a simple four-stepwise ECG algorithm to discriminate the AVs from different sites of LVOT, and our algorithm demonstrated good predictive value in the prospective cohort. Further studies are warranted to verify our results.

Author Contributions: Conceptualization, H.-W.T.; methodology, H.-W.T. and W.-D.G.; formal analysis, W.-D.G. and Z.-S.C.; data curation, H.-W.T., W.-D.G., X.-H.W., Z.-S.C. and X.-B.L.; writing—original draft preparation, H.-W.T. and X.-H.W.; writing—review and editing, X.-B.L.; supervision, X.-B.L.; project administration, X.-B.L. All authors have read and agreed to the published version of the manuscript.

Funding: This research received no external funding.

Institutional Review Board Statement: The study was conducted according to the guidelines of the Declaration of Helsinki, and approved by the Ethics Committee of Tongji Hospital, Tongji University School of Medicine, Shanghai, China (No. 2019-157), 19 April 2019.

Informed Consent Statement: Informed consent was obtained from all subjects involved in the study.

Data Availability Statement: The data underlying this article will be shared upon reasonable request to the corresponding author.

Conflicts of Interest: The authors declare no conflict of interest.

References

1. Prystowsky, E.N.; Padanilam, B.J.; Joshi, S.; Fogel, R.I. Ventricular arrhythmias in the absence of structural heart disease. *J. Am. Coll. Cardiol.* **2012**, *59*, 1733–1744. [CrossRef] [PubMed]
2. Chun, K.R.; Satomi, K.; Kuck, K.H.; Ouyang, F.; Antz, M. Left ventricular outflow tract tachycardia including ventricular tachycardia from the aortic cusps and epicardial ventricular tachycardia. *Herz* **2007**, *32*, 226–332. [CrossRef] [PubMed]
3. Anderson, R.D.; Kumar, S.; Parameswaran, R.; Wong, G.; Voskoboinik, A.; Sugumar, H.; Watts, T.; Sparks, P.B.; Morton, J.B.; McLellan, A.; et al. Differentiating Right- and Left-Sided Outflow Tract Ventricular Arrhythmias: Classical ECG Signatures and Prediction Algorithms. *Circ. Arrhythm. Electrophysiol.* **2019**, *12*, e007392. [CrossRef] [PubMed]
4. Reithmann, C.; Fiek, M. Left ventricular outflow tract arrhythmias with divergent QRS morphology: Mapping of different exits and ablation strategy. *J. Interv. Card. Electrophysiol.* **2018**, *51*, 61–69. [CrossRef]
5. Cheung, J.W.; Anderson, R.H.; Markowitz, S.M.; Lerman, B.B. Catheter Ablation of Arrhythmias Originating From the Left Ventricular Outflow Tract. *JACC Clin. Electrophysiol.* **2019**, *5*, 1–12. [CrossRef]
6. Xie, S.; Kubala, M.; Liang, J.J.; Hayashi, T.; Park, J.; Padros, I.L.; Garcia, F.C.; Santangeli, P.; Supple, G.E.; Frankel, D.S.; et al. Lead I R-wave amplitude to differentiate idiopathic ventricular arrhythmias with left bundle branch block right inferior axis originating from the left versus right ventricular outflow tract. *J. Cardiovasc. Electrophysiol.* **2018**, *29*, 1515–1522. [CrossRef]
7. Cheng, D.; Ju, W.; Zhu, L.; Chen, K.; Zhang, F.; Chen, H.; Yang, G.; Li, X.; Li, M.; Gu, K.; et al. V3R/V7 Index: A Novel Electrocardiographic Criterion for Differentiating Left From Right Ventricular Outflow Tract Arrhythmias Origins. *Circ. Arrhythm. Electrophysiol.* **2018**, *11*, e006243. [CrossRef]
8. Yoshida, N.; Yamada, T.; McElderry, H.T.; Inden, Y.; Shimano, M.; Murohara, T.; Kumar, V.; Doppalapudi, H.; Plumb, V.J.; Kay, G.N. A novel electrocardiographic criterion for differentiating a left from right ventricular outflow tract tachycardia origin: The V2S/V3R index. *J. Cardiovasc. Electrophysiol.* **2014**, *25*, 747–753. [CrossRef]
9. Di, C.; Wan, Z.; Tse, G.; Letsas, K.P.; Liu, T.; Efremidis, M.; Li, J.; Lin, W. The V1-V3 transition index as a novel electrocardiographic criterion for differentiating left from right ventricular outflow tract ventricular arrhythmias. *J. Interv. Card. Electrophysiol.* **2019**, *56*, 37–43. [CrossRef]
10. Igarashi, M.; Nogami, A.; Sekiguchi, Y.; Kuroki, K.; Yamasaki, H.; Machino, T.; Yui, Y.; Ogawa, K.; Talib, A.K.; Murakoshi, N.; et al. The QRS morphology pattern in V5R is a novel and simple parameter for differentiating the origin of idiopathic outflow tract ventricular arrhythmias. *Europace* **2015**, *17*, 1107–1116. [CrossRef]
11. Enriquez, A.; Baranchuk, A.; Briceno, D.; Saenz, L.; Garcia, F. How to use the 12-lead ECG to predict the site of origin of idiopathic ventricular arrhythmias. *Heart Rhythm.* **2019**, *16*, 1538–1544. [CrossRef]
12. Ouyang, F.; Mathew, S.; Wu, S.; Kamioka, M.; Metzner, A.; Xue, Y.; Ju, W.; Yang, B.; Zhan, X.; Rillig, A.; et al. Ventricular arrhythmias arising from the left ventricular outflow tract below the aortic sinus cusps: Mapping and catheter ablation via transseptal approach and electrocardiographic characteristics. *Circ Arrhythm. Electrophysiol.* **2014**, *7*, 445–455. [CrossRef] [PubMed]
13. Yamada, T.; McElderry, H.T.; Doppalapudi, H.; Murakami, Y.; Yoshida, Y.; Yoshida, N.; Okada, T.; Tsuboi, N.; Inden, Y.; Murohara, T.; et al. Idiopathic ventricular arrhythmias originating from the aortic root: Prevalence, electrocardiographic and electrophysiologic characteristics, and results of radiofrequency catheter ablation. *J. Am. Coll. Cardiol.* **2008**, *52*, 139–147. [CrossRef] [PubMed]
14. Yamada, T.; Lau, Y.R.; Litovsky, S.H.; Thomas McElderry, H.; Doppalapud, I.H.; Osorio, J.; Plumb, V.J.; Neal Kay, G. Prevalence and clinical, electrocardiographic, and electrophysiologic characteristics of ventricular arrhythmias originating from the noncoronary sinus of Valsalva. *Heart Rhythm.* **2013**, *10*, 1605–1612. [CrossRef] [PubMed]
15. Anter, E.; Frankel, D.S.; Marchlinski, F.E.; Dixit, S. Effect of electrocardiographic lead placement on localization of outflow tract tachycardias. *Heart Rhythm.* **2012**, *9*, 697–703. [CrossRef]
16. Betensky, B.P.; Park, R.E.; Marchlinski, F.E.; Hutchinson, M.D.; Garcia, F.C.; Dixit, S.; Callans, D.J.; Cooper, J.M.; Bala, R.; Lin, D.; et al. The V(2) transition ratio: A new electrocardiographic criterion for distinguishing left from right ventricular outflow tract tachycardia origin. *J. Am. Coll. Cardiol.* **2011**, *57*, 2255–2262. [CrossRef]
17. Hasdemir, C.; Aktas, S.; Govsa, F.; Aktas, E.O.; Kocak, A.; Bozkaya, Y.T.; Demirbas, M.I.; Ulucan, C.; Ozdogan, O.; Kayikcioglu, M.; et al. Demonstration of ventricular myocardial extensions into the pulmonary artery and aorta beyond the ventriculo-arterial junction. *Pacing Clin. Electrophysiol.* **2007**, *30*, 534–549. [CrossRef]
18. Chen, J.; Hoff, P.I.; Rossvoll, O.; De Bortoli, A.; Solheim, E.; Sun, L.; Schuster, P.; Larsen, T.; Ohm, O.J. Ventricular arrhythmias originating from the aortomitral continuity: An uncommon variant of left ventricular outflow tract tachycardia. *Europace* **2012**, *14*, 388–395. [CrossRef]
19. Steven, D.; Roberts-Thomson, K.C.; Seiler, J.; Inada, K.; Tedrow, U.B.; Mitchell, R.N.; Sobieszczyk, P.S.; Eisenhauer, A.C.; Couper, G.S.; Stevenson, W.G. Ventricular tachycardia arising from the aortomitral continuity in structural heart disease: Characteristics and therapeutic considerations for an anatomically challenging area of origin. *Circ. Arrhythm. Electrophysiol.* **2009**, *2*, 660–666. [CrossRef]
20. Chung, F.P.; Lin, C.Y.; Shirai, Y.; Futyma, P.; Santangeli, P.; Lin, Y.J.; Chang, S.L.; Lo, L.W.; Hu, Y.F.; Chang, H.Y.; et al. Outcomes of catheter ablation of ventricular arrhythmia originating from the left ventricular summit: A multicenter study. *Heart Rhythm.* **2020**, *17*, 1077–1083. [CrossRef]
21. Szili-Torok, T.; van Malderen, S.; de Groot, N. 'Born' with a 'dead'-end-tract resulting in arrhythmias in the aorto-mitral continuity: Coincidence, causation, and 'commensuration'. *Europace* **2012**, *14*, 308–389. [CrossRef] [PubMed]

22. Ouyang, F.; Fotuhi, P.; Ho, S.Y.; Hebe, J.; Volkmer, M.; Goya, M.; Burns, M.; Antz, M.; Ernst, S.; Cappato, R.; et al. Repetitive monomorphic ventricular tachycardia originating from the aortic sinus cusp: Electrocardiographic characterization for guiding catheter ablation. *J. Am. Coll. Cardiol.* **2002**, *39*, 500–508. [CrossRef]
23. Lin, D.; Ilkhanoff, L.; Gerstenfeld, E.; Dixit, S.; Beldner, S.; Bala, R.; Garcia, F.; Callans, D.; Marchlinski, F.E. Twelve-lead electrocardiographic characteristics of the aortic cusp region guided by intracardiac echocardiography and electroanatomic mapping. *Heart Rhythm.* **2008**, *5*, 663–669. [CrossRef] [PubMed]
24. Komatsu, Y.; Nogami, A.; Shinoda, Y.; Masuda, K.; Machino, T.; Kuroki, K.; Yamasaki, H.; Sekiguchi, Y.; Aonuma, K. Idiopathic Ventricular Arrhythmias Originating From the Vicinity of the Communicating Vein of Cardiac Venous Systems at the Left Ventricular Summit. *Circ. Arrhythm. Electrophysiol.* **2018**, *11*, e005386. [CrossRef] [PubMed]

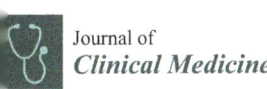

Journal of Clinical Medicine

Article

Angiographic Characteristics of the Vein of Marshall in Patients with and without Atrial Fibrillation

Lei Ding, Hongda Zhang, Fengyuan Yu, Lijie Mi, Wei Hua, Shu Zhang, Yan Yao and Min Tang *

Department of Cardiology, State Key Laboratory of Cardiovascular Disease, Cardiovascular Institute, Fuwai Hospital, National Center for Cardiovascular Diseases, Chinese Academy of Medical Sciences, and Peking Union Medical College, Beijing 100037, China
* Correspondence: doctortangmin@yeah.net

Abstract: Background: Ethanol infusion into the vein of Marshall (Et-VOM) is a novel therapeutic treatment for atrial fibrillation (AF). However, few studies have focused on the difference between AF and non-AF patients (presented other types of arrhythmias) regarding the characteristics of the vein of Marshall (VOM). Objective: This study sought to investigate the incidence, morphology, and angiographic characteristics of the VOM. Methods: Coronary sinus (CS) angiography was performed in all patients. The baseline, angiographic characteristics and measurements of VOM dimensions were compared between the AF and non-AF group. Results: CS angiography was performed in 290 patients. The VOM detection rate was higher in the AF group than in the non-AF group (91.8% vs. 84.1%, p = 0.044). In the right anterior oblique (RAO) projection, AF patients had significant larger VOM ostium, CS ostium, and CS diameter at VOM ostium than non-AF patients (1.9 ± 0.9 vs. 1.7 ± 0.7 mm, p = 0.015; 12.8 ± 4.1 vs. 11.4 ± 3.7 mm, p = 0.016; 9.1 ± 3.1 vs. 8.2 ± 2.9 mm, p = 0.028, respectively). There was a slight linear correlation between the VOM ostium and the CS ostium diameter as well as left atrial volume (LAV). Conclusion: AF patients seem to have a higher incidence of the VOM, larger VOM ostium, CS ostium, and CS lumen in RAO view. Meanwhile, the VOM ostium may correlate with the CS ostium and LAV.

Keywords: atrial fibrillation (AF); vein of Marshall (VOM); ethanol infusion; coronary sinus (CS); coronary sinus ostium (CSo)

1. Introduction

Radiofrequency catheter ablation (RFCA) has been a well-established treatment for atrial fibrillation (AF) [1–3]. Pulmonary veins (PVs) are the most common ectopic triggers for initiating AF, and the treatment strategy mainly consists of PV isolation (PVI). However, only PVI are inadequate when dealing with persistent AF. Many patients suffer recurrent AF and atrial tachycardia which need a redo procedure.

The vein of Marshall (VOM) is an embryological remnant of the left superior vena cava and has been recognized as an important factor for AF initiation and maintenance [4,5]. In addition, the VOM is an epicardial substrate for maintaining perimitral atrial tachycardia [6]. Previous studies have reported the efficacy and safety of ethanol infusion in the VOM [7–10]. Chemical ablation by ethanol infusion could eliminate non-PV AF triggers and facilitate a bidirectional block of the mitral isthmus [11,12]. However, there are no detailed reports in a large cohort of patients with and without AF on the characteristics of the VOM. Meanwhile, the influence of VOM morphology on Et-VOM is also absent.

This study aimed to investigate the incidence, morphology, and angiographic characteristics of the VOM in patients with and without AF by angiography.

2. Materials and Methods

2.1. Population

This was a prospective, cohort study enrolling all patients with tachyarrhythmias who underwent RFCA in Fuwai Hospital between November 2021 and April 2022. No specific exclusion criteria were used. Clinical data, echocardiographic, and imaging data were documented in the study. All patients provided informed consent prior to the procedure. The study protocols were approved by the Ethics Committee of Fuwai Hospital, Chinese Academy of Medical Sciences and were in accordance with the Declaration of Helsinki (No. 2022-1810). Antiarrhythmic drugs were discontinued for at least five half-life periods prior to the procedure.

2.2. Electrophysiology Study and Catheter Ablation

All catheters were inserted percutaneously by the Seldinger technique and were advanced into position under fluoroscopic guidance. A 6F decapolar steerable catheter (Triguy, APT Medical, CHN) was inserted into the coronary sinus (CS) through the left femoral vein. Two quadripolar catheters (6F, Triguy, APT Medical, CHN) were advanced into the His bundle position and the right ventricle in patients with supraventricular tachycardia (SVT). The surface electrocardiogram and intracardiac electrograms were continuously monitored and stored in a recording system (C. R. Bard, Inc., Lowell, MA, USA). Left atrial access was attempted by transseptal puncture when needed, and heparin was given. The mapping catheter was advanced via a SL1 long sheath. Each patient underwent the standard electrophysiology study, including programmed stimulation and diagnostic pacing maneuvers [13]. Isoproterenol was administered for patients who could not induce tachycardia by standard procedures. Radiofrequency (RF) energy was delivered from a generator (Stockert, Freiburg, Germany). The RF power setting followed the standards of the different procedures, ranging from 25 to 45 W.

AF ablation mainly consisted of antral PVI and was performed under sedation using midazolam and fentanyl. For persistent AF patients and paroxysmal AF patients who were in AF rhythm before ablation, VOM angiography and ethanol infusion were performed. After ethanol infusion, mitral isthmus was ablated to achieve a bidirectional conduction block. The end points of the procedure were as follows: (1) atrioventricular nodal reentrant tachycardia (AVNRT)—either a slow pathway blocked or a single atrial echo beat at baseline and during isoproterenol infusion without inducing tachycardia; (2) atrioventricular reentrant tachycardia (AVRT)—appearance of decremental antegrade and retrograde atrioventricular conduction and could not induce tachycardia; (3) atrial flutter (AFL)—a bidirectional conduction block confirmed by differential pacing; (4) AF—absence of ostial PV potentials on a circumferential mapping catheter and no atrial capture from multiple pacing sites within the PV ostium. End points had to be fulfilled after a waiting period of 20 min after the last ablation. Additionally, for patients diagnosed with paroxysmal AF, 40 mg of adenosine triphosphate (ATP) and isoproterenol were given to verify the block of PVs and induce AF.

2.3. VOM Angiography and Ethanol Infusion

After pulmonary vein isolation, the CS was canulated with a SL1 long sheath (8.5F, St. Jude Medical, Inc., St Paul, MN, USA) or a steerable long sheath (8.5-F, Agilis NxT; Abbott) inserted from the right femoral vein. A guiding catheter (6-F Judkins Right [JR] 4; Medtronic, Minneapolis, MN, USA) was proximally positioned inside the CS lumen and contrast was injected to perform CS angiography. Details of stepwise angiography to identify the VOM were shown in Figure 1. First, the CS angiography in the right anterior oblique (RAO) 30° was used. The proximal portion of the valve of Vieussens was targeted and the JR 4 guiding catheter was rotated posteriorly and superiorly to find the ostium of the VOM [14]. In addition, at each location, a small amount of contrast was injected through the guiding catheter to confirm the VOM. Second, if the operator found the suspected VOM, the left anterior oblique (LAO) 30° was performed to identify. However, if there was no suspected VOM, the LAO 30° or LAO 30° with cranial 30° was used to find the VOM. For patients in non-AF group, the VOM angiography was conducted during the waiting period of 20 min.

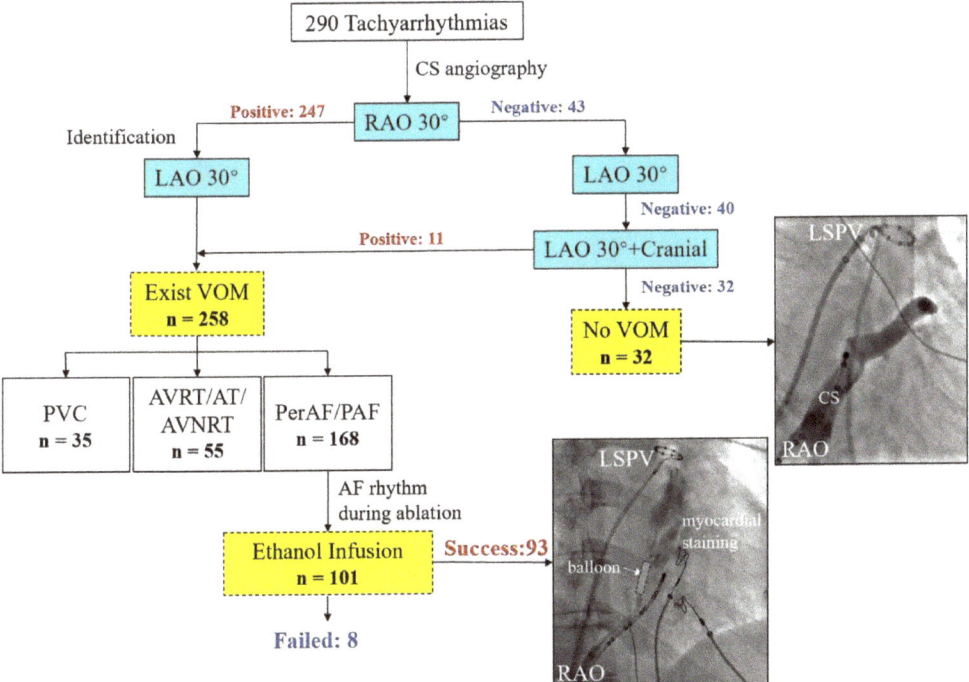

Figure 1. Flowchart of CS angiography, VOM angiography, and ethanol infusion procedure. AF = atrial fibrillation; AT = atrial tachycardia; AVNRT = atrioventricular nodal reentrant tachycardia; AVRT = atrioventricular reentrant tachycardia; CS = coronary sinus; LAO = left anterior oblique; LSPV = left superior pulmonary vein; RAO = right anterior oblique; PAF = paroxysmal atrial fibrillation; PerAF = persistent atrial fibrillation; PVC = premature ventricular contraction; VOM = vein of Marshall.

After identifying the VOM, an angioplasty guidewire (Sion Blue 0.014 inch, Asahi) was advanced into the lumen of the VOM with an over-the-wire balloon preload at the distal portion. An appropriately sized balloon (1.5–2 mm diameter and 8–15 mm length; Boston Scientific, USA) was used depending on the size of the VOM. Subsequently, the balloon was inflated, starting at 1–2 atm, until the operator felt some resistance on the inflator with a maximum of 8–10 atm, and the guidewire was removed. After confirming balloon occlusion, 2 mL of ethanol (95%) was slowly administered over one minute, and the selective angiogram of the VOM was repeated to confirm the myocardial lesion created by ethanol [15]. Following every injection, the balloon was deflated and retracted 1 cm towards the proximal VOM; in the same way, another injection was performed with 2 mL of ethanol. The balloon was retracted until it reached the VOM ostium and a total of 10–12 mL of ethanol was used as a maximum dose.

2.4. Measurements and Definitions

Measurements of the VOM were performed in the RAO 30° and LAO 30° or LAO 30° with cranial 30° (Figure 2). The diameters of the CS ostium (CSo), the VOM ostium, and CS lumen at the VOM ostium were measured in all views. In addition, in the LAO 30° or LAO 30° with cranial 30° (Figure 2A), the distance between the VOM ostium and the CSo, and the angle between the VOM lumen and proximal CS lumen, were measured. Subsequently in the RAO 30° (Figure 2B), operators measured the angle between the VOM lumen and distal CS lumen. According to the number of branches at the VOM ostium, we classified all VOM into two categories (Figure 3). Type I VOM was defined as only one branch and Type II VOM was defined as more than one branch within 1 mm around the VOM ostium.

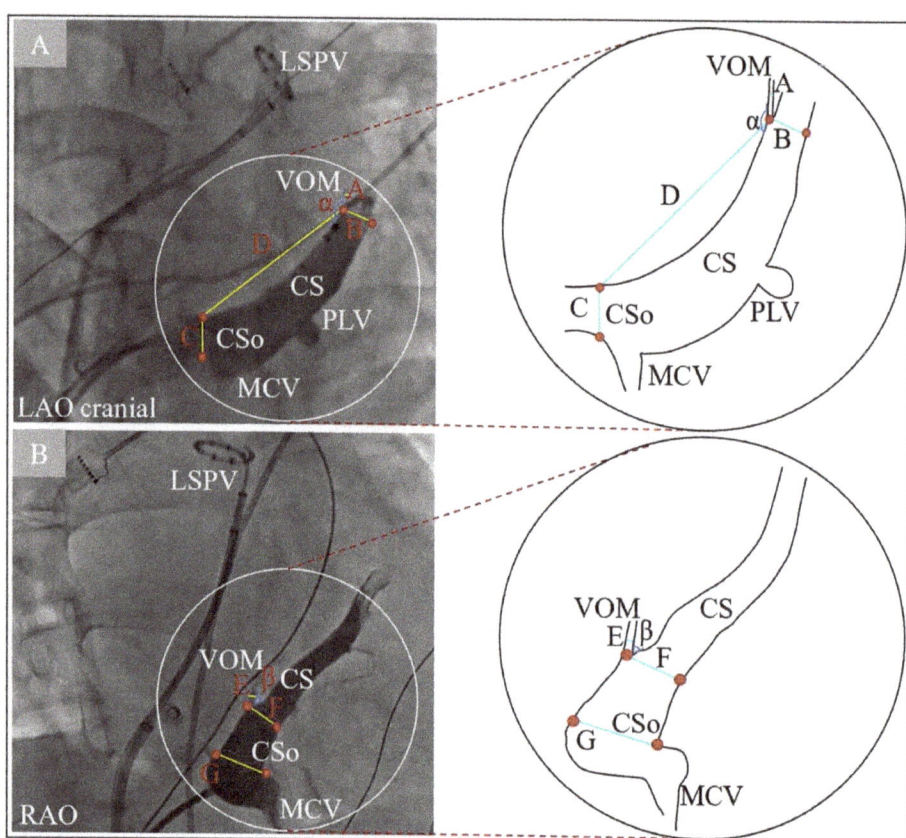

Figure 2. Measurements of the VOM in the LAO/LAO cranial (**A**) and RAO (**B**) views by CS angiography. Segment A and E = diameter of VOM; segment B and F = diameter of the CS at VOM level; segment C and G = diameter of CSo; segment D = distance between VOM ostium and CSo; angle α = angle between VOM and proximal CS; angle β = angle between VOM and distal CS CS = coronary sinus; CSo = coronary sinus ostium; LAO = left anterior oblique; LSPV = left superior pulmonary vein; MCV = middle cardiac vein; PLV = posterior lateral vein; RAO = right anterior oblique; VOM = vein of Marshall.

2.5. Statistical Analysis

Statistical analysis and graphing were performed by SPSS IBM 22 (IBM Co., Armonk, NY, USA) and GraphPad Prism 8.0 (GraphPad Software Inc., La Jolla, CA, USA). Continuous data are presented as means ± standard deviation (SD) or the median and interquartile range, depending on the normality of the distribution. Categorical variables are described as frequency counts and percentages. For continuous data, either the student *t*-test or Mann-Whiney *U*-test was carried out for statistical comparisons. For comparisons of categorical data, the chi-squared test was performed. A *p* value less than 0.05 indicated statistical significance.

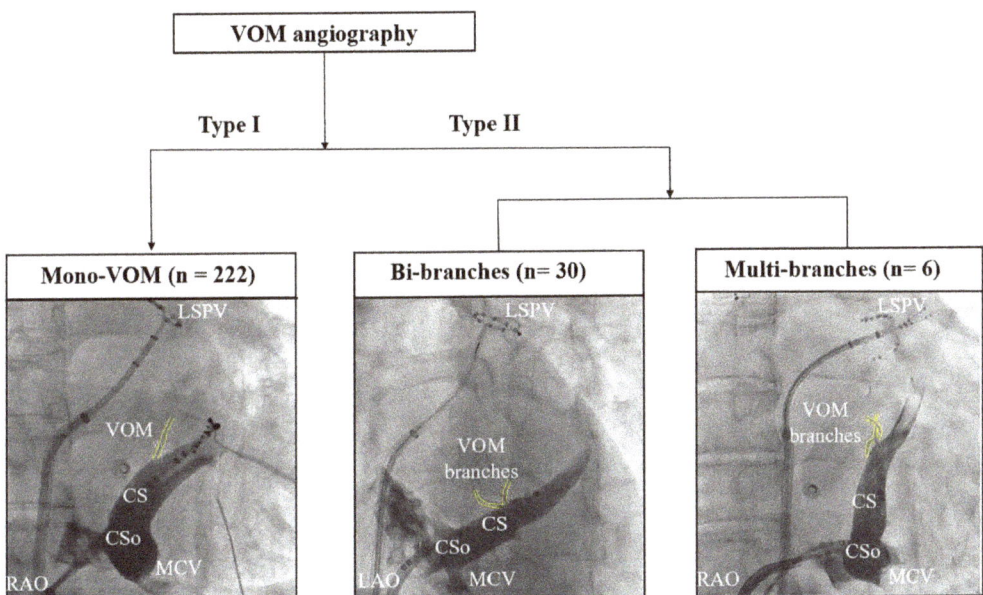

Figure 3. Morphologic classification of the VOM. CS = coronary sinus; CSo = coronary sinus ostium; LAO = left anterior oblique; LSPV = left superior pulmonary vein; MCV = middle cardiac vein; RAO = right anterior oblique; VOM = vein of Marshall.

3. Results

CS angiography was performed in 290 consecutive patients (age 55.2 ± 13.2 years; 114 females) scheduled for RFCA between November 2021 and April 2022. Of these, 183 (63.1%) patients had AF, 36 (12.4%) had AFL, 29 (10.0%) had AVNRT, 20 (6.9%) had AVRT, 20 (6.9%) had AT, and 47 (16.2%) had ventricular arrhythmias. The AF group consisted of 183 patients, whereas the non-AF group consisted of 107 patients. In the non-AF group, there were no patients that presented previous AF episodes. The baseline characteristics of all patients are summarized in Table 1. Of all the AF patients, there were 85 paroxysmal AF (PAF), 98 persistent AF (PerAF), and 14 patients also had AFL. Patients with AF were significantly older, had a higher rate of hypertension and heart failure, and a higher left atrial volume (LAV) than non-AF patients. Similarly, left ventricular ejection fraction (LVEF's) were significantly lower in the AF group compared with the non-AF group. Meanwhile, the CHA_2DS_2-VASc score and the HAS-BLED score were 2.0 ± 1.5 and 0.6 ± 0.7, respectively, in AF patients. Other clinical characteristics are detailed in Table 1.

There were 101 patients that underwent ethanol infusion into the VOM (Et-VOM); a total of 8 patients failed Et-VOM and the success rate of Et-VOM was 92.1% (Figure 1). Measurements of angiographic images are shown in Table 2. The VOM detection rate was significantly higher in the AF group than in the non-AF group (91.8% vs. 84.1%, $p = 0.044$). Of all undetectable cases (n = 32), four patients were diagnosed as persistent left superior vena cava (PLSVA) with no statistically significant difference between the two groups (1.1% vs. 1.9%, $p = 0.584$). There was no significant difference between patients with and without AF in morphologic classifications of VOM ($p = 0.477$). In measurements in the RAO view, AF patients had a significantly larger VOM ostium diameter, CSo diameter, and CS diameter at the VOM ostium than non-AF patients (1.9 ± 0.9 vs. 1.7 ± 0.7 mm, $p = 0.015$; 12.8 ± 4.1 vs. 11.4 ± 3.7 mm, $p = 0.016$; 9.1 ± 3.1 vs. 8.2 ± 2.9 mm, $p = 0.028$, respectively), while the VOM-CS angle was similar in both groups. For measurements in the LAO view, AF patients had a smaller VOM-CS angle and larger CSo diameter as well as CS diameter at the VOM level (144.2 ± 36.8° vs. 156.0 ± 12.6°, p = 0.036; 11.7 ± 5.8 vs. 10.1 ± 5.4 mm p = 0.022; 7.2 ± 2.9 vs. 6.5 ± 2.0 mm, p = 0.047). Other details are shown in Table 2.

Table 1. Clinical characteristics of all patients.

	AF (n = 183)	Non-AF (n = 107)	p Value
Age onset, y	53.9 ± 11.6	45.4 ± 16.5	<0.001 *
Age at admission, y	58.5 ± 11.0	50.5 ± 15.1	<0.001 *
Female, n (%)	57 (31.1)	57 (53.3)	0.001 *
BMI, kg/m^2	25.8 ± 3.6	25.0 ± 3.5	0.059
Comorbidities, n (%)			
Hypertension	95 (51.9)	35 (32.7)	0.002 *
Diabetes mellitus	36 (19.7)	18 (16.8)	0.547
Coronary heart disease	31 (16.9)	13 (12.1)	0.273
Heart failure	25 (13.7)	4 (3.7)	0.007 *
Stroke	24 (13.1)	7 (6.5)	0.080
Vascular disease	19 (10.4)	5 (4.7)	0.089
CHA$_2$DS$_2$-VASc score	2.0 ± 1.5	-	-
HAS-BLED score	0.6 ± 0.7	-	-
Open heart surgery, n (%)	7 (3.8)	2 (1.9)	0.354
NYHA-FC, n (%)			
I/II	177 (96.7)	107 (100.0)	0.058
III/IV	6 (3.3)	0	0.058
LAV, mL	68.2 ± 25.8	49.7 ± 18.1	<0.001 *
LVEF, %	62.3 ± 7.0	64.0 ± 5.3	0.023 *

BMI = body mass index; LAV = left atrial volume; LVEF = left ventricular ejection fraction; NYHA-FC = New York Heart Association functional class. * Variables with p value < 0.05.

Table 2. Assessment of angiography images.

	AF (n = 183)	Non-AF (n = 107)	p Value
Undetectable VOM on venography in all views, n (%)	15 (8.2)	17 (15.9)	0.044 *
Detectable PLSVA, n (%)	2 (1.1)	2 (1.9)	0.584
Number of branches at VOM ostium			
Type I	143 (78.1)	79 (73.8)	0.477
Type II	25 (13.7)	11 (10.3)	0.477
RAO			
Undetectable VOM on venography in RAO	20 (10.9)	23 (21.5)	0.015 *
VOM-CS angle, °	45.3 ± 20.5	41.4 ± 18.5	0.237
VOM ostium diameter, mm	1.9 ± 0.9	1.7 ± 0.7	0.015 *
CSo diameter, mm	12.8 ± 4.1	11.4 ± 3.7	0.016 *
CS diameter at VOM level, mm	9.1 ± 3.1	8.2 ± 2.9	0.028 *
LAO			
Undetectable VOM on venography in LAO	53 (29.0)	45 (42.1)	0.023 *
VOM-CS angle, °	144.2 ± 36.8	156.0 ± 12.6	0.036 *
VOM-to-CSo distance, mm	37.8 ± 15.6	36.8 ± 13.1	0.684
VOM ostium diameter, mm	1.7 ± 1.0	1.7 ± 0.7	0.664
CSo diameter, mm	11.7 ± 5.8	10.1 ± 5.4	0.022 *
CS diameter at VOM level, mm	7.2 ± 2.9	6.5 ± 2.0	0.047 *
LAO cranial			
Undetectable VOM on venography in LAO + Cranial	39 (21.3)	27 (25.2)	0.442
VOM-CS angle, °	127.9 ± 57.5	109.2 ± 70.7	0.087
VOM-to-CSo distance, mm	39.6 ± 16.6	37.8 ± 13.8	0.419
VOM ostium diameter, mm	1.9 ± 1.1	1.6 ± 0.8	0.069
CSo diameter, mm	13.1 ± 5.0	12.4 ± 4.8	0.263
CS diameter at VOM level, mm	8.1 ± 3.2	7.4 ± 2.4	0.141

AF = atrial fibrillation; CS = coronary sinus; CSo = coronary sinus ostium; LAO = left anterior oblique; PLSVA = persistent left superior vena cava; RAO = right anterior oblique; VOM = vein of Marshall. Other abbreviations as Table 1. * Variables with p value < 0.05.

The non-AF patients (n = 76) and AF patients (n = 76) were then matched in a ratio of 1:1 based on age and gender. As a result, there were no significant differences between the two groups except LAV (68.7 ± 25.3 mL vs. 52.2 ± 19.5 mL, $p < 0.001$, Supplementary Table S2). Patients in the AF group still have a significantly higher incidence of the VOM, larger VOM ostium diameter, and CSo diameter in the RAO view (Supplementary Table S3).

We initially investigated the linear correlation between the VOM ostium and age as AF patients were significantly older. We did not find a linear correlation between the VOM ostium and age in the AF group, non-AF group, or the total patient group (Figure 4). Meanwhile, we found that there were no significant differences of detection rate of the VOM, diameter of the VOM, VOM-CS angle, and VOM-to-CSo distance in all views between different genders (Supplementary Table S1). We also found that male patients have a significantly larger CSo diameter in RAO and LAO cranial views (11.6 ± 4.0 vs. 12.7 ± 4.0 mm, $p = 0.025$; 12.0 ± 4.2 vs. 13.4 ± 5.4 mm, $p = 0.041$). In addition, patients with a higher LAV may have a larger VOM in the AF group, while there was no obvious linear correlation in the non-AF group (Figure 4). We also found that patients with a larger CSo or CS diameter at the VOM ostium had a larger VOM ostium in both groups and had a slight linear correlation ($p < 0.001$, Figure 5).

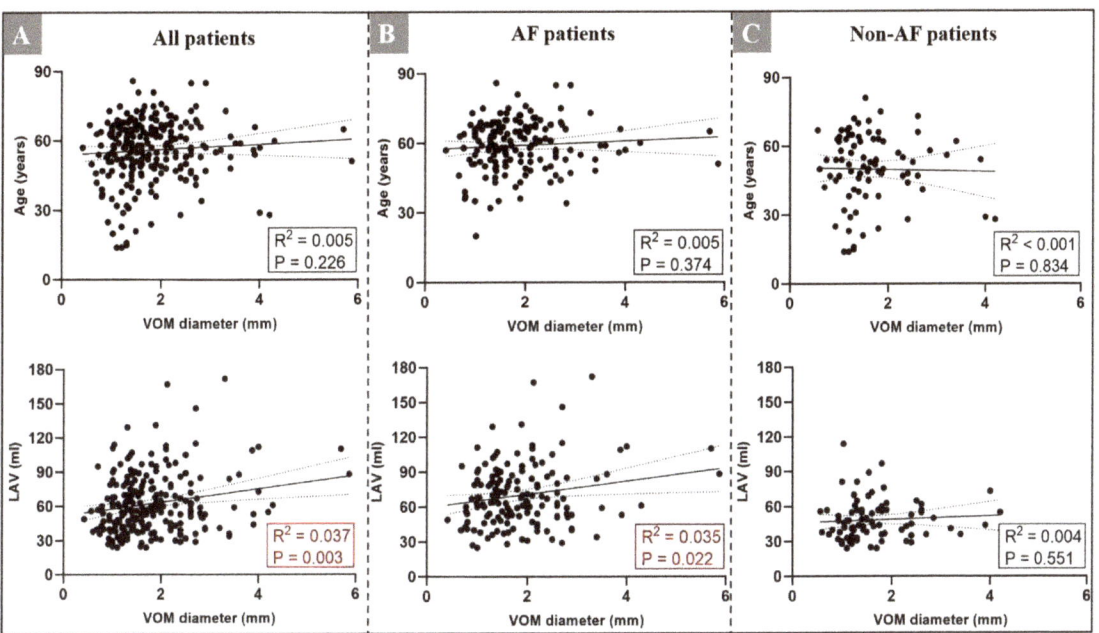

Figure 4. (A) Correlation between the VOM ostium diameter and age as well as LAV in all patients (n = 290); (B) correlation between the VOM ostium diameter and age as well as LAV in AF patients (n = 183); (C) correlation between the VOM diameter and age as well as LAV in non-AF patients (n = 107). AF = atrial fibrillation; CS = coronary sinus; CSo = coronary sinus ostium; LAV = left atrial volume; VOM = vein of Marshall.

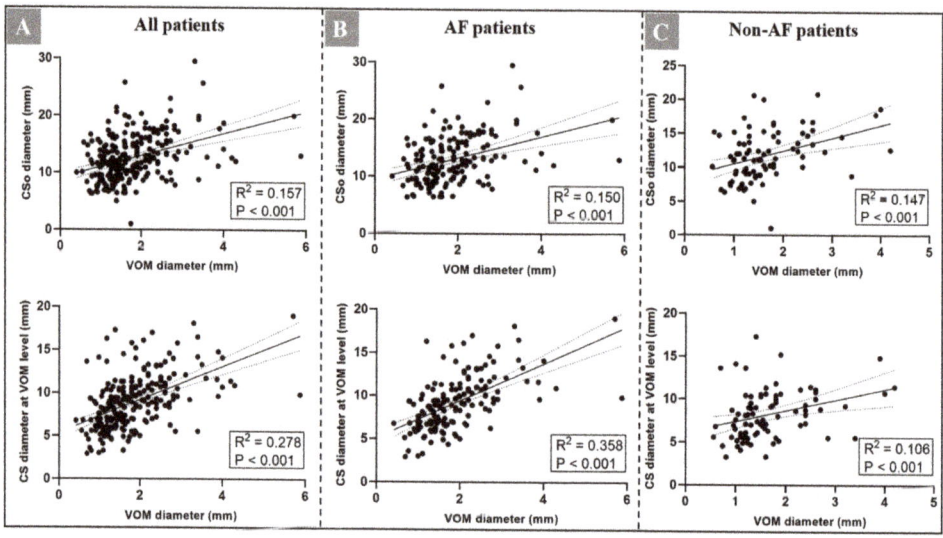

Figure 5. (**A**) Correlation between the VOM ostium diameter and the CSo diameter as well as CS diameter at the VOM level in the RAO plane in all patients (n = 290); (**B**) correlation between the VOM ostium diameter and the CSo diameter as well as CS diameter at the VOM level in the RAO plane in AF patients (n = 183); (**C**) correlation between the VOM ostium diameter and the CSo diameter as well as CS diameter at the VOM level in the RAO plane in non-AF patients (n = 107) AF = atrial fibrillation; CS = coronary sinus; CSo = coronary sinus ostium; RAO = right anterior oblique; VOM = vein of Marshall.

4. Discussion

In summary, the present study illustrated the difference between AF and non-AF patients regarding the VOM dimensions. The main findings of this study are as follows: (1) AF patients were associated with a significantly higher incidence of the VOM, larger VOM ostium, CSo, and CS lumen at the VOM ostium; (2) there was a slight linear correlation between the diameter of the VOM ostium and CSo as well as the diameter of CS at the VOM level; (3) patients with a larger LAV tend to have a larger VOM ostium.

4.1. Characteristics of the VOM and Difference between Patients with and without AF

According to previous reports, the incidence of the VOM varied from 21% to 98% in anatomical studies [16,17]. The presence of the VOM ranged from 63% in a study of optimized VOM-CT protocol to 73% [18] in a study of 100 patients undergoing CS angiography [19]. By contrast, in the present study, the overall incidence of the VOM is 89% under the workflow of angiography (Figure 1). As Et-VOM has been proved to benefit outcomes of AF and will be widely used [7,9], the angiography of workflow should be undergone before Et-VOM to identify the VOM, especially for centers that are in the early stage of operating Et-VOM. In addition, we found that patients with AF have a significantly larger VOM ostium, CSo, and CS lumen at the VOM ostium. The CSo diameter is comparable with previous studies [20–22]. Ortale et al. [22] reported that the CSo ranged from 4.0 to 16.0 mm in 37 adult human heart specimens. Another study [21] involved measurements of CSo by angiography and showed that the median diameter of CSo was 10–11 mm in non-AF patients. However, few studies compare the VOM between patients with and without AF. Our study demonstrated that the VOM ostium and the CSo are larger in AF patients and there may be a correlation between them. Results of the present study suggest that anatomic factors may contribute to the genesis of AF. Larger VOM may produce more atrial connections into the left atrium, thus, giving rise to AF. Although the pathogeneses of AF are complicated, other large scale, prospective cohort studies need to be conducted to prove these hypotheses.

4.2. The Morphology Characteristics of the VOM

Some studies have investigated the morphology of the VOM. Valderrábano et al. [23] pointed that the VOM was varied in branching patterns and 88.6% of patients present venous plexus at the VOM ostium or variable branches into small venules. Kamakura et al. [8] further classified the VOM into three morphologies according to the numbers of branches in the trunk. They found multiple branches in 92%, a large trunk in 5.0%, and no branches in 3.0%. In the present study, we classified the VOM as two categories according to the numbers of branches within 1 mm of the VOM ostium. Type I was over 70% (222/76.6%), while Type II only counts for 23.4%. However, there was no difference between AF and non-AF patients.

4.3. Correlation between the VOM and LAV

Many studies had reported that the LAV contributes to the pathogenesis of AF [24–28]. An echocardiographic measurement of LAV was shown to be a predictor of new-onset AF in 574 subjects, and prospectively followed for a mean of 1.9 years [24]. Tan et al. [25] also pointed that the LAV index is associated with new-onset AF in embolic strokes of an undetermined source in patients. However, few studies have investigated the correlation between the LAV and left atrial veins. In our study, we found that AF patients tend to have a larger LAV, and there was a weak linear correlation between the LAV and the size of the VOM ostium. As Njoku et al. [26] concluded, a larger LAV may present structural remodeling, atrial hypertrophy, and stretch peri-LA tissues. In this way, an increased LAV may result in a larger VOM ostium. This morphologic variation may be the anatomic substrate for AF pathogenesis, but still needs to be investigated in other large-scaled, prospective cohort studies.

4.4. Limitations

There are some limitations of this study. First, it is possible that the left atrial appendage (LAA) vein was mistaken as the VOM because it also drains into the CS. However, the LAA vein extends toward the anterior and we confirmed the course of the vein both at RAO and LAO views. Second, the incidence of the VOM remains unclear in the anatomical study; for patients who could not find the VOM, we changed at least two different sites and fluorography angles for angiography. Third, this study consisted of a small sample size, whereas a prospective cohort study with a larger population is necessary to evaluate the correlation between the VOM and LAV. Fourth, the two-dimensional (2D) imaging of angiography may could not assess a 3D structure, including the VOM, adequately; we used as many angiography views as possible to illustrate the characteristics of the VOM. Other techniques, such as 3D quantitative angiography, may mitigate against this limitation.

5. Conclusions

AF patients appear to have a higher incidence of the VOM, larger VOM ostium, CSo, and CS lumen in the RAO view compared to non-AF patients. Meanwhile, the VOM ostium may correlate with the CS ostium and LAV.

Supplementary Materials: The following are available online at https://www.mdpi.com/article/10.3390/jcm11185384/s1, Table S1: Assessment of angiography images according to gender, Table S2: Clinical characteristics after propensity score matching, Table S3: Assessment of angiography images after propensity score matching.

Author Contributions: Conceptualization, M.T.; Data curation, L.M.; Formal analysis, L.D.; Funding acquisition, M.T. and H.Z.; Investigation, F.Y.; Methodology, H.Z. and M.T.; Project administration, W.H. and M.T.; Resources, S.Z. and Y.Y.; Writing—original draft, L.D.; Writing—review & editing, H.Z. All authors have read and agreed to the published version of the manuscript.

Funding: National Natural Science Foundation of China (Grant No. U1913210 and No. 82000064).

Institutional Review Board Statement: The study was conducted in accordance with the Declaration of Helsinki, and approved by the Ethics Committee of Fuwai Hospital, Chinese Academy of Medical Sciences (No. 2022-1810).

Informed Consent Statement: Informed consent was obtained from all subjects involved in the study.

Data Availability Statement: The datasets presented in this article are not readily available because research data is confidential. Data sharing requests are required to meet the policies of the hospital and the funder. Requests to access the datasets should be directed to doctortangmin@yeah.net.

Conflicts of Interest: The authors declare no conflict of interest.

References

1. Calkins, H.; Hindricks, G.; Cappato, R.; Kim, Y.H.; Saad, E.B.; Aguinaga, L.; Akar, J.G.; Badhwar, V.; Brugada, J.; Camm, J.; et al. 2017 HRS/EHRA/ECAS/APHRS/SOLAECE expert consensus statement on catheter and surgical ablation of atrial fibrillation. *Heart Rhythm* **2017**, *14*, e275–e444. [CrossRef]
2. Poole, J.E.; Bahnson, T.D.; Monahan, K.H.; Johnson, G.; Rostami, H.; Silverstein, A.P.; Al-Khalidi, H.R.; Rosenberg, Y.; Mark, D.B.; Lee, K.L.; et al. Recurrence of Atrial Fibrillation After Catheter Ablation or Antiarrhythmic Drug Therapy in the CABANA trial. *J. Am. Coll. Cardiol.* **2020**, *75*, 3105–3118. [CrossRef] [PubMed]
3. Morillo, C.A.; Verma, A.; Connolly, S.J.; Kuck, K.H.; Nair, G.M.; Champagne, J.; Sterns, L.D.; Beresh, H.; Healey, J.S.; Natale A.; et al. Radiofrequency ablation vs antiarrhythmic drugs as fisrt-line treatment of paroxysmal atrial fibrillation (RAAFT-2): A randomized trial. *JAMA* **2014**, *311*, 692–699. [CrossRef]
4. Lee, S.H.; Tai, C.T.; Hsieh, M.H.; Tsao, H.M.; Lin, Y.J.; Chang, S.L.; Huang, J.L.; Lee, K.T.; Chen, Y.J.; Cheng, J.J.; et al. Predictors of non-pulmonary vein ectopic beats initiating paroxysmal atrial fibrillation: Implication for catheter ablation. *J. Am. Coll. Cardiol.* **2005**, *46*, 1054–1059. [CrossRef] [PubMed]
5. Choi, J.I.; Pak, H.N.; Park, J.H.; Choi, E.J.; Kim, S.K.; Kwak, J.J.; Jang, J.K.; Hwang, C.; Kim, Y. Clincal significance of complete conduction block of the left lateral isthmus and its relationship with anatomical variation of the vein of Marshall in patients with nonparoxysmal atrial fibrillation. *J. Cardiovasc. Electrophysiol.* **2009**, *20*, 616–622. [CrossRef] [PubMed]
6. Ulphani, J.S.; Arora, R.; Cain, J.H.; Villuendas, R.; Shen, S.; Gordon, D.; Inderyas, F.; Harvey, L.A.; Morris, A.; Goldberger, J.J.; et al. The ligament of Marshall as a parasympathetic conduit. *Am. J. Physiol. Heart Circ. Physiol.* **2007**, *293*, H1629–H1635. [CrossRef] [PubMed]
7. Valderrábano, M.; Peterson, L.E.; Swarup, V.; Schurmann, P.A.; Makkar, A.; Doshi, R.N.; DeLurgio, D.; Athill, C.A.; Ellenbogen, K.A.; Natale, A.; et al. Effect of Catheter Ablation With Vein of Marshall Ethanol Infusion vs Catheter Ablation Alone on Persistent Atrial Fibrillation: The VENUS Randomized Clinical Trial. *JAMA* **2020**, *324*, 1620–1628. [CrossRef]
8. Kamakura, T.; Derval, N.; Duchateau, J.; Denis, A.; Nakashima, T.; Takagi, T.; Ramirez, F.D.; André, C.; Krisai, P.; Nakatani, Y.; et al. Vein of Marshall Ethanol Infusion: Feasibility, Pitfalls, and Complications in Over 700 Patients. *Circ. Arrhythm. Electrophysiol.* **2021**, *14*, e010001. [CrossRef]
9. Derval, N.; Duchateau, J.; Denis, A.; Ramirez, F.D.; Mahida, S.; André, C.; Krisai, P.; Nakatani, Y.; Kitamura, T.; Takigawa, M.; et al. Marhshall bundle elimination, Pulmonary vein isolation, and Line completion for ANtomical ablation of persistent atrial fibrillation (Marhall-PLAN): Prospective, single-center study. *Heart Rhythm* **2021**, *18*, 529–537. [CrossRef]
10. Gillis, K.; O'Neill, L.; Wielandts, J.Y.; Hilfiker, G.; Almorad, A.; Lycke, M.; El Haddad, M.; de Waroux, J.B.; Tavernier, R.; Duytschaever, M.; et al. Vein of Marshall Ethanol Infusion as First Step for Mitral Ishthmus Linear Ablation. *JACC Clin. Electrophysiol.* **2022**, *8*, 367–376. [CrossRef]
11. Baez-Escudero, J.L.; Morales, P.F.; Dave, A.S.; Sasaridis, C.M.; Kim, Y.H.; Okishige, K.; Valderrabano, M. Ethanol infusion in the vein of Marshall facilitates mitral isthmus ablation. *Heart Rhythm* **2012**, *9*, 1207–1215. [CrossRef] [PubMed]
12. Dave, A.S.; Baez-Escudero, J.L.; Sasaridis, C.; Hong, T.E.; Rami, T.; Valderrabano, M. Role of the vein of Marshall in atrial fibrillation recurrences after catheter ablation: Therapeutic effect of ethanol infusion. *J. Cardiovasc. Electrophysiol.* **2012**, *23*, 583–591. [CrossRef] [PubMed]
13. Knight, B.P.; Ebinger, M.; Oral, H.; Kim, M.H.; Sticherling, C.; Pelosi, F.; Michaud, G.F.; Strickberger, S.A.; Morady, F. Diagnostic value of tachycardia features and pacing maneuvers during paroxysmal supraventricular tachycardia. *J. Am. Coll. Cardiol.* **2000**, *36*, 574–582. [CrossRef]
14. Saremi, F.; Muresian, H.; SánchezQuintana, D. Coronary veins: Comprehensive CT-anatomic classification and review of variantsand clinical implications. *Radiographics* **2012**, *32*, E1–E32. [CrossRef] [PubMed]
15. Kitamura, T.; Vlachos, K.; Denis, A.; Andre, C.; Martin, R.; Pambrun, T.; Duchateau, J.; Frontera, A.; Takigawa, M.; Thompson, N.; et al. Ethanol infusion for Marshall bundle epicardial connections in Marshall bundle-related atrial tachycardias following atrial fibrillation ablation: The accessibility and success rate of ethanol infusion by using a femoral approach. *J. Cardiovasc. Electrophysiol.* **2019**, *30*, 1443–1451. [CrossRef]
16. Lfjllinghausen, M.V.; Ohmachi, N.; Besch, S.; Mettenleiter, A. Atrial Veins of the Human Heart. *Clin. Anat.* **1995**, *8*, 169–189.
17. Ludinghausen, M. The venous drainage of the human myocardium. *Anat. Embryol. Cell Biol.* **2003**, *168*, 1–104.

8. Takagi, T.; Derval, N.; Pambrun, T.; Nakatani, Y.; André, C.; Ramirez, F.D.; Nakashima, T.; Krisai, P.; Kamakura, T.; Pineau, X.; et al. Optimized Computed Tomography Acquisition Protocol for Ethanol Infusion Into the Vein of Marshall. *JACC Clin. Electrophysiol.* **2022**, *8*, 168–178. [CrossRef]
9. Kurotobi, T.; Ito, H.; Inoue, K.; Iwakura, K.; Kawano, S.; Okamura, A.; Date, M.; Fujii, K. Marshall vein as arrhythmogenic source in patients with atrial fibrillation: Correlation between its anatomy and electrophysiological findings. *J. Cardiovasc. Electrophysiol.* **2006**, *17*, 1062–1067. [CrossRef]
10. Habib, A.; Lachman, N.; Christensen, K.N.; Asirvatham, S.J. The anatomy of the coronary sinus venous system for the cardiac electrophysiologist. *Europace* **2009**, *11* (Suppl. 5), v15–v21. [CrossRef]
11. Hummel, J.D.; Strickberger, S.A.; Man, K.C.; Daoud, E.; Nibeauer, M.; Morady, F. A quantitative fluoroscopic comparison of the coronary sinus ostium in patients with and without AV nodal reentrant tachycardia. *J. Cardiovasc. Electrophysiol.* **1995**, *6*, 681–686. [CrossRef] [PubMed]
12. Ortale, J.R.; Gabriel, E.A.; Iost, C.; Márquez, C.Q. The anatomy of the coronary sinus and its tributaries. *Surg. Radiol. Anat.* **2001**, *23*, 15–21. [CrossRef] [PubMed]
13. Valderrabano, M.; Morales, P.F.; Rodriguez-Manero, M.; Lloves, C.; Schurmann, P.A.; Dave, A.S. The Human Left Atrial Venous Circulation as a Vascular Route for Atrial Pharmacological Therapies: Effects of Ethanol Infusion. *JACC Clin. Electrophysiol.* **2017**, *3*, 1020–1032. [CrossRef] [PubMed]
14. Abhayaratna, W.P.; Fatema, K.; Barnes, M.E.; Seward, J.B.; Gersh, B.J.; Bailey, K.R.; Casaclang-Verzosa, G.; Tsang, T.S. Left atrial reservoir function as a potent marker for first atrial fibrillation or flutter in persons > or = 65 years of age. *Am. J. Cardiol.* **2008**, *101*, 1626–1629. [CrossRef]
15. Tan, B.Y.; Ho, J.S.; Sia, C.H.; Boi, Y.; Foo, A.S.; Dalakoti, M.; Chan, M.Y.; Ho, A.F.; Leow, A.S.; Chan, B.P.; et al. Left Atrial Volume Index Predicts New-Onset Atrial Fibrillation and Stroke Recurrence in Patients with Embolic Stroke of Undetermined Source. *Cerebrovasc. Dis.* **2020**, *49*, 285–291. [CrossRef]
16. Njoku, A.; Kannabhiran, M.; Arora, R.; Reddy, P.; Gopinathannair, R.; Lakkireddy, D.; Dominic, P. Left atrial volume predicts atrial fibrillation recurrence after radiofrequency ablation: A meta-analysis. *Europace* **2018**, *20*, 33–42. [CrossRef]
17. Flaker, G.C.; Fletcher, K.A.; Rothbart, R.M.; Halperin, J.L.; Hart, R.G. Clinical and echocardiographic features of intermittent atrial fibrillation that predict recurrent atrial fibrillation. Stroke Prevention in Atrial Fibrillation (SPAF) investigators. *Am. J. Cardiol.* **1995**, *76*, 355–358. [CrossRef]
18. Tsang, T.S.; Barnes, M.E.; Bailey, K.R.; Leibson, C.L.; Montgomery, S.C.; Takemoto, Y.; Diamond, P.M.; Marra, M.A.; Gersh, B.J.; Wiebers, D.O.; et al. Left atrial volume: Important risk marker of incident atrial fibrillation in 1655 older men and women. *Mayo Clin. Proc.* **2001**, *76*, 467–475. [CrossRef]

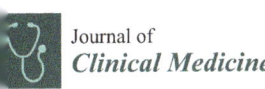

Article

Clinical Efficacy of Catheter Ablation in the Treatment of Vasovagal Syncope

Longping Xu [1,2], Yixin Zhao [3], Yichao Duan [2], Rui Wang [2], Junlong Hou [2], Jing Wang [2], Bin Chen [2], Ye Yang [2], Xianjun Xue [2], Yongyong Zhao [2], Bo Zhang [2], Chaofeng Sun [1,*] and Fengwei Guo [4,*]

1. Department of Cardiovascular Medicine, The First Affiliated Hospital of Xi'an Jiaotong University, Xi'an 710061, China
2. Department of Cardiovascular Medicine, Syncope Center, Xianyang Central Hospital, Xianyang 712000, China
3. Department of Neurology, The First Affiliated Hospital of Xi'an Jiaotong University, Xi'an 710061, China
4. Department of Cardiovascular Surgery, The First Affiliated Hospital of Xi'an Jiaotong University, Xi'an 710061, China
* Correspondence: cfsun1@xjtu.edu.cn (C.S.); guofengwei@xjtu.edu.cn (F.G.)

Abstract: Catheter ablation of ganglionated plexi (GPs) performed as cardioneuroablation in the left atrium (LA) has been reported previously as a treatment for vasovagal syncope (VVS). However, the efficacy and safety of catheter ablation in the treatment of VVS remains unclear. The objective of this study is to explore the efficacy and safety of catheter ablation in the treatment of VVS and to compare the different ganglion-mapping methods for prognostic effects. A total of 108 patients with refractory VVS who underwent catheter ablation were retrospectively enrolled. Patients preferred to use high-frequency stimulation (HFS) ($n = 66$), and anatomic landmark ($n = 42$) targeting is used when HFS failed to induce a positive reaction. The efficacy of the treatment is evaluated by comparing the location and probability of the intraoperative vagal reflex, the remission rate of postoperative syncope symptoms, and the rate of negative head-up tilt (HUT) results. Adverse events are analyzed, and safety is evaluated. After follow-up for 8 (5, 15) months, both HFS mapping and anatomical ablation can effectively improve the syncope symptoms in VVS patients, and 83.7% of patients no longer experienced syncope (<0.001). Both approaches to catheter ablation in the treatment of VVS effectively inhibit the recurrence of VVS; they are safe and effective. Therefore, catheter ablation can be used as a treatment option for patients with symptomatic VVS.

Keywords: syncope; vasovagal syncope; catheter ablation; ganglionated plexus; high-frequency stimulation

Citation: Xu, L.; Zhao, Y.; Duan, Y.; Wang, R.; Hou, J.; Wang, J.; Chen, B.; Yang, Y.; Xue, X.; Zhao, Y.; et al. Clinical Efficacy of Catheter Ablation in the Treatment of Vasovagal Syncope. *J. Clin. Med.* **2022**, *11*, 5371. https://doi.org/10.3390/jcm11185371

Academic Editor: Tong Liu

Received: 7 August 2022
Accepted: 5 September 2022
Published: 13 September 2022

Publisher's Note: MDPI stays neutral with regard to jurisdictional claims in published maps and institutional affiliations.

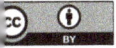

Copyright: © 2022 by the authors. Licensee MDPI, Basel, Switzerland. This article is an open access article distributed under the terms and conditions of the Creative Commons Attribution (CC BY) license (https://creativecommons.org/licenses/by/4.0/).

1. Introduction

Vasovagal syncope (VVS), a neuro-mediated syndrome, is a disorder of cardiovascular autonomic regulation and is the most common cause of sudden and transient loss of consciousness caused by cerebral hypoperfusion [1]. Although syncope itself has a good prognosis, VVS causes physical injuries and poor quality of life [2]. The difference in heart rate and blood pressure with a positive HUT indicates that VVS can be divided into cardioinhibitory, vasodepressive, and mixed according to the pattern of hemodynamic changes during syncope attacks [3]. Treatment for VVS has been challenging. Conventional interventions (education, avoiding precipitating factors, and maintaining fluid and salt intake), orthostatic training, pharmacological treatments, and implantable rhythm devices have failed to show good clinical outcomes (25–65% recurrent syncope) [4–6]. The pathophysiological mechanisms that underlie VVS are complex and far from being fully elucidated. Pathological increases in vagal tone may play a significant role in VVS [2]. Posterior vagus ganglion neurons of the heart are mainly distributed in the epicardial fat pad, which transmits information between preganglionic and postganglionic nerve fibers and regulates cardiac rhythm and conduction [7,8]. The search for a more effective therapy aimed at achieving long-term suppression of vagal reflexes is therefore justified. Preliminary studies have shown that catheter ablation of the LA endocardial parasympathetic ganglion is effective in the treatment of refractory VVS and can achieve a good long-term prognosis [9–11]. Here, we describe 108 patients with VVS who underwent LAGP catheter ablation; in this study, we compared high-frequency stimulation (HFS) with anatomic markers and analyzed ablation safety and efficacy.

2. Materials and Methods

2.1. Patients

In total, 1425 patients with VVS were diagnosed by the syncope center from January 2018 to January 2021 in Xianyang Central Hospital, China, including 125 patients with VVS who received catheter ablation, in which 8 patients who were lost to follow-up and 9 patients with missing postoperative follow-up data. Finally, a total of 108 patients in our syncope center were retrospectively enrolled.

All patients had (1) fulfilled the diagnostic criteria of VVS proposed by the 2015 Heart Rhythm Society Guideline and underwent cardioneuroablation [4]; (2) there was no improvement in symptoms after drug treatment through optimal salt and liquid intake and physical back pressure training; (3) positive response to HUT; (4) the patients or their family members agreed to accept the study protocol and signed their informed consent.

Exclusion criteria were (1) structural cardiac or cardiopulmonary diseases (cardiac valvular diseases, severe aortic stenosis, acute myocardial infarction within 6 months, pulmonary embolism, pulmonary hypertension, and hypertrophic obstructive cardiomyopathy); (2) cerebrovascular diseases (vascular steal syndromes and seizures); (3) medication-related syncope (vasodilators, antipsychotics, and antidiabetics); (4) disease that affected autonomic nerve (diabetes mellitus and nervous system–related diseases) and (5) terminal diseases or New York Heart Association Class III or IV heart failure.

The protocols involving human participants were reviewed and approved by the Institutional Ethics Committee for Biomedical Research of Xianyang Central Hospital. The patients and participants provided written informed consent to participate in this study.

2.2. HUT

HUT was performed in the morning in patients in a fasting state. A SHUT-100 tilt table (SHUT-100, Standard Healthcare, Jiangsu Province, China) with a footboard for weight bearing and restraining belts was used for the procedure. Subjects underwent a passive phase (tilted at 70° for 30 min, if under 18 or over 75 years of age tilted at 60°). If no symptoms occurred during the passive phase, participants further underwent an additional provocative phase (0.5 mg sublingually administered nitroglycerin and continued to be tilted for an additional 20 min). Continuous ECG monitoring and noninvasive blood pressure measurements were performed. If after diagnosis by 2 or more experienced clinicians, the physician believed that the clinical presentation was consistent with VVS and the HUT nitroglycerin stimulation test result was negative, isoproterenol stimulation of HUT was added (starting with 1 µg/min and increasing by 1 µg/min every 5 min until reaching 3 µg/min, and ending when the average heart rate exceeded 20–25% of the baseline level; the maximum heart rate was not allowed to exceed 150 bpm). A positive response of HUT was defined when syncope or presyncope occurred in the presence of bradycardia (heart rate < 40 bpm) or abrupt hypotension (systolic blood pressure < 70 mmHg or diastolic blood pressure < 40 mmHg) as well as reproduction of the patient's relevant clinical symptoms [3].

2.3. Preablation Preparation

Before the procedure, all medications were discontinued for at least 5 half-lives. All procedures were performed under local anesthesia. Pulse oximetry and blood pressure were monitored during the procedure. Routinely, the subclavian vein and femoral vein were punctured to place electrodes in the coronary sinus (CS) and right ventricle. Then we used the annular pulmonary vein catheter puncture into the LA through the atrial septum. The 3-dimensional geometry of the LA was conducted under the guidance of the Ensite-Navx Velocity 5.0 system (Abbott) or Carto3 Version 6.0 system (Johnson & Johnson). Target mapping and ablation were performed in the LA using a cold saline irrigated-tip ablation catheter. Patients were preferred to use HFS, and anatomic landmark targeting was used when HFS failed to induce a positive reaction. Patients were divided into an HFS group and an anatomic ablation group according to different operation modes. In the HFS group, HFS mapping was performed on the endocardial surface of the LA to search for positive response points and radiofrequency ablation. In the anatomical ablation group, the ablation endpoint was the disappearance of the vagal response in all GP anatomical regions (i.e., repeated stimulation or ablation in GP no longer showed a positive response).

During the operation, ventricular pacing was automatically output by a temporary pacemaker to avoid ventricular electrode connection with an EP4 stimulator or HFS by ventricular electrode output accidentally caused by the operator. To ensure cerebral perfusion, ablation was stopped when the blood pressure was lower than 70/40 mmHg as assessed by invasive blood pressure monitoring of the radial artery.

2.4. High-Frequency Stimulation-Guided Endocardial Catheter Ablation of GPs in the LA

HFS (50 Hz, 10–20 mA, 5 s) was applied by an electrophysiological stimulator (St Jude Medical EP4 electrophysiological stimulator) to identify five common GP distribution areas in the LA. GPs site could be anatomically located as follows: left superior GP (located in the superolateral area around the root of the left superior pulmonary vein, LSGP); left inferior GP (located in the inferoposterior area around the root of the left inferior pulmonary vein, LIGP); right anterior GP (located in the superoanterior area around the root of the right superior pulmonary vein, RAGP); right inferior GP (located in the inferoposterior area around the root of the right inferior pulmonary vein, RIGP) and coronary sinus electrodes from 3.4 to 5.6 corresponding to the CSMGP of the endocardial region of the LA [12]. In some patients, GP was widely distributed or displaced, and LIGP was extended to the anterior crest of the left upper pulmonary vein and the anterior wall between the left two lungs (Figure 1). RAGP extends to the top of the right superior pulmonary vein vestibule. The middle of the CS covers the coronal sinus electrode 1.2–7.8 corresponding to the endocardium (Figure 2). When GPs were stimulated by high frequency, an RR interval prolonged by more than 50% and a radial artery invasive pressure decreased by more than 5 mmHg were defined as positive reaction points (Figure 3). These positive reaction points were then ablated (power 35 W, temperature limit 43 °C, target force-time integral 400 gs). Each positive point was ablated for 30 s, which was repeated until reached the endpoint. HFS often induces atrial fibrillation. A temporary pacemaker was used if cardiac arrest occurred during the process (heart rate below 40 bpm). After marking positive reaction points, discharge ablation was performed one by one until the endpoint was reached (Figure 4).

2.5. Anatomically Guided Endocardial Catheter Ablation of GP in LA

The above GP distribution areas were located by ablation, and the 5 GP anatomical positions of the LA chamber were tested and ablated successively from the upper left to the left lateral left, lower left, right front, and lower right (power 35 W, temperature limit 43 °C, target force-time integral 400 gs). Each positive point was ablated for 30 s, which was repeated until all five GPs reached the endpoint.

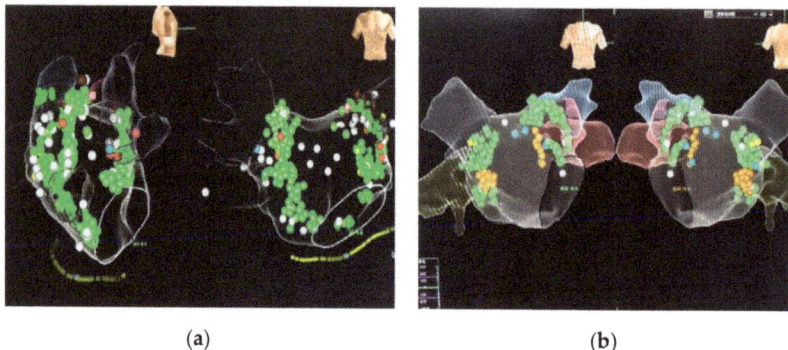

Figure 1. Distribution of GP. (**a**) High-frequency stimulation group. The green dots represent positive spots. The blood pressure and heart rate decreased significantly during high-frequency stimulation which was widely distributed in the pulmonary vein vestibule. The white dots are negative spots the heart rate and blood pressure did not change significantly during stimulation. The red dots represent cardiac arrest for >4 s at the time of stimulation. (**b**) Anatomical group. The green points are positive reaction points for anterior wall GP ablation, the yellow points are positive reaction points for posterior wall GP ablation, and the white and blue points are negative points.

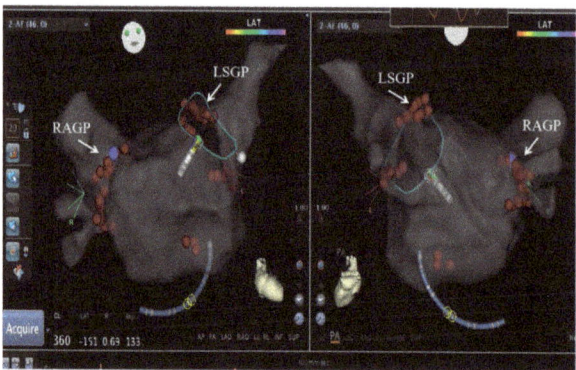

Figure 2. Distribution of ablation sites for anatomic ablation: LSG, RAGP, LIGP, RIGP, and CSMGP.

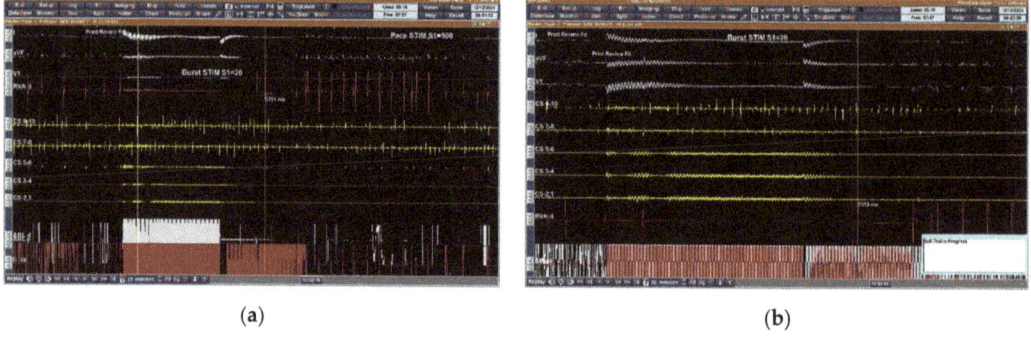

Figure 3. Ventricular arrest induced by high-frequency stimulation. (**a**) Upper left GPHFS induced 5251 ms of asystole. (**b**) Right anterior GPHFS induced 4350 ms of asystole.

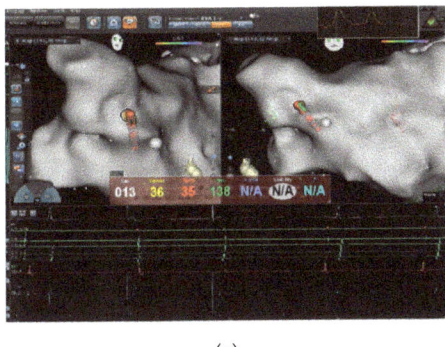 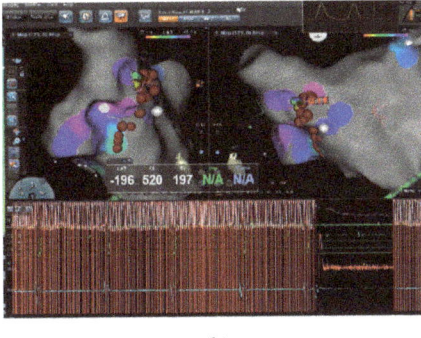

(a) (b)

Figure 4. (a) During RAGP ablation, the heart rate decreased, the temporary pacemaker started pacing below the set frequency, and ablation continued until the positive reaction disappeared. (b) Repeated high-frequency stimulation verification after ablation showed no heart rate decline, reaching the ablation endpoint.

2.6. Postablation Follow-Up

Rivaroxaban 20 mg was taken daily after surgery. Previous medications, including beta blockers, fludrocortisones, and midodrine, were discontinued after the procedure. At a follow-up of 8 (5, 15) months after surgery, an outpatient review of ECG, cardiac ultrasound, 24 h ambulatory ECG monitoring, and HUT was performed. Syncope symptoms were assessed, and recurrent syncope and any associated physical impairment were recorded. Both recurrent syncope and any related physical injuries were carefully documented. Prodromes including transient dizziness, diaphoresis, or fatigue without loss of consciousness were not considered recurrent episodes of syncope. During the follow-up period, a change in HUT from positive (preoperatively) to negative, the lack of recurrence of syncope, or the presence of syncope with 50% fewer episodes than before was considered effective. Any associated perioperative adverse events were recorded in detail to assess safety.

2.7. Statistical Analysis

All data are reported as the mean ± SD for continuous variables and as the number of subjects (%) for categorical variables. Measurement data of skewness distribution are represented by Median (Q1, Q3). Independent sample t-tests were used to analyze differences between the two groups. Paired T-tests or Wilcoxon rank sum tests were used for comparisons of pre- and post-ablation measures. Categorical variables were compared using Pearson χ^2 analysis. A two-sided p value < 0.05 indicated statistical significance. Data were analyzed using the SPSS statistical package for Windows, version 22.0 (IBM Corp., Armonk, NY, USA).

3. Results

3.1. Patient Characteristics

Comparison of baseline data between the two groups (Table 1). In total, 108 patients participated in this retrospective clinical study. There were no significant differences between the anatomic ablation group (n = 42) and the HFS group (n = 66). All patients successfully completed catheter ablation. The mean age of the patients was 51.2 ± 15.3 years, and 44.4% of them were males. The 108 patients were classified into the mixed depression type (62.0%), vascular depression type (38.0%), and cardiac depression type (0%) according to the preoperative HUT. Concurrent arrhythmias were as follows: atrial arrhythmias (paroxysmal atrial fibrillation, sustained atrial fibrillation, atrial premature beats, atrial tachycardia, atrial flutter): 41.7%; sinus bradycardia: 5.6%; intermittent atrioventricular block: 1.9%; ventricular arrhythmias (ventricular premature beat, ventricular tachycardia):

25.0%; supraventricular tachycardia (atrioventricular nodule reentrant tachycardia, atrioventricular reentrant tachycardia): 17.6%.

Table 1. Baseline characteristics of the study patients between the two groups.

	Anatomical Ablation Group (n = 42)	High-Frequency Stimulation Group (n = 66)	p Value
Age, years	47.9 ± 13.8	53.4 ± 15.8	0.066
Sex, female (%)	15 (35.7)	33 (50.0)	0.145
Diabetes, n	16	26	0.893
Serum creatinine, μmol/L	71.7 (61.3, 80.2)	70.0 (61.0, 81.9)	0.944
Left atrial diameter, mm	35.0 (31.0, 43.0)	38.0 (33.0, 46.0)	0.605
Left ventricular end diastolic diameter, mm	43.0 ± 7.3	45.0 ± 8.8	0.742
Left ventricular ejection fraction, %	63.7 ± 7.0	62.8 ± 7.6	0.749
Syncope burden			
Number of syncopal episodes in the preceding year	2.7 ± 1.9	2.5 ± 1.7	0.437
Number of precursory symptoms of syncope	23 (54.7)	36 (54.5)	0.982
Number of symptoms of syncope, n (%)	19 (45.2)	30 (45.5)	0.982
Complications			
Atrial arrhythmia*, n (%)	17 (40.5)	28 (42.4)	0.841
Sinus bradycardia, n (%)	2 (4.8)	4 (6.1)	1
Intermittent atrioventricular block, n (%)	1 (2.4)	1 (1.5)	1
Ventricular arrhythmias*, n (%)	12 (28.6)	15 (22.7)	0.494
Supraventricular tachycardia (AVRT, AVNRT), n (%)	7 (16.7)	12 (18.2)	0.84
Coronary atherosclerotic heart disease, n (%)	7 (16.7)	9 (13.6)	0.666
Hypertension, n (%)	6 (14.3)	15 (22.7)	0.28
Congenital heart disease, n (%)	1 (2.4)	5 (7.6)	0.401
Coronary artery spasm, n (%)	2 (4.8)	1 (1.5)	0.559
VVS types			
Mixed type	27 (64.3)	40 (60.6)	0.701
Vasodepressor type	15 (35.7)	26 (39.4)	0.701
Cardioinhibitory type	0	0	-

Data are expressed as the mean (SD), number (%), or n. Atrial arrhythmia*: paroxysmal atrial fibrillation, persistent atrial fibrillation, atrial premature beat, atrial tachycardia, atrial flutter. Ventricular arrhythmias*: Premature ventricular beat, ventricular tachycardia.

3.2. Catheter Ablation

Detailed information about the procedures for the following sites is listed in Table 2: LSGP (71.3%), LIGP (17.6%), RAGP (53.7%), RIGP (19.4%), CSMGP (20.4%), no positive reaction (8.3%). The immediate heart rate increased by 15 (3, 30) bpm before and after intraoperative ablation. The recovery time of the sinoatrial node (SNRT) was shortened by 264 (140,359) ms, and the SNRT shortening rate was 19.4%. The invasive pressure of the radial artery decreased by 31.8 ± 22.7 mmHg during ablation, which indicates that there is a positive reaction to ablation.

Table 2. Comparison of procedure parameter changes between the two groups.

	Anatomical Ablation Group n = 42	High-Frequency Stimulation Group n = 66	p Value
LSGP, n (%)	29 (69.0)	48 (72.7)	0.68
LIGP, n (%)	4 (9.5)	15 (22.7)	0.119
RAGP, n (%)	20 (47.6)	38 (57.6)	0.312
RIGP, n (%)	5 (11.9)	16 (24.2)	0.114
CSMGP, n (%)	4 (9.5)	18 (27.3)	0.029
Negative vagal response, n (%)	9 (21.4)	0 (0)	-
The ablation endpoint was defined and reached, n (%)	33 (78.6)	66 (100.0)	-

3.3. Clinical Outcomes

At a follow-up of 8 (5, 15) months, the patients' symptoms of syncope improved significantly after catheter ablation; 83.7% of patients had no recurrence of syncope (<0.001), and 81.5% had HUT results that turned negative Subgroup analysis showed that anatomical ablation and HFS ablation could effectively improve syncope symptoms (Table 3). During the 8 (5, 15) month follow-up, eight patients (11.9%) underwent a conversion from mixed suppression to vascular suppression (absence of heart rate inhibition and residual blood pressure inhibition). The number of syncope symptoms decreased in 76.9% of the patients compared with the previous attacks (Table 4). At 1-year follow-up, the number of syncope symptoms decreased in 84.3% of the patients compared with the previous attacks (Table 5). Both HFS mapping and anatomical ablation can effectively improve the syncope symptoms in VVS patients (Table 4). A Holter monitoring comparison of 108 VVS patients before and after catheter ablation showed that the mean heart rate (SDNN) of the slowest heart rate was statistically different (Table 6).

Table 3. Clinical data of the patients pre- and postablation.

	Preoperative n = 108	Postoperative n = 108	p Value
Total (n = 108)			
HUT, n (%)			
Mixed type	67	6	<0.001
Vasodepressor type	41	14	<0.001
Negative type	0	88	<0.001
Syncope, n (%)	49	8	<0.001
HFS-Guided Ablation (n = 42)			
HUT, n (%)			
Mixed type	40	2	<0.001
Vasodepressor type	26	14	0.023
Negative type	0	50	<0.001
Syncope, n (%)	30	0	<0.001
Anatomically Guided Ablation (n = 66)			
HUT, n (%)			
Mixed type	27	4	<0.001
Vasodepressor type	15	0	<0.001
Negative type	0	38	<0.001
Syncope, n (%)	19	8	0.01

Table 4. Short-term follow-up results of syncope symptoms in the two groups.

	Anatomical Ablation Group	High-Frequency Stimulation Group	p Value
No recurrence of syncope, n (%)	11(26.2)	30(45.5)	
Reduced syncope attacks, n (%)	8(19.0)	0(0)	0.002
Improvement of precursory symptoms of syncope, n (%)	13(31.0)	21(31.8)	
No improvement, n (%)	10(23.8)	15(22.7)	

Table 5. One-year follow-up results of syncope symptoms in the two groups.

	Anatomical Ablation Group	High-Frequency Stimulation Group	p Value
No recurrence of syncope, n (%)	10(23.8)	28(42.4)	
Reduced syncope attacks, n (%)	9(21.4)	2(3.0)	0.007
Improvement of precursory symptoms of syncope, n (%)	18(42.9)	24(36.4)	
No improvement, n (%)	5(11.9)	12(18.2)	

Table 6. Changes in HR and HR variation after ablation during follow-up.

	Preoperative n = 108	Postoperative 8 (5, 15) Months n = 108	p Value
SDNN (ms)	107.5 ± 57.8	91.5 ± 44.8	0.046
Minimum HR, bpm	52.5 ± 10.9	62.1 ± 11.5	<0.001
Maximum HR, bpm	119.5 ± 21.6	115.9 ± 17.7	0.23
Mean HR, bpm	73.7 ± 12.5	78.3 ± 10.7	0.009

Two patients in the HFS group developed postoperative bradycardia with a ventricular rate of 45–55 bpm and hypotension of 80/50 mmHg. Dopamine and atropine were used to improve the blood pressure and heart rate, and sinus rhythm was restored 72 h later with blood pressures above 90/60 mmHg. During the follow-up period, syncope or with recurrent precursory symptoms of syncope, such as dizziness, palpitation, and sweating, disappeared, and the HUT turned negative. There were no other surgery-related complications, including malignant arrhythmias, cardiac tamponade, pericarditis, symptoms associated with delayed gastric emptying, or death.

4. Discussion

The results revealed the following findings: (1) Symptoms associated with syncope were improved by both HFS and anatomic ablation-guided LA ganglion ablation in patients. A total of 83.7% of patients did not experience a recurrence of syncope or any related physical injury during a mean follow-up period of 8 (5, 15) months. (2) Catheter ablation has shown some effectiveness in the treatment of mixed inhibitory VVS, which can effectively relieve heart rate inhibition. (3) Many patients with VVS also have atrial fibrillation, idiopathic premature ventricular beats, and supraventricular tachycardia, and these patients should pay attention to preoperative screening of VVS. In this study, the sample size was significantly increased. Moreover, preoperative and postoperative HUT changes were added to the evaluation of efficacy. Patients with arrhythmias had no hemodynamic disorders and no malignant arrhythmias at the time of the arrhythmia attack. Moreover, no malignant arrhythmias were detected during the syncope episode. HUT induces a decrease in heart rate and/or blood pressure consistent with the patient's clinical symptoms. Therefore, the patient's symptoms were considered to be caused by VVS. Although two patients in our study developed arrhythmias after the invasive procedure, both recovered after drug treatment; consequently, catheter ablation of LAGP did not increase the incidence of sympathetic-related malignant arrhythmias. This unreproduced and non-controlled study is our preliminary experience demonstrating the efficacy and safety of LAGP ablation for the prevention of VVS.

The autonomic nervous system affects the function of the cardiovascular system by regulating the delicate balance between sympathetic and parasympathetic tension. VVS is caused by the imbalance of sympathetic and parasympathetic tension and the negative effect of pathologically increased vagal tone on cardiac conduction and vascular tension [2]. Therefore, some scholars have proposed achieving permanent endocardial denervation by catheter ablation of the epicardial ganglion of the atrial wall from the endocardial surface to treat patients with VVS [13,14]. Professor Pachon published articles in 2005 and 2011 demonstrating that catheter ablation can significantly improve the symptoms of patients with VVS [10,11]. The parasympathetic nerves were found to be more densely distributed in the atrial than the sympathetic nerves, with a proportion between 1.3:1 and 1.6:1, mainly located in the subendocardium of the myocardium [15]. Second, anatomical studies of the internal cardiac nervous system show that GP in the LA is mainly located around the root of the pulmonary veins [16]. Subsequently, Sun Wei reported that LAGP ablation showed good long-term clinical outcomes in a protocol that was performed only on the LA and not the right atrium or atrial septum [9].

In our study, the target and end points of catheter ablation were clear and feasible. A total of 91.7% of patients achieved a clear ablation endpoint. Patients followed up after ablation showed significant improvement in syncope or syncope-related symptoms such as dizziness and chest tightness, which severely affected daily life. The HUT review showed that 81.5% of patients changed from positive to negative; 79.1%, from mixed inhibition to negative; 11.9%, from mixed inhibition to vascular inhibition, suggesting that catheter ablation is more effective in the treatment of mixed inhibition of VVS and can effectively relieve the inhibition of heart rate. Some patients with VVS do not experience a syncope attack but have symptoms such as chest tightness, dizziness, blaumosis, palpitation, fatigue, sweating, etc., or have a simultaneous arrhythmia, which seriously affects daily life. Combined with the inducement, clinical manifestation, and positive HUT result, VVS can be diagnosed. For arrhythmias requiring catheter ablation, VVS should be routinely examined before surgery. For patients with obvious symptoms, modified LAGP ablation can be performed simultaneously [17]. This study showed that many patients with VVS also had atrial fibrillation, idiopathic premature ventricular beats, and supraventricular tachycardia. Therefore, attention should be given to the preoperative screening of VVS in these patients. In this study, 11.1% of patients had had a definite diagnosis of VVS without complications and received catheter ablation.

After the modified ablation of LAGP, sympathetic nerve tension increased, and there was a possibility of increased malignant arrhythmias. However, in this study, only part of the LA vagus nerve received the intervention, namely, modified ablation. The results of dynamic ECG showed that SDNN, the heart rate variability index, was shortened. After ablation of left atrial vagal ganglion, vagal tone decreased, and heart rate may increase. There was no difference in the maximum heart rate before and after the operation, and no malignant arrhythmia was observed after the operation. It is suggested that catheter ablation of LAGP does not increase the incidence of sympathetic-related malignant arrhythmias.

The comparison between the anatomical ablation group and the HFS group showed that there was no difference between the two groups in the intraoperative mapping of the LSGP, RAGP, LIGP, and RIGP, and the high positive rate of HFS mapping in the CSMGP [9]. The reason may be that the CSMGP is related to the location of the Marshall vein opening, and the location varies greatly. In the anatomical ablation group, $CS_{3, 4-5, 6}$ and six electrodes were ablated and mapped, and the positions were relatively fixed. The HFS group had an advantage because repeated HFSn mapping was performed in a wide area involving $CS_{1,2-9,0}$. In both groups, the positive rates of the LSGP and RAGP were significantly higher than those of the other GPs. Due to individual differences in GP distribution, the intraoperative mapping of these two GPs should be carefully expanded. Our center summarized the experience of catheter ablation in the treatment of VVS and suggested routine intervention of the LSGP and RAGP regardless of the positive results of the map. In addition, after the intervention of the RAGP, the incidence of vagal reflex in other parts of the ablation region decreased or ceased, which affected the clarity of the ablation endpoint. Therefore, ablation of the RAGP should be performed last to ensure that each GP can reach the definite endpoint.

There was no significant difference in most parameters between the anatomic ablation group and the HFS group, and both methods were optional. The advantages of HFS are that the mapping range is wide, the damage is small, the repeatability is high, and the mapping is accurate, but the stimulation intensity is weaker than the rf energy.

5. Conclusions

Catheter ablation may be a safe and effective in the treatment of VVS. Both HFS mapping and anatomical ablation can effectively improve the symptoms of patients with VVS, and LAGP ablation may be more effective in improving the components of cardiac inhibition.

6. Study Limitations

This study was a retrospective single-center sample. Although the sample size was large, it still had some limitations, and further multicenter, prospective, large-sample randomized controlled studies should provide evidence-based information for catheter ablation in the treatment of VVS. In addition, there is a selection bias as follows: patients who failed with HFS underwent the anatomical approach. Long-term follow-up is needed to determine whether nerve regeneration leads to the recurrence of syncope symptoms.

Author Contributions: Writing—original draft preparation, L.X., Y.Z. (Yixin Zhao); writing—review and editing, C.S., F.G.; methodology, Y.D., R.W., and L.X.; formal analysis, J.H., J.W., and B.C.; investigation, Y.Y., X.X.; data curation, Y.Z. (Yongyong Zhao), B.Z.; supervision, F.G.; project administration C.S. All authors have read and agreed to the published version of the manuscript.

Funding: This work was funded by the Natural Science Foundation of Shaanxi Province (2020JM-373).

Institutional Review Board Statement: The study was conducted in accordance with the Declaration of Helsinki and approved by the ethics committee of Xianyang Central Hospital approved this study (No.20180022, 4 January 2018). No potentially identifiable human images or data is presented in this study.

Informed Consent Statement: Written informed consent to participate in this study was provided by the participants or the participants' legal guardians/next of kin.

Data Availability Statement: The raw data supporting the conclusions of this article will be made available by the authors, without undue reservation. Requests to access the datasets should be directed to cfsun1@xjtu.edu.cn; guofengwei@xjtu.edu.cn.

Acknowledgments: We acknowledge and appreciate the effort of all physicians and nurses in the collaborative care of these patients.

Conflicts of Interest: The authors declare no conflict of interest.

References

1. Grubb, B.P. Neurocardiogenic syncope. *N. Engl. J. Med.* **2005**, *352*, 1004–1010. [CrossRef]
2. Chen-Scarabelli, C.; Scarabelli, T.M. Neurocardiogenic syncope. *BMJ* **2004**, *329*, 336–341. [CrossRef]
3. Brignole, M.; Moya, A.; de Lange, F.J.; Deharo, J.-C.; Elliott, P.M.; Fanciulli, A.; Fedorowski, A.; Furlan, R.; Kenny, R.A.; Martín, A. et al. 2018 ESC Guidelines for the diagnosis and management of syncope. *Eur. Heart J.* **2018**, *39*, 1883–1948. [CrossRef] [PubMed]
4. Sheldon, R.S.; Grubb, B.P.; Olshansky, B.; Shen, W.-K.; Calkins, H.; Brignole, M.; Raj, S.R.; Krahn, A.D.; Morillo, C.A.; Stewart, J.M. et al. 2015 heart rhythm society expert consensus statement on the diagnosis and treatment of postural tachycardia syndrome inappropriate sinus tachycardia, and vasovagal syncope. *Heart Rhythm.* **2015**, *12*, e41–e63. [CrossRef] [PubMed]
5. Brignole, M.; Menozzi, C.; Moya, A.; Andresen, D.; Blanc, J.J.; Krahn, A.D.; Wieling, W.; Beiras, X.; Deharo, J.C.; Russo, V.; et al Pacemaker therapy in patients with neurally mediated syncope and documented asystole: Third International Study on Syncope of Uncertain Etiology (ISSUE-3): A randomized trial. *Circulation* **2012**, *125*, 2566–2571. [CrossRef] [PubMed]
6. Tan, M.P.; Newton, J.L.; Chadwick, T.J.; Gray, J.C.; Nath, S.; Parry, S.W. Home orthostatic training in vasovagal syncope modifies autonomic tone: Results of a randomized, placebo-controlled pilot study. *Europace* **2010**, *12*, 240–246. [CrossRef] [PubMed]
7. Stavrakis, S.; Po, S. Ganglionated Plexi Ablation: Physiology and Clinical Applications. *Arrhythmia Electrophysiol. Rev.* **2017**, *6*, 186–190. [CrossRef] [PubMed]
8. Xia, Y.; Zhao, W.; Yang, Z.-J.; Zhang, J.-Y.; Zhao, L.; Gu, X.-J.; Zhao, X.; Lu, F.; Wu, Z.-G.; Liao, D.-N. Catheter Ablation of Cardiac Fat Pads Attenuates Bezold-Jarisch Reflex in Dogs. *J. Cardiovasc. Electrophysiol.* **2011**, *22*, 573–578. [CrossRef] [PubMed]
9. Sun, W.; Zheng, L.; Qiao, Y.; Shi, R.; Hou, B.; Wu, L.; Guo, J.; Zhang, S.; Yao, Y. Catheter Ablation as a Treatment for Vasovagal Syncope: Long-Term Outcome of Endocardial Autonomic Modification of the Left Atrium. *J. Am. Heart Assoc.* **2016**, *5*, e003471 [CrossRef] [PubMed]
10. Pachon, J.C.; Pachon, E.I.; Pachon, J.C.; Lobo, T.J.; Pachon, M.Z.; Vargas, R.N.A.; Jatene, A.D. "Cardioneuroablation"—New treatment for neurocardiogenic syncope, functional AV block and sinus dysfunction using catheter RF-ablation. *Europace* **2005**, *7*, 1–13. [CrossRef] [PubMed]
11. Pachon, J.C.M.; Pachon, E.I.M.; Cunha Pachon, M.Z.; Lobo, T.J.; Pachon, J.C.M.; Santillana, T.G.P. Catheter ablation of severe neurally meditated reflex (neurocardiogenic or vasovagal) syncope: Cardioneuroablation long-term results. *Europace* **2011**, *13*, 1231–1242. [CrossRef] [PubMed]
12. Yao, Y.; Shi, R.; Wong, T.; Zheng, L.; Chen, W.; Yang, L.; Huang, W.; Bao, J.; Zhang, S. Endocardial autonomic denervation of the left atrium to treat vasovagal syncope: An early experience in humans. *Circ. Arrhythmia Electrophysiol.* **2012**, *5*, 279–286. [CrossRef] [PubMed]

3. Tu, B.; Wu, L.; Hu, F.; Fan, S.; Liu, S.; Liu, L.; Ding, L.; Zheng, L.; Yao, Y. Cardiac Deceleration Capacity as an Indicator for Cardioneuroablation in Patients with Refractory Vasovagal Syncope. *Heart Rhythm* **2021**, *19*, 562–569. [CrossRef] [PubMed]
4. Hu, F.; Zheng, L.; Liu, S.; Shen, L.; Liang, E.; Liu, L.; Wu, L.; Ding, L.; Yao, Y. The impacts of the ganglionated plexus ablation sequence on the vagal response, heart rate, and blood pressure during cardioneuroablation. *Auton. Neurosci.-Basic Clin.* **2021**, *233*, 102812. [CrossRef] [PubMed]
5. Kawano, H.; Okada, R.; Yano, K. Histological study on the distribution of autonomic nerves in the human heart. *Heart Vessels* **2003**, *18*, 32–39. [CrossRef] [PubMed]
6. Tan, A.Y.; Li, H.; Wachsmann-Hogiu, S.; Chen, L.S.; Chen, P.-S.; Fishbein, M.C. Autonomic innervation and segmental muscular disconnections at the human pulmonary vein-atrial junction: Implications for catheter ablation of atrial-pulmonary vein junction. *J. Am. Coll. Cardiol.* **2006**, *48*, 132–143. [CrossRef] [PubMed]
7. Komatsu, S.; Sumiyoshi, M.; Miura, S.; Kimura, Y.; Shiozawa, T.; Hirano, K.; Odagiri, F.; Tabuchi, H.; Hayashi, H.; Sekita, G.; et al. A proposal of clinical ECG index "vagal score" for determining the mechanism of paroxysmal atrioventricular block. *J. Arrhythmia* **2017**, *33*, 208–213. [CrossRef] [PubMed]

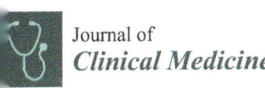

Journal of Clinical Medicine

Article

Deep-Learning-Based Detection of Paroxysmal Supraventricular Tachycardia Using Sinus-Rhythm Electrocardiograms

Lei Wang [1,†], Shipeng Dang [2,†], Shuangxiong Chen [1], Jin-Yu Sun [3], Ru-Xing Wang [2,*] and Feng Pan [1,*]

1. Key Laboratory of Advanced Process Control for Light Industry (Ministry of Education), Jiangnan University, Wuxi 214122, China
2. Department of Cardiology, The Affiliated Wuxi People's Hospital of Nanjing Medical University, Wuxi 214023, China
3. Department of Cardiology, The Affiliated Hospital of Nanjing Medical University, Nanjing 210011, China
* Correspondence: ruxingw@aliyun.com (R.-X.W.); pan_feng_63@jiangnan.edu.cn (F.P.)
† These authors contributed equally to this work.

Abstract: Background: Paroxysmal supraventricular tachycardia (PSVT) is a common arrhythmia associated with palpitation and a decline in quality of life. However, it is undetectable with sinus-rhythmic ECGs when patients are not in the symptomatic onset stage. Methods: In the current study, a convolution neural network (CNN) was trained with normal-sinus-rhythm standard 12-lead electrocardiographs (ECGs) of negative control patients and PSVT patients to identify patients with unrecognized PSVT. PSVT refers to atrioventricular nodal reentry tachycardia or atrioventricular reentry tachycardia based on a concealed accessory pathway as confirmed by electrophysiological procedure. Negative control group data were obtained from 5107 patients with at least one normal sinus-rhythmic ECG without any palpitation symptoms. All ECGs were randomly allocated to the training, validation and testing datasets in a 7:1:2 ratio. Model performance was evaluated on the testing dataset through F1 score, overall accuracy, area under the curve, sensitivity, specificity and precision. Results: We retrospectively enrolled 407 sinus-rhythm ECGs of PSVT procedural patients and 1794 ECGs of control patients. A total of 2201 ECGs were randomly divided into training (n = 1541), validation (n = 220) and testing (n = 440) datasets. In the testing dataset, the CNN algorithm showed an overall accuracy of 95.5%, sensitivity of 90.2%, specificity of 96.6% and precision of 86.0%. Conclusion: Our study reveals that a well-trained CNN algorithm may be a rapid, effective, inexpensive and reliable method to contribute to the detection of PSVT.

Keywords: deep learning; convolution neural network; paroxysmal supraventricular tachycardia; electrocardiography; detection

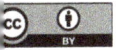

1. Introduction

Paroxysmal supraventricular tachycardia (PSVT) is one of the common types of arrhythmia, a clinical syndrome characterized by the presence of regular and rapid tachycardia with abrupt onset and termination and an incidence of 35 per 100,000 patient-years [1,2]. The most frequent symptoms of PSVT are rapid heart rate, palpitations, lightheadedness, shortness of breath, chest pain, anxiety, and potentially syncope [3,4]. The primary consequence of PSVT in most patients is a decline in quality of life. In some rare cases, incessant PSVT can cause tachycardia-induced cardiomyopathy and sudden death [5]. PSVT is also a novel risk-factor for cryptogenic stroke [3,6,7]. Most patients with PSVT can be temporarily managed using physiological maneuvers, medications and occasionally even electrical cardioversion [5]. Catheter ablation is a permanent method for patients who want to cure the arrhythmia [8].

In the present study, the term "PSVT" mainly refers to atrioventricular nodal reentry tachycardia (AVNRT) or atrioventricular reentry tachycardia (AVRT) excluding atrial fibrillation, atrial flutter and atrial tachycardia. The occurrence of AVRT is based on an overt (Wolff–Parkinson–White (WPW) syndrome) or concealed accessory pathway [8,9]. A confirmatory diagnosis of PSVT can be made via electrocardiogram (ECG) or other rhythm-recording devices during tachycardia. Except for WPW syndrome, confirming a diagnosis of PSVT can be challenging because of its variable duration and sporadic nature [4]. Furthermore, patients with unrecognized AVNRT or AVRT based on a concealed accessory pathway cannot be diagnosed when they are not in the PSVT onset stage via sinus-rhythmic ECGs. Currently, most medical image detection relies on the classical approach, which follows a three-step procedure (hand-crafted feature extraction, study and recognition) [10,11]. However, deep learning is an end-to-end deep neural network that can extract even subtle features automatically to achieve identification, classification and prediction [12]. It is unlike conventional machine learning, which needs manual feature extraction. In recent years, deep neural networks, especially convolutional neural networks (CNNs) have been shown to outperform classical machine learning approaches in most medical image analysis tasks. The application of a CNN to an ECG can predict cardiovascular diseases and even non-cardiovascular diseases such as serum potassium aberrations, anemia and sleep apnea [13–17]. CNN-enabled ECGs could identify patients with left ventricle dysfunction using a threshold of LVEF $\leq$ 35% or 50% according to transthoracic echocardiogram [18,19]. A previous study also reported that a well-trained CNN could detect patients with the electrocardiographic signature of atrial fibrillation present during normal sinus rhythm, which has practical implications for atrial fibrillation screening [20]. However, the application of CNN to screen patients for PSVT from normal sinus rhythmic ECGs has not been investigated.

In the current study, we hypothesized that a deep neural network could identify PSVT patients even if they were not in the PSVT onset stage. To test and verify our hypothesis, we trained, validated and tested a CNN model using patients with standard 12-lead normal sinus rhythmic ECGs.

2. Materials and Methods

2.1. Data Sources and Collection

Under the approval of the Ethics Committee of The Affiliated Wuxi People's Hospital of Nanjing Medical University, 1714 ECGs of 1143 patients with PSVT were collected from 1 January 2013 to 31 August 2021, and 5365 ECGs of 5107 patients were also collected between 1 January, 2020 and 10 March, 2020 as a control group. All ECG images in both control and PSVT groups were digital, standard 10-s, 12-lead ECGs acquired at a sampling rate of 500 Hz using MAC 800 or 1200ST ECG machines (GE Healthcare). The bandwidth of filter setting was 0.16–40 Hz. All ECG images used in this study were overread and analyzed by two cardiologists, who corrected diagnostic labels as needed. This study was carried out in accordance with The Code of Ethics of the World Medical Association (Declaration of Helsinki).

2.2. Identifying Study Groups and Processing ECG Data

We used ECG data to classify patients into two groups: patients positive for PSVT and patients without any symptoms, signs or records of PSVT. For the PSVT group, the inclusion criteria were as follows: (1) Patients were included if they had abrupt onset and termination of palpitation symptoms or they were diagnosed with PSVT clinically. (2) Patients were diagnosed and confirmed with PSVT by electrophysiological study and radiofrequency ablation; (3) Patient were included if they had a sinus rhythmic ECG before an electrophysiological procedure. For the control group, patients who were evaluated without evidence of PSVT in the outpatient clinic by cardiologist via history collection, medical records or telephone follow-up were included. The exclusion criteria for the control group were: patients with signs of PSVT and general exclusion criteria. The general exclusion criteria were as follows: non-sinus-rhythm ECGs, WPW syndrome, serious atrioventricular bundle block, wide QRS tachycardias, acute myocardial infarction,

HR > 130 bpm, HR < 45 bpm and age < 14 years for both groups (Figure 1). The patients in both groups did not receive any anti-arrhythmic drugs. It is worth mentioning that a complete ECG not only contains a physiological signal waveform diagram but also some metadata such as sex, age, heart rate, P–R interval and QT interval, which will interfere with the feature extraction of the model. Therefore, the metadata part of the ECG images was cut out from the original ECG images (resolution of 6786 × 4731); only the physiological signal waveform diagram was kept, with a resolution of 6600 × 3347.

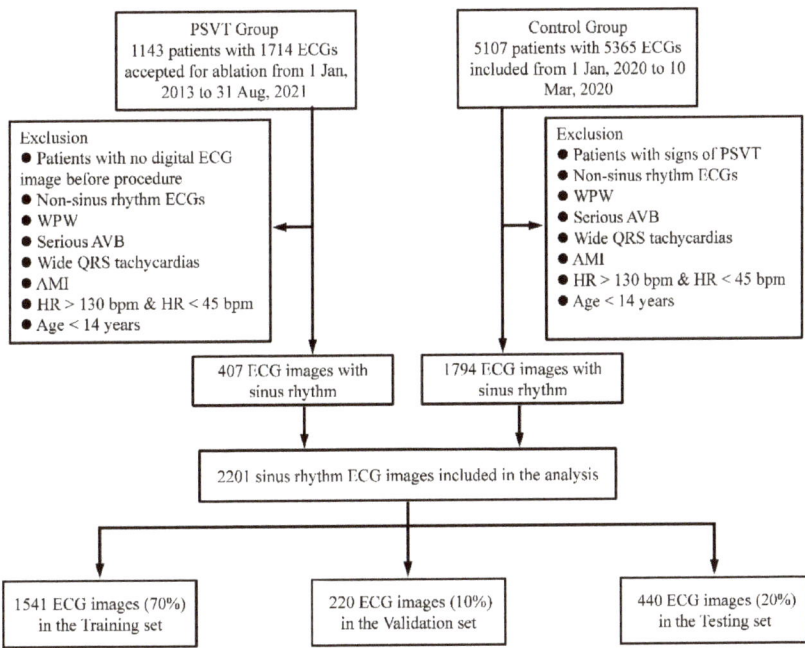

Figure 1. Flowchart of data collection and dataset creation. A total of 1714 ECGs of 1143 patients with PSVT and 5365 ECGs of 5107 control patients were collected. After exclusion of non-sinus-rhythm ECGs, WPW syndrome, serious AVB, wide QRS tachycardias, acute myocardial infarction, HR > 130 bpm, HR < 45 bpm and age < 14 years, a total of 2201 ECGs (407 ECGs for PSVT group and 1794 ECGs for control group) were included in this study. These ECGs were randomly divided into three datasets: a training set (n = 1541), validation set (n = 220) and testing set (n = 440).

In total, 2201 ECG images were randomly allocated to the training set, validation set and testing set at a ratio of 7:1:2. None of the patients overlapped among these three groups. ECGs in the training set were used for training the model, ECGs in the validation set were used to adjust parameters and optimize the model, and the remaining 20% of ECGs comprised the testing set, which was used to assess the generalization ability of the model and evaluate the ability of a CNN-based model to detect PSVT. A schematic representation of the proposed method is given in Figure 2.

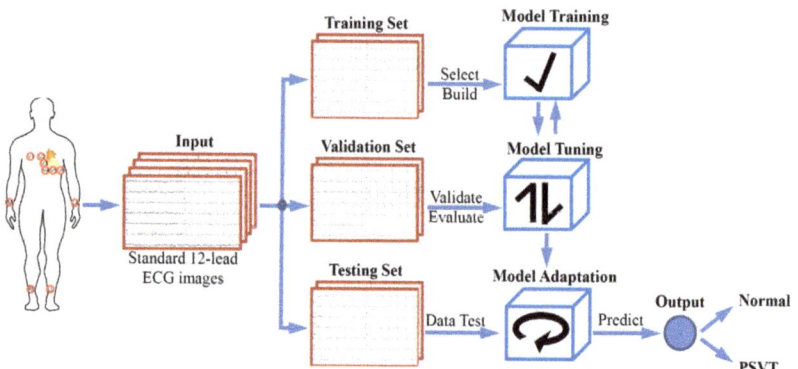

Figure 2. The comprehensive process of the creation and evaluation of the CNN model. The ECG images were acquired and allocated to the training set, validation set, or testing set. ECG images in the training set were used as the input of the CNN, whereas the testing set was used to evaluate the screening performance of the CNN model.

2.3. The Proposed Deep Neural Network

The CNN was implemented by using PyTorch backend with Python, and all the experiments were conducted on a Windows Server 2012 R2 with an NVIDIA Tesla V100 (16 GB). Numpy, matplotlib and other deep learning libraries were used for deep learning algorithms.

All ECG images were resized to 1600 × 800 as inputs for the model through a quadratic linear interpolation scaling algorithm, with the aim of retaining as much waveform information as possible to help detect the subtle features. The batch size was set to 8. Adam optimizer and categorical cross entropy loss function were selected. For the hyperparameters of the proposed model, the initial learning rate was set to 10^{-4}. Meanwhile, cosine annealing was adopted for learning rate decay.

Considering the ECG images consisted of multiple waves, we paid more attention to edge detection, and we set three convolution layers in the initial stage of the network to extract waveform features, as the early layers of the neural network was aimed at detecting edges. Each convolution layer was followed by a batch-normalization layer, which was used to eliminate distribution differences between layers while preserving the sample distribution characteristics. Following the third batch-normalization layer, there was a nonlinear ReLU function and a max-pooling layer [21,22]. Then, the samples had better sparsity and the dimension of the array was reduced on the premise of preserving the characteristics of the sample. Moreover, the SE–ResNet bottleneck module was applied to extract subtle features that were not readily apparent to the naked eye from ECG images. The design of the bottleneck not only reduced the network parameters but also deepened the network depth to study more features. Meanwhile, an attention mechanism that allowed the network to emphasize informative features and to suppress less useful ones was introduced into the bottleneck. To avoid gradient disappearance, between the input of the SE–ResNet Bottleneck module and its output, a 1 × 1 convolution layer was used to adjust the number of channels if the module was at the top of its stage; otherwise, an identity shortcut link was used to allow gradient propagation [23]. Following the last SE–ResNet Bottleneck module, the image was fed to a global pooling layer and a dropout layer, which helped to avoid overfitting. The final output layer (fully connected layer) was activated by using the softmax function, which provided a probability of PSVT. The architecture of the model is shown in Figure 3.

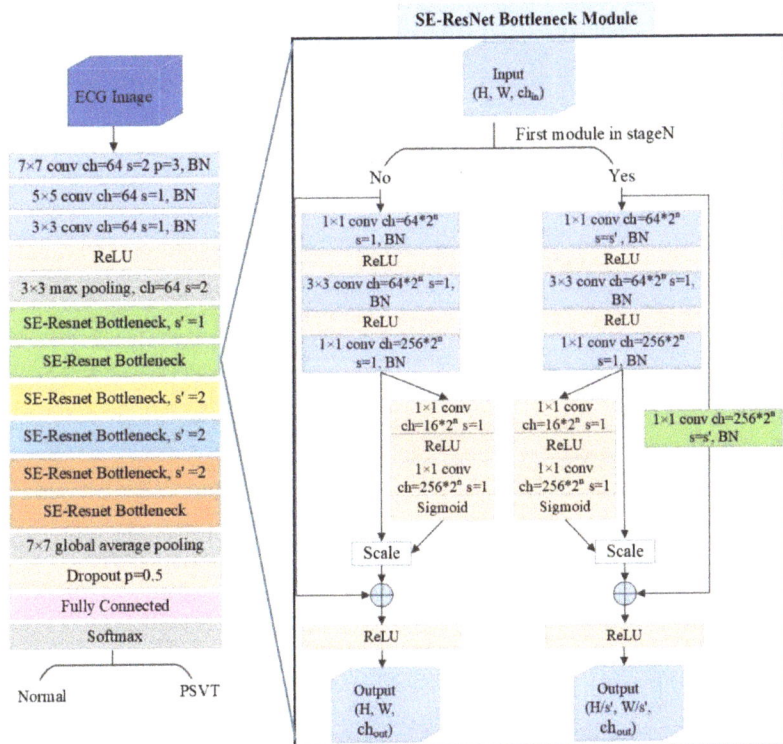

Figure 3. The architecture of the artificial intelligence model. The SE–ResNet Bottleneck contained 4 stages (State N: Stage 0, green; Stage 1, yellow; Stage 2, blue; and Stage 3, orange). Stage 0 and Stage 3 had two SE–ResNet Bottleneck modules each, and Stage 1 and Stage 2 had only one SE–ResNet Bottleneck module each. The value of N ranged from 0 to 3, which also determined the number of channels per module.

2.4. Outcomes of Interest

In addition, we created ROC curves and measured the corresponding AUCs for the validation and testing sets to assess the classification performance of the proposed CNN to screen patients for PSVT based on ECG images during normal sinus rhythm. We selected a suitable probability threshold on the ROC curve for the validation set and applied the same threshold to the testing set to calculate the F1 score, accuracy, sensitivity, specificity and precision. Moreover, we created receiver–operator curves and measured the corresponding AUCs to assess the network strength of the proposed CNN model to screen patients for PSVT based on ECG data alone.

2.5. Statistical Analysis

Descriptive statistics were applied to report the clinical characteristics of patients included in this study. Continuous variables were expressed as mean values ± standard deviation. Categorical variables were expressed as ratios or percentages. Levene's test was used to check the homogeneity of variance. Normally distributed data were compared using independent student's *t*-test. Chi-square was used for categorical variables. Statistical optimization of the CNN was performed through iterative training using the Keras package. Measures of diagnostic performance included the ROC AUC, accuracy, sensitivity, specificity and the F1 score. We used two-sided 95% CIs to summarize the sample variability in the estimates. SPSS version 19.0 (Armonk, NY, USA: IBM Corp) was used for statistical analysis. All tests were performed with a two-tailed significance level of 0.05.

3. Results

3.1. Dataset Characteristics

We screened 407 ECG images in the PSVT group and 1794 ECG images in the control group according to the inclusion and exclusion criteria. The mean age of patients was 48.2 ± 16.4 years, and 46.3% of patients were male. There were no statistically significant differences in ECG characteristics between the control group and the PSVT group in terms of P–R interval, QRS interval or QT interval. However, the heart rates and QTc were slightly higher in the control group than in the PSVT group. The clinical characteristics of these patients are shown in Table 1.

Table 1. Baseline characteristics of patients and ECGs.

Parameters	Control (n = 1794)	PSVT (n = 407)	Total (n = 2201)	p-Value
Age (years)	47.2 ± 16.5	52.7 ± 14.9	48.2 ± 16.4	<0.001
Gender (male, %)	835 (46.5)	183 (45.0)	1018 (46.3)	0.564
Heart rate	80.6 ± 14.7	78.0 ± 18.8	80.1 ± 14.6	0.001
P–R interval	149.5 ± 19.1	151.0 ± 22.3	149.8 ± 19.7	0.189
QRS interval	84.7 ± 11.7	85.1 ± 11.7	84.8 ± 11.7	0.466
QT interval	363.6 ± 32.0	361.0 ± 33.1	363.1 ± 32.2	0.134
QTc	416.7 ± 25.9	411.3 ± 26.7	415.8 ± 26.1	<0.001

3.2. Model Screening Performance

Receiver–operator curves (ROCs) were created, and the areas under the curves (AUCs) were measured to assess the network. The AUC for detecting PSVT was 0.956 (0.917–0.996) when using the validation set and 0.975 (0.959–0.991) when using the testing set (Figure 4). The probability value that yielded preferable sensitivity, specificity and accuracy of 95.5% on the validation set was applied to the testing set and yielded an F1 score of 88.0%, sensitivity of 90.2% (81.2–95.4), specificity of 96.6% (94.0–98.2), precision of 86.0% (76.5–92.3) and an overall accuracy of 95.5%. The proposed CNN model provided a low-cost, non-invasive and feasible method to diagnose PSVT in patients with palpitations.

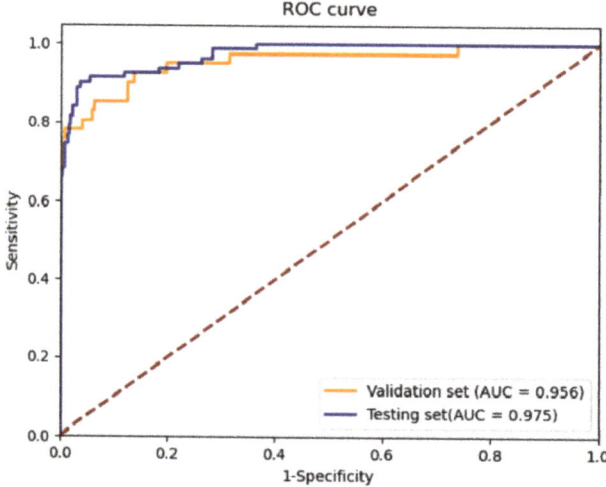

Figure 4. ROC of the screening performance on the validation set and testing set: AUC, area under the curve; ROC, receiver–operating characteristic curve.

4. Discussion

In the past 10 years, several studies have been conducted attempting to detect arrhythmias and cardiac arrest based on CNN-enabled ECG, and have shown promising performance. In the present study, we trained a CNN model that automatically extracts the hidden features from ECG images to diagnose unrecognized PSVT based on sinus-rhythm ECGs. This model demonstrated an overall accuracy of 95.5%, sensitivity of 90.2%, and specificity of 96.6% to predict pre-onset PSVT from ECGs. Our results provide an effective and convenient method for the early detection of PSVT from palpitation patients, which could help these patients receive timely intervention and improve their quality of life.

PSVT is a clinical syndrome characterized by the presence of a regular and rapid heart rhythm with abrupt onset and termination [2]. By virtue of its episodic nature, confirming a diagnosis of PSVT can be challenging [4]. Patients may be initially misdiagnosed with anxiety or other rhythm disorders. Consequently, PSVT can go undiagnosed for years, and patients may be diagnosed with other cardiac conditions or arrhythmias before obtaining a formal diagnosis of PSVT [2]. Furthermore, some patients need invasive electrophysiological study to confirm PSVT. Developing low-cost and non-invasive methods to detect PSVT has important diagnostic and therapeutic implications.

ECG is a common, noninvasive examination method to detect cardiovascular diseases. With the rapid advances in artificial intelligence (AI) in ECG interpretation, AI cannot only make classification based on ECGs, but it can also detect the subtle signals in the ECG that might be invisible to the human eye, yet which contain important information to predict diseases [13,24]. An AI-enabled ECG using a convolutional neural network could detect the electrocardiographic signature of atrial fibrillation present during normal sinus rhythm using standard 10-s, 12-lead ECGs with an AUC of 0.87, sensitivity of 79.0%, specificity of 79.5%, F1 score of 39.2% and overall accuracy of 79.4% [20]. Jo et al. trained a deep learning model (DLM) that could identify PSVT during normal sinus rhythm. During accuracy testing, the ROC of the DLM was 0.966, the accuracy, sensitivity, specificity, positive predictive value and negative predictive value of the DLM were 0.970, 0.868, 0.972, 0.255 and 0.998, respectively. They also found that the QT interval is highly correlated with the development of PSVT using sensitivity map [25]. In the present study, we trained a CNN with sinus-rhythmic ECGs of PSVT patients and control patients with no signs of PSVT. This CNN algorithm showed an AUC of 0.975, overall accuracy of 95.5%, sensitivity of 90.2%, specificity of 96.6%, precision of 86.0% and F1 score of 88.0%, which was consistent with the DLM. Our data also support the idea that QT interval is highly correlated with the development of PSVT, as there was a statistical difference of QTc between the control group and the PSVT group. Our study is also different from Jo's study. Firstly, only AVNRT and concealed accessory-pathway-induced AVRT, which could not be diagnosed with sinus-rhythmic ECGs, were included, and overt accessory-pathway-induced AVRT (WPW syndrome), which could be diagnosed with sinus-rhythmic ECGs by a cardiologist, was excluded in our study. Secondly, in the present study, the cases in the PSVT group were confirmed by electrophysiological study and radiofrequency ablation to exclude atrial tachycardia. However, both of these models could benefit clinicians in the future application of sinus-rhythmic ECGs to diagnose unrecognized PSVT in a timely manner, and would also avoid unnecessary invasive electrophysiology studies, which would ease the pain of patients and reduce medical expenditure.

In previous studies, raw data of ECGs were utilized for artificial intelligence-based ECGs to identify cardiovascular diseases [19,20,25]. Our group developed an AI-based method to screen patients with left ventricular ejection fraction (LVEF) of 50% or less using ECG data alone. The CNN algorithm showed an overall accuracy of 73.9%, sensitivity of 69.2%, specificity of 70.5%, positive predictive value of 70.1% and precision of 69.9%, which demonstrates that a well-trained CNN algorithm may be used as a low-cost and noninvasive method to identify patients with left ventricular dysfunction [18]. In the present study, we used images of standard 10-s, 12-lead ECGs for input of training, validation and testing. Our data demonstrated that ECG images and not only raw ECG data from the ECG management system could be applied for deep learning training to predict arrhythmias with sinus-rhythm ECGs. Contrary to ECG raw data, ECG images are much more easily acquired for patients examined at different hospitals with different ECG machines. Once a CNN network is trained, it can be applied to any standard 12-lead ECG images from a mobile device. In the future, patients with suspected PSVT could use this low-cost and noninvasive tool to exclude or confirm pre-onset PSVT, which is especially beneficial for patients from rural areas or developing countries.

Limitations

This study has several limitations. Firstly, we cannot know exactly what features are extracted by the algorithm, which is known as a "black box" system. Secondly, the number of ECGs for PSVT patients was relatively small, which might limit the model performance and reduce model robustness. Finally, this is a single-center retrospective study. Prospective large-scale and multi-center studies are required to validate the performance of the model.

5. Conclusions

An artificial-intelligence-enabled ECG acquired during normal sinus rhythm can identify individuals with a high likelihood of PSVT. The results of this study could have useful implications for PSVT screening and diagnosis.

Author Contributions: Conceptualization, L.W. and S.D.; methodology, L.W.; software, L.W. and S.C.; validation, L.W. and S.C.; formal analysis, L.W., S.D. and J.-Y.S.; investigation, L.W. and S.C.; data curation, L.W., S.D. and S.C.; writing—original draft preparation, L.W. and S.D.; writing—review and editing, J.-Y.S., R.-X.W. and F.P.; supervision, R.-X.W. and F.P.; project administration, R.-X.W. and F.P.; funding acquisition, R.-X.W. and S.D. All authors have read and agreed to the published version of the manuscript.

Funding: This study was funded by grants from the National Natural Science Foundation of China (81770331), the Jiangsu province Young Medical Talents (QNRC2016185), the Top Talent Support Program for young and middle-aged people of Wuxi Health Committee (BJ016) and the Program of Wuxi Translational Medicine Center (2020ZHYB14).

Institutional Review Board Statement: The study was conducted in accordance with the Declaration of Helsinki and was approved by the Institutional Review Board of the Affiliated Wuxi People's Hospital of Nanjing Medical University.

Informed Consent Statement: Informed consent was obtained from all the subjects involved in the study.

Data Availability Statement: The data that support the findings of this study are available from the corresponding author upon reasonable request.

Conflicts of Interest: The authors declare no conflict of interest.

References

1. Orejarena, L.A.; Vidaillet, H.; DeStefano, F., Jr.; Nordstrom, D.L.; Vierkant, R.A.; Smith, P.N.; Hayes, J.J. Paroxysmal supraventricular tachycardia in the general population. *J. Am. Coll. Cardiol.* **1998**, *31*, 150–157. [CrossRef]
2. Rehorn, M.; Sacks, N.C.; Emden, M.R.; Healey, B.; Preib, M.T.; Cyr, P.L.; Pokorney, S.D. Prevalence and incidence of patients with paroxysmal supraventricular tachycardia in the United States. *J. Cardiovasc. Electrophysiol.* **2021**, *32*, 2199–2206. [CrossRef]
3. Chiang, J.K.; Kao, H.H.; Kao, Y.H. Association of paroxysmal supraventricular tachycardia with ischemic stroke: A national case-control study. *J. Stroke Cerebrovasc. Dis.* **2017**, *26*, 1493–1499. [CrossRef] [PubMed]
4. Sacks, N.C.; Everson, K.; Emden, M.R.; Cyr, P.L.; Wood, D.R.; Raza, S.; Wood, K.A.; Pokorney, S.D. Disparities in the management of newly diagnosed paroxysmal supraventricular tachycardia for women versus men in the United States. *J. Am. Heart Assoc.* **2020**, *9*, e015910. [CrossRef]
5. Page, R.L.; Joglar, J.A.; Caldwell, M.A.; Calkins, H.; Conti, J.B.; Deal, B.J.; Estes, N.A., III; Field, M.E.; Goldberger, Z.D.; Hammill, S.C.; et al. Evidence Review Committee Chairdouble d. 2015 ACC/AHA/HRS Guideline for the management of adult patients with supraventricular tachycardia: A report of the American College of Cardiology/American Heart Association Task Force on Clinical Practice Guidelines and the Heart Rhythm Society. *Circulation* **2016**, *133*, e506–e574.

Kamel, H.; Elkind, M.S.; Bhave, P.D.; Navi, B.B.; Okin, P.M.; Iadecola, C.; Devereux, R.B.; Fink, M.E. Paroxysmal supraventricular tachycardia and the risk of ischemic stroke. *Stroke* **2013**, *44*, 1550–1554. [CrossRef] [PubMed]

Sharma, S.P.; Kondur, A.; Gopinathannair, R.; Kamerzell, T.; Mansour, M.; Mahapatra, S.; Bartus, K.; Lakkireddy, D. Is paroxysmal supraventricular tachycardia truly benign? Insightful association between PSVT and stroke from a National Inpatient Database Study. *J. Interv. Card. Electrophysiol.* **2020**, *59*, 35–41. [CrossRef]

Geczy, T.; RamdatMisier, N.L.; Szili-Torok, T. Contact-force-sensing-based radiofrequency catheter ablation in paroxysmal supraventricular tachycardias (COBRA-PATH): A randomized controlled trial. *Trials* **2020**, *21*, 321. [CrossRef] [PubMed]

Kadish, A.; Passman, R. Mechanisms and management of paroxysmal supraventricular tachycardia. *Cardiol. Rev.* **1999**, *7*, 254–264. [CrossRef]

Teplitzky, B.A.; McRoberts, M.; Ghanbari, H. Deep learning for comprehensive ECG annotation. *Heart Rhythm* **2020**, *17 Pt B*, 881–888. [CrossRef]

Al'Aref, S.J.; Anchouche, K.; Singh, G.; Slomka, P.J.; Kolli, K.K.; Kumar, A.; Pandey, M.; Maliakal, G.; van Rosendael, A.R.; Beecy, A.N.; et al. Clinical applications of machine learning in cardiovascular disease and its relevance to cardiac imaging. *Eur. Heart J.* **2019**, *40*, 1975–1986. [CrossRef] [PubMed]

Baloglu, U.B.; Talo, M.; Yildirim, O.; Tan, R.S.; Acharya, U.R. Classification of myocardial infarction with multi-lead ECG signals and deep CNN. *Pattern Recognit. Lett.* **2019**, *122*, 23–30. [CrossRef]

Hannun, A.Y.; Rajpurkar, P.; Haghpanahi, M.; Tison, G.H.; Bourn, C.; Turakhia, M.P.; Ng, A.Y. Cardiologist-level arrhythmia detection and classification in ambulatory electrocardiograms using a deep neural network. *Nat. Med.* **2019**, *25*, 65–69. [CrossRef] [PubMed]

Siontis, K.C.; Noseworthy, P.A.; Attia, Z.I.; Friedman, P.A. Artificial intelligence-enhanced electrocardiography in cardiovascular disease management. *Nat. Rev. Cardiol.* **2021**, *18*, 465–478. [CrossRef]

Kwon, J.M.; Cho, Y.; Jeon, K.H.; Cho, S.; Kim, K.H.; Baek, S.D.; Jeung, S.; Park, J.; Oh, B.H. A deep learning algorithm to detect anaemia with ECGs: A retrospective, multicentre study. *Lancet Digit. Health* **2020**, *2*, e358–e367. [CrossRef]

Sridhar, N.; Shoeb, A.; Stephens, P.; Kharbouch, A.; Shimol, D.B.; Burkart, J.; Ghoreyshi, A.; Myers, L. Deep learning for automated sleep staging using instantaneous heart rate. *NPJ Digit. Med.* **2020**, *3*, 106. [CrossRef]

Feeny, A.K.; Chung, M.K.; Madabhushi, A.; Attia, Z.I.; Cikes, M.; Firouznia, M.; Friedman, P.A.; Kalscheur, M.M.; Kapa, S.; Narayan, S.M.; et al. Artificial intelligence and machine learning in arrhythmias and cardiac electrophysiology. *Circ. Arrhythm. Electrophysiol.* **2020**, *13*, e007952. [CrossRef]

Sun, J.Y.; Qiu, Y.; Guo, H.C.; Hua, Y.; Shao, B.; Qiao, Y.C.; Guo, J.; Ding, H.L.; Zhang, Z.Y.; Miao, L.F.; et al. A method to screen left ventricular dysfunction through ECG based on convolutional neural network. *J. Cardiovasc. Electrophysiol.* **2021**, *32*, 1095–1102. [CrossRef]

Attia, Z.I.; Kapa, S.; Lopez-Jimenez, F.; McKie, P.M.; Ladewig, D.J.; Satam, G.; Pellikka, P.A.; Enriquez-Sarano, M.; Noseworthy, P.A.; Munger, T.M.; et al. Screening for cardiac contractile dysfunction using an artificial intelligence-enabled electrocardiogram. *Nat. Med.* **2019**, *25*, 70–74. [CrossRef]

Attia, Z.I.; Noseworthy, P.A.; Lopez-Jimenez, F.; Asirvatham, S.J.; Deshmukh, A.J.; Gersh, B.J.; Carter, R.E.; Yao, X.; Rabinstein, A.A.; Erickson, B.J.; et al. An artificial intelligence-enabled ECG algorithm for the identification of patients with atrial fibrillation during sinus rhythm: A retrospective analysis of outcome prediction. *Lancet* **2019**, *394*, 861–867. [CrossRef]

Ioffe, S.; Szegedy, C. Batch normalization: Accelerating deep network training by reducing internal covariate shift. *Proc. Int. Conf. Mach. Learn.* **2015**, *37*, 448–456.

Nagi, J.; Ducatelle, F.; Di Caro, G.; Meier, C.U.; Giusti, A.; Nagi, F.; Schmidhuber, J.L.G. Max-pooling convolutional neural networks for vision-based hand gesture recognition. In Proceedings of the 2011 IEEE International Conference on Signal and Image Processing Applications (ICSIPA), Kuala Lumpur, Malaysia, 16–18 November 2011; pp. 342–347.

Hu, J.; Shen, L.; Albanie, S.; Sun, G.; Wu, E.H. Squeeze-and-Excitation Networks. *IEEE Trans. Pattern Anal. Mach. Intell.* **2020**, *42*, 2011–2023. [CrossRef] [PubMed]

Somani, S.; Russak, A.J.; Richter, F.; Zhao, S.; Vaid, A.; Chaudhry, F.; De Freitas, J.K.; Naik, N.; Miotto, R.; Nadkarni, G.N.; et al. Deep learning and the electrocardiogram: Review of the current state-of-the-art. *Europace* **2021**, *23*, 1179–1191. [CrossRef] [PubMed]

Jo, Y.-Y.; Kwon, J.-M.; Jeon, K.-H.; Cho, Y.-H.; Shin, J.-H.; Lee, Y.-J.; Jung, M.-S.; Ban, J.-H.; Kim, K.-H.; Lee, S.Y.; et al. Artificial intelligence to diagnose paroxysmal supraventricular tachycardia using electrocardiography during normal sinus rhythm. *Eur. Heart J. Digit. Health* **2021**, *2*, 290–298. [CrossRef]

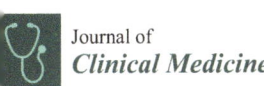

Safety and Efficacy of Left Atrial Catheter Ablation in Patients with Left Atrial Appendage Occlusion Devices

Binhao Wang, Bin He, Guohua Fu, Mingjun Feng, Xianfeng Du, Jing Liu, Yibo Yu and Huimin Chu *

Arrhythmia Center, Ningbo First Hospital, Ningbo 315000, China; wangbinhao0504@163.com (B.W.); socrates_he@126.com (B.H.); eagle1002@126.com (G.F.); fmj76@126.com (M.F.); drduxianfeng@126.com (X.D.); nblight6@126.com (J.L.); mubird@foxmail.com (Y.Y.)
* Correspondence: epnbheart@163.com

Abstract: Background: Left atrial appendage occlusion (LAAO) is an alternative to oral anticoagulation for thromboembolic prevention in patients with atrial fibrillation (AF). Left atrial (LA) catheter ablation (CA) in patients with LAAO devices has not been well investigated. Here, we report on the safety and efficacy of LA CA in patients with nitinol cage or plug LAAO devices. Methods: A total of 18 patients (aged 67 ± 11 years; 14 males; 5 paroxysmal AF) with LAAO devices (nitinol cage, $n = 10$; nitinol plug, $n = 8$) and symptomatic LA tachyarrhythmias were included. Periprocedural and follow-up data were assessed. Results: A total of 20 LA CA procedures were performed at a median of 130 (63, 338) days after LAAO. The strategy of CA consisted of circumferential pulmonary vein isolation ($n = 16$), linear lesions ($n = 14$) and complex fractionated atrial electrogram ablation ($n = 6$). No major adverse events occurred periprocedurally. Repeated transesophageal echocardiography showed no device-related thrombus, newly developed peridevice leakage or device dislodgement. After a median follow-up period of 793 (376, 1090) days, four patients (22%) experienced LA tachyarrhythmias recurrence and two received redo LA CA. No patients suffered stroke or major bleeding events during follow-up. Conclusions: LA CA in patients with LAAO devices (either nitinol cages or nitinol plugs) seems to be safe and efficient in our single-center experience.

Keywords: atrial fibrillation; catheter ablation; left atrial appendage occlusion

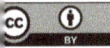

1. Introduction

Atrial fibrillation (AF) is the most common arrhythmia in the clinical setting and significantly increases the risk of stroke [1]. The majority of thrombi originate from the left atrial appendage (LAA) [2]. Oral anticoagulation (OAC) is recommended for nonvalvular AF patients with CHA_2DS_2-VASc scores ≥ 2 in males or ≥ 3 in females [1]. However, some patients have contraindications for long-term OAC (e.g., major bleeding events under OAC). Recently, left atrial appendage occlusion (LAAO) was proven to be noninferior to warfarin [3] and the nonvitamin antagonist oral anticoagulant (NOAC) [4] in stroke prevention. Left atrial (LA) catheter ablation (CA) is effective in maintaining sinus rhythm in patients with symptomatic AF [5]. However, the long-term influence of LA CA on stroke prevention remains unclear. Therefore, combining LA CA and LAAO in a single procedure has emerged as a successful strategy [6–8].

However, some patients may undergo LAAO first for stroke prevention. They may require LA CA for symptomatic LA tachyarrhythmias in the future. Data regarding this issue are limited. A small number of case reports [8–10] and case series [11–15] with small samples have been carried out to investigate the feasibility and efficacy of LA CA in patients with LAAO devices. However, most patients in prior studies were implanted with nitinol cage devices (e.g., Watchman). Investigations concerning LA CA in patients with nitinol plug devices (e.g., Amplatzer Cardiac Plug, ACP) are rare. We report on the safety and efficacy of LA CA for the treatment of LA tachyarrhythmias in patients with nitinol cage or plug LAAO devices.

2. Materials and Methods

2.1. Study Population

This was a retrospective, single-center study to assess the safety and efficacy of LA CA in 18 consecutive patients (aged 67 ± 11 years; 14 males; 5 exhibiting paroxysmal AF) with previously implanted LAAO devices (Watchman, $n = 10$; ACP, $n = 4$; LAmbre, $n = 4$) to treat symptomatic and drug-refractory LA tachyarrhythmias (AF, $n = 15$; atrial flutter (AFL), $n = 1$; atrial tachycardia (AT), $n = 2$) from March 2016 to October 2019 at Ningbo First Hospital. Patient characteristics were collected to calculate the individual CHA_2DS_2 VASc score [16] and HAS-BLED score [17]. Transesophageal echocardiography (TEE) was performed before LA CA to exclude LA thrombi and evaluate the LAAO devices for device-related thrombus (DRT) and peridevice leakage (PDL). Transthoracic echocardiography was also conducted to measure the LA diameter and left ventricular ejection fraction (LVEF). This study was approved by the Ethics Committee of Ningbo First Hospital and complies with the Declaration of Helsinki. Informed consent was obtained from all study participants.

2.2. LA CA Procedure

Antiarrhythmic drugs were stopped five half-lives before the procedure. Warfarin with a therapeutic international normalized ratio was continued uninterrupted, while NOACs were ceased 12~24 h preprocedurally. Patients were placed under deep sedation for LA CA. A decapolar diagnostic catheter was positioned in the coronary sinus through left femoral venous access. Double transseptal accesses were obtained for the placement of two sheaths via right femoral venous access. Intravenous heparin was administered prior to the first transseptal puncture with a target activated clotting time ≥ 350 s [1]. A circular mapping catheter and an irrigated tip ablation catheter were utilized for mapping and LA CA. Three-dimensional reconstruction of the LA and pulmonary veins (PV) was performed from the CT scan using electroanatomic mapping systems (CARTO, Biosense Webster, Diamond Bar CA, USA; or Ensite NavX Verismo software, St. Jude Medical, St. Paul, MN, USA). A maximum temperature cutoff of 43 °C and maximum power cutoff of 35 W were chosen, with a catheter infusion rate of 17–25 mL/min. Circumferential pulmonary vein isolation (CPVI) was performed in patients with AF. Additional linear lesions and/or complex fractionated atrial electrograms (CFAEs) were targeted if necessary. For macroreentrant LA tachyarrhythmias, ablation of linear lesions was performed. During all procedures within the LA, catheter impedance was closely monitored to avoid device-related complications. After the procedures, all patients underwent TEE to exclude pericardial effusion and evaluate the LAAO devices. Periprocedural adverse events included thromboembolic events (stroke, transient ischemic attack (TIA), or systemic embolism), pericardial effusion, bleeding events, interference with the device and device dislodgement. Major bleeding was defined according to the BARC (Bleeding Academic Research Consortium) criteria (type 3 or higher) [18].

2.3. Follow-Up

Antiarrhythmic drugs and OACs were recommended for 3 months after the procedure. OAC was then discontinued and displaced by a recommended postimplant regimen for LAAO devices [1]. TEE follow-up was arranged to determine the presence of device dislodgement, DRT or newly developed PDL. Clinical follow-up for LA tachyarrhythmias recurrence was performed at 3, 6 and 12 months using 24 h Holter monitoring. Arrhythmia recurrence was defined as documented LA tachyarrhythmias (AF, AFL, and AT) that lasted at least 30 s after a 3 month blanking period. Thromboembolic events (stroke, TIA, or systemic embolism) and bleeding events (major or minor) were also recorded during follow-up.

2.4. Statistical Analysis

The study patients were divided into two groups according to the type of LAAO devices: a nitinol cage group ($n = 10$) and a nitinol plug group ($n = 8$). The nitinol cage group included patients with previously implanted Watchman devices. The nitinol plug group consisted of subjects with ACP or LAmbre devices. Continuous variables were expressed as the median (interquartile range). Categorical variables were expressed as absolute numbers (percentages). Continuous variables were compared using the Mann–Whitney U test. Categorical variables were compared using the chi-square test or Fisher's exact test where appropriate. Survivor functions were estimated using the Kaplan–Meier method to assess the cumulative event-free curves of LA tachyarrhythmias for each group and statistically evaluated using a log-rank test of trend. Statistical analyses were performed with SPSS 19.0 (IBM, Armonk, NY, USA), and a p value < 0.05 was considered statistically significant.

3. Results

3.1. Patient Characteristics

Patient characteristics are displayed in Table 1. The median CHA_2DS_2-VASc and HAS-BLED scores were 4.5 (3, 6) and 3 (2.5, 4), respectively. Five patients (28%) had prior LA CA. The numbers of patients with prior stroke/TIA and bleeding were 16 (89%) and 7 (39%), respectively. The characteristics were comparable between the nitinol cage group and the nitinol plug group.

Table 1. Baseline characteristics.

Variable	Total	Nitinol Cage	Nitinol Plug	p Value
n	18	10	8	-
Age, years	70 (60, 74)	64 (57, 78)	71 (68, 74)	0.450
Male, n (%)	14 (78)	9 (90)	5 (63)	0.275
Type of arrhythmias, n (%)				
Paroxysmal AF	5 (28)	3 (30)	2 (25)	1.000
Persistent AF	10 (56)	6 (60)	4 (50)	1.000
AFL	1 (6)	0	1 (13)	0.444
AT	2 (11)	1 (10)	1 (13)	1.000
CHA_2DS_2-VASc score, points	4.5 (3, 6)	4 (3, 6)	4.5 (4, 6)	0.752
HAS-BLED score, points	3 (2.5, 4)	3 (2, 4)	3 (3, 5)	0.483
Prior stroke/TIA, n (%)	16 (89)	10 (100)	6 (75)	0.183
Prior bleeding, n (%)	7 (39)	5 (50)	2 (25)	0.367
Prior LA CA, n (%)	5 (28)	3 (30)	2 (25)	1.000
LA diameter, mm	42 (39, 45)	41 (36, 47)	43 (40, 45)	0.532
LVEF, %	64 (63, 67)	65 (63, 68)	64 (63, 67)	0.788

AF—atrial fibrillation; AFL—atrial flutter; AT—atrial tachycardia; CA—catheter ablation; LA—left atrium; LVEF—left ventricular ejection fraction; TIA—transient ischemic attack.

3.2. Periprocedural Data

The periprocedural data are shown in Table 2. The median time from LAAO to CA was 130 (63, 338) days. Twenty procedures (index procedure, $n = 18$; redo procedure, $n = 2$) were performed. During the index procedure in patients with AF or AFL, CPVI was targeted in all patients ($n = 16$), followed by linear lesions ($n = 10$) and CFAE ($n = 5$). The patient with AFL was mitral isthmus-dependent and was terminated by linear ablation at the mitral isthmus. One patient's case of AT was terminated by creating a linear lesion at the ridge between the left PV and LAA. Another patient with AT underwent prior ablation with CPVI, and all PVs were confirmed to be isolated. Two types of AT were detected and terminated by linear lesions (roof line plus anterior line). No LAA isolation was performed.

Two patients received redo ablation. One had AF recurrence 346 days after the index procedure. All PVs were still isolated, and linear lesions (roof line, posterior line, and superior vena cava line) and CFAE ablation were targeted to restore sinus rhythm. Another patient showed AFL recurrence 378 days after the index procedure. Activation mapping revealed localized reentry at the ridge between the LAA and left superior PV, and ablation at this region terminated the AFL (Figure 1).

The procedural time, ablation time, X-ray exposure time and X-ray exposure dose were similar between the two groups. At the end of all procedures, all PVs were successfully isolated, and bidirectional block was achieved at all lines that were applied. No thromboembolic events, pericardial effusion, major bleeding events, interference with the device and device dislodgement occurred periprocedurally. Two patients experienced minor bleeding events at the puncture site (one in the nitinol cage group and one in the nitinol plug group).

Table 2. Periprocedural data.

Variable	Total	Nitinol Cage	Nitinol Plug	*p* Value
No. of LA CA	20	11	9	-
Strategy of CA, *n* (%)				
CPVI	16 (80)	9 (82)	7 (78)	1.000
Linear lesions	14 (70)	6 (55)	8 (89)	0.157
CFAE	6 (30)	3 (27)	3 (33)	1.000
Procedural time, min	119 (89, 130)	112 (99, 126)	122 (79, 131)	0.894
Ablation time, min	34 (23, 46)	31 (20, 39)	40 (25, 52)	0.328
X-ray exposure time, min	5.0 (4.0, 6.1)	5.0 (3.8, 6.1)	4.9 (4.1, 6.0)	1.000
X-ray exposure dose, mGy	25 (20, 36)	23 (19, 40)	28 (24, 34)	0.534
Complications, *n* (%)				
Stroke/TIA	0	0	0	1.000
Systemic embolism	0	0	0	1.000
Pericardial effusion	0	0	0	1.000
Major bleeding events	0	0	0	1.000
Minor bleeding events	2 (10)	1 (9)	1 (11)	1.000
Interference with device	0	0	0	1.000
Device dislodgement	0	0	0	1.000

CA—catheter ablation; CFAE—complex fractionated atrial electrogram; CPVI—circumferential pulmonary vein isolation; LA—left atrium; TIA—transient ischemic attack.

3.3. Follow-Up Results

Follow-up results are shown in Table 3. OAC therapy was prescribed for all patients (two with warfarin, eight with dabigatran and eight with rivaroxaban) for 3 months. After 3 months, five patients switched to dual antiplatelet therapy (100 mg/d aspirin plus 75 mg/d clopidogrel) until 6 months post-LAAO, followed by single antiplatelet therapy (100 mg/d aspirin or 75 mg/d clopidogrel) indefinitely. The remaining 13 patients beyond 6 months after the LAAO procedure changed to single antiplatelet therapy. Repeated TEE was performed in 14 patients (78%). No DRT, newly developed PDL or device dislodgement was documented.

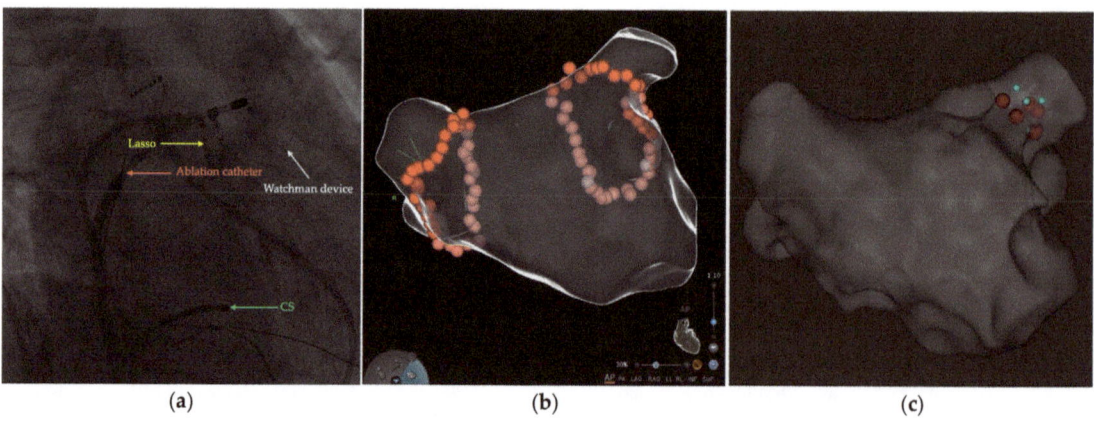

(a) (b) (c)

Figure 1. *Cont.*

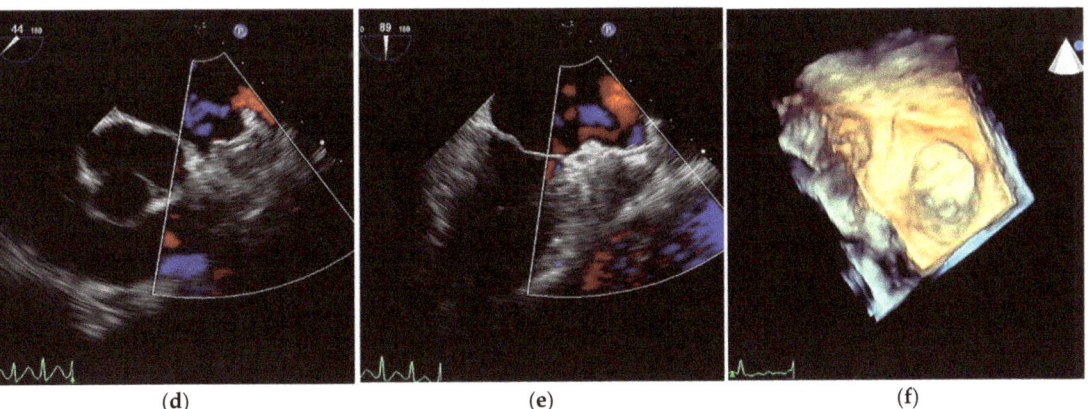

Figure 1. The LA CA procedure (index and redo) and TEE follow-up in a patient with an implanted LAAO device. (**a**) Fluoroscopic image showed the position of Watchman device (white arrow), coronary sinus catheter (green arrow), circular mapping catheter (yellow arrow) and ablation catheter (red arrow); (**b**) during the index procedure for paroxysmal AF, CPVI was successfully performed; (**c**) during the redo procedure for AFL, the ridge between the LAA and left superior PV were targeted (red dots) to restore sinus rhythm; (**d–f**) TEE follow-up after LA CA showed no device dislodgement, PDL, or DRT. AF—atrial fibrillation; AFL—atrial flutter; CA—catheter ablation; CPVI—circumferential pulmonary vein isolation; DRT—device-related thrombus; LA—left atrium; LAAO—left atrial appendage occlusion; PDL—peridevice leakage; PV—pulmonary vein.

After a median follow-up period of 793 (376, 1090) days, four patients (22%) experienced LA tachyarrhythmias recurrence (Figure 2a). The recurrence rates between the two groups showed no statistical significance (nitinol cage group, one AF and one AFL; nitinol plug group, two AF; Figure 2b). In addition, no patient suffered thromboembolic or major bleeding events. Only one patient in the nitinol cage group experienced gingival bleeding.

Table 3. Follow-up results.

Variable	Total	Nitinol Cage	Nitinol Plug	p Value
n	18	10	8	-
Recurrent LA tachyarrhythmias, n (%)	4 (22)	2 (20)	2 (25)	1.000
Redo ablation, n (%)	2 (11)	1 (10)	1 (13)	1.000
Stroke/TIA/systemic embolism, n (%)	0	0	0	1.000
Major bleeding events, n (%)	0	0	0	1.000
Minor bleeding events, n (%)	1 (6)	1 (10)	0	1.000
TEE follow-up, n (%)	14 (78)	8 (80)	6 (75)	1.000
DRT	0	0	0	1.000
Newly developed PDL	0	0	0	1.000
LAAO device dislodgement	0	0	0	1.000
OAC therapy, n (%)				
Warfarin	2 (11)	2 (20)	0	0.477
Dabigatran	8 (44)	4 (40)	4 (50)	1.000
Rivaroxaban	8 (44)	4 (40)	4 (50)	1.000

DRT—device-related thrombus; LA—left atrium; LAAO—left atrial appendage occlusion; OAC—oral anticoagulation; PDL—peridevice leakage; TEE—transesophageal echocardiography; TIA—transient ischemic attack.

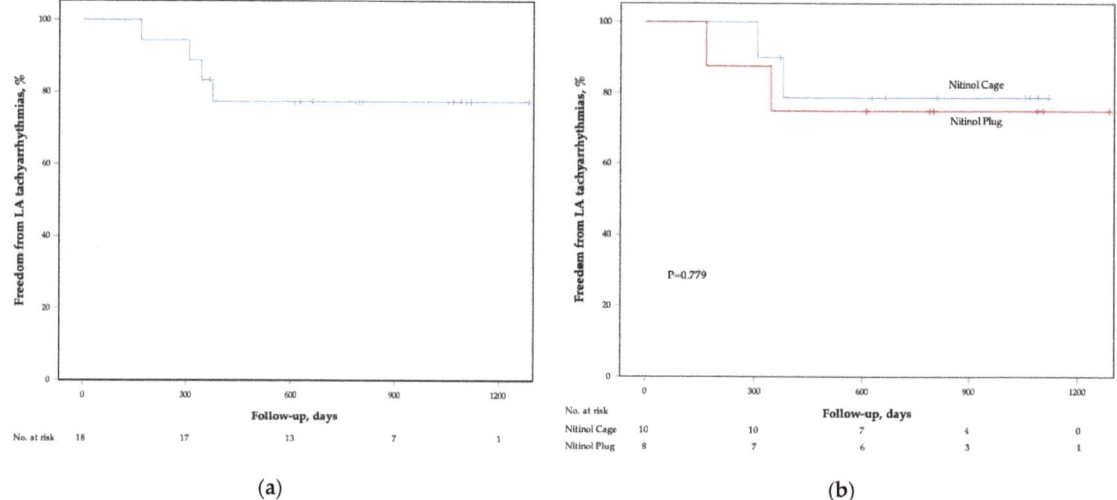

Figure 2. Kaplan–Meier cumulative event-free curves of LA tachyarrhythmias. (**a**) Total study population; (**b**) nitinol cage vs. nitinol plug. LA—left atrium.

4. Discussion

We present a single-center study on the safety and efficacy of LA CA in patients with LAAO devices. To the best of our knowledge, the present investigation is the first case series report including patients with nitinol plug devices to date. Our main finding is that LA CA in patients with either nitinol cage or nitinol plug devices seems to be safe and efficient.

An animal study showed that endothelial cells covered the endocardial surface with smooth muscle cells within 45 days of Watchman device implantation [19]. In another canine study, there was complete coverage of the ACP atrial surface by stable mature neointima in the device and within the surface neointima within 90 days of implantation [20]. No occurrence of late Watchman device embolization has been reported in previous investigations thus far [12]. In addition, late device embolization of ACP devices was also rare, with only a few case reports [21,22]. The minimum timeframe from Watchman device implantation to LA CA ranged from 41 days to 190 days [11–13]. In the present study, the minimum time-points of LA CA following LAAO device implantation were 47 days and 63 days in the nitinol cage group and nitinol plug group, respectively. It remained unclear how soon after LAAO device implantation LA CA could be considered according to the limited data.

Impedance-measurement errors may occur during LA CA. A case reported indicated that delivery of radiofrequency energy near the ACP device resulted in automatic generator shut-off with impedance-measurement errors [8]. However, impedance-measurement errors did not occur in previous investigations or in our study. One patient with a Watchman device had thrombus formation at the site of the device after LA CA [11]. In a multicenter AF registry, a higher proportion (10%) of severe PDLs after LAA isolation in patients with Watchman devices was indicated [14]. However, there were no newly developed PDLs in most patients without LAA isolation. Cryoballoon ablation may be an optional choice to avoid the contact with the LAAO device. Huang et al. [15] performed PVI in patients with Watchman device implantation by cryoballoon ablation. The study showed that cryoballoon ablation was feasible and safe in patients with preexisting LAAO devices. The above findings may have resulted from the damage of endothelial tissue covering the endocardial surface of the LAAO devices caused by the application of LA CA. No LAA isolation was targeted in our study, and no new PDL or DRT was detected after LA CA. Therefore, several points must be addressed: (1) TEE and/or cardiac CT should be arranged before the LA CA procedure to evaluate the anatomic characteristics of the LAAO device and left PV. (2) During procedure, satisfied LA anatomic mapping should be performed to guide ablation. The ablation points at the ridge between LAA and left PV should be chosen nearer to the left PV side to avoid the contact with LAAO device. Additionally, close monitoring of catheter impedance should be performed to avoid device-related complications. (3) OAC may be necessary after the LA CA procedure due to the potential damage of endothelial tissue on the LAAO devices. Most patients in the prior investigations and in our study received OAC therapy for at least 3 months. (4) Follow-up TEE should be performed before discontinuation of OACs to assess the presence of DRT and PDL.

CPVI is the cornerstone for the treatment of AF [23]. However, additional linear lesions and CFAE ablation are often required for persistent AF [24]. In our study, CPVI plus additional ablation was successfully performed in all patients. One patient with AT for index CA and one with AFL for redo CA (both had a Watchman device) had their arrhythmias successfully terminated by targeting the ridge between the LAA and left PV. The LAA has been recognized as a potential arrhythmogenic source in AF [25]. The BELIEF trial demonstrated that LAA isolation improved long-term freedom from atrial arrhythmias without increasing complications in patients with longstanding persistent AF [26]. In the study by Turagam et al., 28% (17/60) of the study population had focal triggered activity from the LAA in patients with Watchman device implantation, and LAA isolation was achieved in 58% (10/17) [14]. LAA isolation is a challenging procedure in patients with LAAO devices. Theoretically, it should be more difficult in patients with nitinol plug devices covering the ostium of the LAA. The nitinol plug devices contain a proximal disc that extends outside the ostium of the LAA toward the LA ridge. Because of the overlap of this disc and the LA ridge, successful LAA isolation in these patients may be technically more difficult than for patients implanted with the nitinol cage devices. In addition, LAA isolation may result in newly developed PDLs, as mentioned above. Therefore, whether LAA isolation is necessary and feasible in patients with LAAO devices still needs further discussion.

No major periprocedural adverse events or thromboembolic or major bleeding events during follow-up occurred in our study. The complications in other studies were rare and mainly occurred at the site of puncture (e.g., hematoma and arteriovenous fistula) [12–14]. Additionally, none of the patients suffered major bleeding events or stroke during follow-up [12–14]. The rate of patients free from LA tachyarrhythmias during follow-up ranged from 42% to 83% in prior studies [12–15]. In the present research, 78% remained in sinus rhythm after a median follow-up period of 793 days. The difference in the recurrence rate in different studies may be attributed to the difference in patient characteristics and the limited number of patients. Therefore, LA CA for the treatment of LA tachyarrhythmias in patients with LAAO devices is likely to be safe and efficient. However, the safety and efficacy should be further assessed in the future in large study populations.

There are several limitations in our study. First, the study sample was relatively small. However, this is the first investigation including a case series with previously implanted nitinol plug devices. Second, all the procedures were performed using radiofrequency energy. The experience from the present investigation cannot be extended to other ablation energies (e.g., cryoablation and pulsed field ablation). Third, four patients refused to finish TEE follow-up after LA CA. Therefore, the presence or absence of DRT and newly developed PDL was unknown in those patients.

5. Conclusions

LA CA in patients with prior implanted LAAO devices (either nitinol cages or nitinol plugs) seems to be safe and efficient in our single-center experience. Further multicenter investigations with a large study population are needed to prove this finding in the future.

Author Contributions: Conceptualization, B.W. and H.C.; methodology, B.W. and H.C.; software, B.W.; formal analysis, B.W. and G.F.; investigation, B.W., B.H., G.F. and H.C.; data curation, B.W. and G.F.; writing—original draft preparation, B.W., B.H. and G.F.; writing—review and editing, M.F., X.D., J.L., Y.Y. and H.C. All authors have read and agreed to the published version of the manuscript.

Funding: This research was funded by the Basic Public Welfare Research Project of Zhejiang Province grant number LGJ20H20001.

Institutional Review Board Statement: The study was conducted according to the guidelines of the Declaration of Helsinki and approved by the Ethics Committee of Ningbo First Hospital (protocol code 2020-R141).

Informed Consent Statement: Informed consent was obtained from all subjects involved in the study.

Data Availability Statement: The data used to support the findings of this study are available from the corresponding author upon reasonable request.

Acknowledgments: We wish to acknowledge all the patients in this study.

Conflicts of Interest: The authors declare no conflict of interest.

References

1. Hindricks, G.; Potpara, T.; Dagres, N.; Arbelo, E.; Bax, J.J.; Blomstrom-Lundqvist, C.; Boriani, G.; Castella, M.; Dan, G.A.; Dilaveris, P.E.; et al. 2020 ESC Guidelines for the diagnosis and management of atrial fibrillation developed in collaboration with the European Association for Cardio-Thoracic Surgery (EACTS). *Eur. Heart J.* **2021**, *42*, 373–498. [CrossRef] [PubMed]
2. Blackshear, J.L.; Odell, J.A. Appendage obliteration to reduce stroke in cardiac surgical patients with atrial fibrillation. *Ann. Thorac. Surg.* **1996**, *61*, 755–759. [CrossRef]
3. Reddy, V.Y.; Doshi, S.K.; Kar, S.; Gibson, D.N.; Price, M.J.; Huber, K.; Horton, R.P.; Buchbinder, M.; Neuzil, P.; Gordon, N.T.; et al. 5-Year Outcomes After Left Atrial Appendage Closure: From the PREVAIL and PROTECT AF Trials. *J. Am. Coll. Cardiol.* **2017**, *70*, 2964–2975. [CrossRef] [PubMed]
4. Osmancik, P.; Herman, D.; Neuzil, P.; Hala, P.; Taborsky, M.; Kala, P.; Poloczek, M.; Stasek, J.; Haman, L.; Branny, M.; et al. 4-Year Outcomes After Left Atrial Appendage Closure Versus Nonwarfarin Oral Anticoagulation for Atrial Fibrillation. *J. Am. Coll. Cardiol.* **2022**, *79*, 1–14. [CrossRef] [PubMed]
5. Wilber, D.J.; Pappone, C.; Neuzil, P.; De Paola, A.; Marchlinski, F.; Natale, A.; Macle, L.; Daoud, E.G.; Calkins, H.; Hall, B.; et al. Comparison of antiarrhythmic drug therapy and radiofrequency catheter ablation in patients with paroxysmal atrial fibrillation: A randomized controlled trial. *JAMA* **2010**, *303*, 333–340. [CrossRef] [PubMed]
6. Du, X.; Chu, H.; Ye, P.; He, B.; Xu, H.; Jiang, S.; Lin, M.; Lin, R.; Liu, J.; Wang, B.; et al. Combination of left atrial appendage closure and catheter ablation in a single procedure for patients with atrial fibrillation: Multicenter experience. *J. Formos. Med. Assoc.* **2019**, *118*, 891–897. [CrossRef]
7. Fassini, G.; Conti, S.; Moltrasio, M.; Maltagliati, A.; Tundo, F.; Riva, S.; Dello Russo, A.; Casella, M.; Majocchi, B.; Zucchetti, M.; et al. Concomitant cryoballoon ablation and percutaneous closure of left atrial appendage in patients with atrial fibrillation. *Europace* **2016**, *18*, 1705–1710. [CrossRef]
8. Steckman, D.A.; Nguyen, D.T.; Sauer, W.H. Catheter ablation of atrial fibrillation and left atrial flutter in a patient with a left atrial appendage occlusion device. *Europace* **2014**, *16*, 651. [CrossRef]
9. Huang, H.D.; Patel, V.M.; Sharma, P.S.; Jameria, Z.; Lazar, S.; Trohman, R.; Wissner, E. Cryoballoon pulmonary vein isolation and voltage mapping for symptomatic atrial fibrillation 9 months after Watchman device implantation. *HeartRhythm Case Rep.* **2018**, *4*, 6–9. [CrossRef]
10. Pietrasik, G.M.; Huang, H.D.; Rodriguez, J.M.; Sharma, P.S.; Trohman, R.G.; Krishnan, K. Safety and feasibility of radiofrequency redo pulmonary vein isolation ablation for atrial fibrillation after Amulet implantation and device electrical characteristics. *HeartRhythm Case Rep.* **2020**, *6*, 415–418. [CrossRef]
11. Heeger, C.H.; Rillig, A.; Lin, T.; Mathew, S.; Deiss, S.; Lemes, C.; Botros, M.; Metzner, A.; Wissner, E.; Kuck, K.H.; et al. Feasibility and clinical efficacy of left atrial ablation for the treatment of atrial tachyarrhythmias in patients with left atrial appendage closure devices. *Heart Rhythm* **2015**, *12*, 1524–1531. [CrossRef] [PubMed]
12. Walker, D.T.; Phillips, K.P. Left atrial catheter ablation subsequent to Watchman(R) left atrial appendage device implantation: A single centre experience. *Europace* **2015**, *17*, 1402–1406. [CrossRef]
13. Wintgens, L.I.S.; Klaver, M.N.; Swaans, M.J.; Alipour, A.; Balt, J.C.; van Dijk, V.F.; Rensing, B.; Wijffels, M.; Boersma, L.V.A. Left atrial catheter ablation in patients with previously implanted left atrial appendage closure devices. *Europace* **2019**, *21*, 428–433. [CrossRef] [PubMed]
14. Turagam, M.K.; Lavu, M.; Afzal, M.R.; Vuddanda, V.; Jazayeri, M.A.; Parikh, V.; Atkins, D.; Bommana, S.; Di Biase, L.; Horton, R.; et al. Catheter Ablation for Atrial Fibrillation in Patients with Watchman Left Atrial Appendage Occlusion Device: Results from a Multicenter Registry. *J. Cardiovasc. Electrophysiol.* **2017**, *28*, 139–146. [CrossRef] [PubMed]

25. Huang, H.D.; Krishnan, K.; Sharma, P.S.; Kavinsky, C.J.; Rodriguez, J.; Ravi, V.; Larsen, T.R.; Trohman, R.G. Cryoballoon Ablation and Bipolar Voltage Mapping in Patients with Left Atrial Appendage Occlusion Devices. *Am. J. Cardiol.* **2020**, *135*, 99–104. [CrossRef] [PubMed]
26. Lip, G.Y.; Nieuwlaat, R.; Pisters, R.; Lane, D.A.; Crijns, H.J. Refining clinical risk stratification for predicting stroke and thromboembolism in atrial fibrillation using a novel risk factor-based approach: The euro heart survey on atrial fibrillation. *Chest* **2010**, *137*, 263–272. [CrossRef]
27. Pisters, R.; Lane, D.A.; Nieuwlaat, R.; de Vos, C.B.; Crijns, H.J.; Lip, G.Y. A novel user-friendly score (HAS-BLED) to assess 1-year risk of major bleeding in patients with atrial fibrillation: The Euro Heart Survey. *Chest* **2010**, *138*, 1093–1100. [CrossRef]
28. Mehran, R.; Rao, S.V.; Bhatt, D.L.; Gibson, C.M.; Caixeta, A.; Eikelboom, J.; Kaul, S.; Wiviott, S.D.; Menon, V.; Nikolsky, E.; et al. Standardized bleeding definitions for cardiovascular clinical trials: A consensus report from the Bleeding Academic Research Consortium. *Circulation* **2011**, *123*, 2736–2747. [CrossRef]
29. Schwartz, R.S.; Holmes, D.R.; Van Tassel, R.A.; Hauser, R.; Henry, T.D.; Mooney, M.; Matthews, R.; Doshi, S.; Jones, R.M.; Virmani, R. Left atrial appendage obliteration: Mechanisms of healing and intracardiac integration. *JACC Cardiovasc. Interv.* **2010**, *3*, 870–877. [CrossRef]
30. Bass, J.L. Transcatheter occlusion of the left atrial appendage–experimental testing of a new Amplatzer device. *Catheter. Cardiovasc. Interv.* **2010**, *76*, 181–185. [CrossRef]
31. Aminian, A.; Chouchane, I.; Compagnie, M.; Decubber, M.; Lalmand, J. Delayed and fatal embolization of a left atrial appendage closure device. *Circ. Cardiovasc. Interv.* **2014**, *7*, 628–630. [CrossRef] [PubMed]
32. Schroeter, M.R.; Danner, B.C.; Hunlich, M.; Schillinger, W. Uncommon delayed and late complications after percutaneous left atrial appendage closure with Amplatzer((R)) Cardiac Plug. *Clin. Res. Cardiol.* **2014**, *103*, 285–290. [CrossRef] [PubMed]
33. Ouyang, F.; Tilz, R.; Chun, J.; Schmidt, B.; Wissner, E.; Zerm, T.; Neven, K.; Kokturk, B.; Konstantinidou, M.; Metzner, A.; et al. Long-term results of catheter ablation in paroxysmal atrial fibrillation: Lessons from a 5-year follow-up. *Circulation* **2010**, *122*, 2368–2377. [CrossRef] [PubMed]
34. Tilz, R.R.; Rillig, A.; Thum, A.M.; Arya, A.; Wohlmuth, P.; Metzner, A.; Mathew, S.; Yoshiga, Y.; Wissner, E.; Kuck, K.H.; et al. Catheter ablation of long-standing persistent atrial fibrillation: 5-year outcomes of the Hamburg Sequential Ablation Strategy. *J. Am. Coll. Cardiol.* **2012**, *60*, 1921–1929. [CrossRef] [PubMed]
35. Di Biase, L.; Burkhardt, J.D.; Mohanty, P.; Sanchez, J.; Mohanty, S.; Horton, R.; Gallinghouse, G.J.; Bailey, S.M.; Zagrodzky, J.D.; Santangeli, P.; et al. Left atrial appendage: An underrecognized trigger site of atrial fibrillation. *Circulation* **2010**, *122*, 109–118. [CrossRef]
36. Di Biase, L.; Burkhardt, J.D.; Mohanty, P.; Mohanty, S.; Sanchez, J.E.; Trivedi, C.; Gunes, M.; Gokoglan, Y.; Gianni, C.; Horton, R.P.; et al. Left Atrial Appendage Isolation in Patients with Longstanding Persistent AF Undergoing Catheter Ablation: BELIEF Trial. *J. Am. Coll. Cardiol.* **2016**, *68*, 1929–1940. [CrossRef]

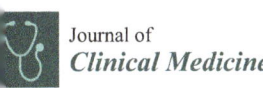

Review

Strategies for Safe Implantation and Effective Performance of Single-Chamber and Dual-Chamber Leadless Pacemakers

Fei Tong and Zhijun Sun *

Department of Cardiology, Shengjing Hospital of China Medical University, Shenyang 110004, China; tongfeimed@163.com
* Correspondence: 18940251218@163.com

Abstract: Leadless pacemakers (LPMs) have emerged as an alternative to conventional transvenous pacemakers to eliminate the complications associated with leads and subcutaneous pockets. However, LPMs still present with complications, such as cardiac perforation, dislodgment, vascular complications, infection, and tricuspid valve regurgitation. Furthermore, the efficacy of the leadless VDD LPMs is influenced by the unachievable 100% atrioventricular synchrony. In this article, we review the available data on the strategy selection, including appropriate patient selection, procedure techniques, device design, and post-implant programming, to minimize the complication rate and maximize the efficacy, and we summarize the clinical settings in which a choice must be made between VVI LPMs, VDD LPMs, or conventional transvenous pacemakers. In addition, we provide an outlook for the technology for the realization of true dual-chamber leadless and battery-less pacemakers.

Keywords: leadless single-chamber pacemaker; complication; atrioventricular synchrony; leadless dual-chamber pacemaker; strategy selection

1. Introduction

Conventional transvenous pacemakers (TPMs) have been the cornerstone of the treatment of bradyarrhythmias. Researchers have estimated that more than one million devices have been implanted annually in recent years [1]. Despite numerous technological advances since the introduction of TPMs, lead- and pocket-related complications are still common. Acute complications involving pneumothorax, cardiac perforation, lead dislodgment, pocket infection, or hematoma occur in 12% of patients [2], and chronic complications such as lead malfunction, lead-related endovascular infection, and tricuspid valve (TV) dysfunction occur at rates of 2.5–5.5%, 0.5–1.3% and 14.5%, respectively, in those who have received TPM implantation [3–6]. With technological advances in device miniaturization, communication, and battery longevity, leadless pacemakers (LPMs) have emerged as an alternative to TPMs to eliminate the complications associated with leads and subcutaneous pockets. However, the LPM usage was restricted by its indication area (single-chamber only) and specific complications, with a short-term complication rate of 4–6.7% [7,8] and a chronic complication rate of 4.6–6.6% [9,10]. Many strategies, including appropriate patient selection, procedure techniques, device design and postimplant programming, have been developed to overcome complicated situations. In this review, we summarize the safety and efficacy of the currently available LPMs, and we discuss strategies to minimize the complication rate and maximize the efficacy, providing an outlook for the technology for the realization of true dual-chamber leadless and battery-less pacemakers.

2. Leadless Ventricular Pacemakers

2.1. Brief History and Current State of Two Leadless Systems

Nanostim (St.Jude, Saint Paul, MN, USA), as the first commercially available LPM capable of the VVI(R) pacing mode, was launched in 2012; however, the use of Nanostim

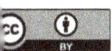

implantation was discontinued due to the detachment of the docking button and premature battery failures, which occurred at two years after implantation [11]. The Aveir VR (Abbot Abbott Park, IL, USA) by Abbott, which is an improvement of the Nanostim LPM, received Food and Drug Administration (FDA) approval on April 2022, and it could provide an expandable platform to support dual-chamber pacing once approved by the FDA [12].

The Micra VR (Medtronic, Minneapolis, MN, USA), which is now widely used over the world, was first implanted in 2013 and it obtained FDA approval in 2016. The main indications for the Micra VR implantation are atrial fibrillation (AF) with slow ventricular response, as well as non-AF with low anticipated ventricular pacing, such as transient atrioventricular (AV) block and sinus node dysfunction [13,14]. The Micra AV (Medtronic) is the only currently available LPM that is capable of delivering the VDD pacing mode [15,16]. With an identical mass, appearance, design, and implant procedure to the Micra VR, the novel algorithm of the Micra AV discerns the signal of atrial mechanical contraction through the intracardiac accelerometer from the device in the right ventricle (RV) and fulfills AV synchrony. Limited by the mechanism of accelerometer-based atrial sensing rather than electric atrial sensing, and the absence of a pacing device in the right atrial (RA), the Micra AV is not suitable for those indicated for conventional DDD-TPMs, such as those with sick sinus syndrome and poor atrial contraction.

Elderly or malnourished patients with high infectious risk are prone to choosing LPMs [17,18]. Patients on haemodialysis would benefit from LPM implantation because it spares the subclavian and superior cava veins for dialysis treatment. The obstruction of the venous route used for TPM and potential pocket issues (e.g., in the case of dementia) are the indications for LPM [17]. Apart from patients with clinical frailty, younger patients also choose LPMs out of esthetical or active lifestyle concerns [19]. However, the scant clinical data regarding the end-of-life strategy and the possibility of implanting two or more LPMs in the same patient limit the routine use of LPMs in patients with a life expectancy of >20 years [17].

2.2. Evaluation of Clinical Performance and Recommendation of Strategies

The success rate of LPM implantation was extraordinarily high for the Micra VR with 99.2% (719/725) in the Micra Investigational Device Exemption (IDE) trial [20] and 99.1% (1801/1817) in a real-world setting [21]. The success rate was 98% (196/200) for the Aveir VR in the LEADLESS II phase 2 IDE study. The mean pacing threshold and R-wave amplitude of the Micra VR were 0.66 ± 0.55 V at 0.24 ms and 11.1 ± 5.2 mV at implantation and the electrical parameters remained stable during 18 months of follow-up [21]. A total of 196 patients were successfully implanted with the Aveir VR. For 95.9% of these patients, the pacing thresholds were less than 2.0 V at 0.4 ms and the R waves were greater than 5.0 mV at the 6 week follow-up [12]. However, no clear consensus has been determined in terms of the complication rate of LPMs when compared to TPMs. The Micra VR was associated with 48% and 63% lower risks of major complications than those of a historical TPM cohort in the Micra IDE trial [20] and the Micra Post-Approval Registry (PAR) [21], respectively during the 12 month follow-up period. The analyses were based on the comparison with a historical TPM cohort and a long-term follow-up period [20,21]. However, a meta-analysis on four studies showed no difference in the incidences of any complications between LPMs and TPMs [22]. Moreover, in a prospective analysis, no significant difference at an almost 2 year complication rate was observed between LPMs and TPMs [23], which could be because the contemporary complication rate of TPMs is significantly lower than the historical one as a result of standard implantation procedures and improved techniques. However, a contemporary prospective propensity-matched analysis also demonstrated that the rate of complication in a TPM cohort was 4.9% vs. 0.9% in a LPM cohort, during 800 days of follow-up and after excluding the pacemaker advisory-related complications [24]. Furthermore, in real-world practice, Micra implantation ($n = 16,825$) is associated with a lower complication rate of 8.6%, which is lower than the 11.2% of contemporary TPM implantation ($n = 564,100$) [25]. A continuous enrollment study and contemporaneous comparison of the

Micra and TPMs in the Micra Coverage with Evidence Development (CED) study observed that the Micra implantation was associated with 23% fewer and 31% fewer complications compared with TPMs over 6 months [26] and 2 years [9], respectively, indicating that the fewer LPM complications were due to a time-dependent effect, which was also manifested by the improved LPM complication rates from the 6 month follow-up to the 2 year follow-up, and the similar 30 day adjusted complication rate of LPMs to that of TPMs [26]. A large and real-world analysis of the national database from the United States showed that, overall, the unadjusted in-hospital complication rate of 16% for LPMs was higher than that of the 6.4% for TPMs; however, it should be noted that the patients with LPMs in this analysis were older and had more sepsis, chronic kidney disease, heart failure and malnutrition [18]. Transvenous lead- and subcutaneous-pocket-related complications account for most of these TPM complications [3,4], and they take time to occur. In contrast, the more frequent incidences of cardiac perforation and pericardial effusion in LPMs than TPMs and the relatively high incidence of vascular complications in LPMs are short-term complications, both of which form a non-conclusive picture of the complications encountered with LPMs vs. TPMs. The discrepancies of the complication percentages between studies are partly because some studies only report complications requiring reinterventions [24], while some studies describe all complications [25].

2.2.1. Cardiac Perforation and Pericardial Effusion

The overall rate of cardiac perforation and pericardial effusion in the Micra IDE, Micra PAR, and Micra Continued Access study was 1.1% (32/2817) [27]. The risk of pericardial effusion after the implantation of Micra decreased from 1.8% to 0.8% over time [27]. The rate of pericardial effusion was 0.8% in the Micra CED study. The Manufacturer and User Facility Device Experience (MAUDE) report also estimated a 1% incidence of cardiac tamponade, and more than three times the cardiac tamponade of the Micra compared with the TPM ventricular lead [28]. In a real-world setting, 1.3% of LPM recipients suffered from cardiac effusion or perforation [18], and the figure was significantly higher than that of TPM recipients [25]. Similarly, as for Aveir VR implantation, the rate of cardiac tamponade was 1.5% (3/200) in the LEADLESS II-phase 2 IDE study [12]. A relatively high rate of cardiac perforation following LPM implantation could be worrying; hence, we recommend measures to be taken and strategies to limit those adverse events:

Patients' characteristics: Apart from the patients' characteristics, such as old age, female gender, and chronic obstructive pulmonary disease (COPD) that easily develops cardiac injury [20], a low body mass index (BMI) and congestive heart failure were also identified by the PAR investigators as predictors of perforation [21]. A novel risk score model, which included similar risk factors such as age of >85 years, BMI of <20, female gender, heart failure, prior myocardial infarction, COPD, haemodialysis, and the absence of previous cardiothoracic surgery, was developed and validated to predict pericardial effusion [27]. Additional attention should be paid to the presence of the abovementioned risk factors.

Procedure technique: The positioning of the Micra at the interventricular septum has been linked to a lower risk of cardiac perforation compared with the apex or free wall [20], and deployment in the mid-septum should be achieved [29], which leads to a narrower-paced QRS complex [30]. However, deploying a Micra near the anterior interventricular groove might increase the risk of perforation [31]. Contrast injection is recommended to ensure a mid-septal position in orthogonal fluoroscopic views prior to deployment [29], and RV trabeculation in front of and inferior to the tip of the delivery catheter suggests the septum location, as opposed to a lack of trabeculation, which suggests the apical location [29] (Figure 1). The combination of orthogonal fluoroscopic views and transthoracic echocardiography in the subxiphoid, parasternal, and apical views without contrast injection significantly reduces inadvertent non-septal implantation compared with ventriculography [32]. The pacing threshold will frequently improve over 2–3 min, and especially when the impedance suggests good myocardial apposition (>500 ohms). Therefore, it is reasonable to allow at least 3 min for the thresholds to improve before deciding on an alternate location [33]. As for the sensed R-wave, a 1.5-mV increase in R-wave amplitude after approximately 13 min since the first deployment is predictive of a reduction of pacing threshold below 1 V/0.24 ms at follow-up, which also suggests that waiting and evaluating a second electrical parameter may be capable to avoid unnecessary device repositioning in case of high pacing threshold recording at implant [34].

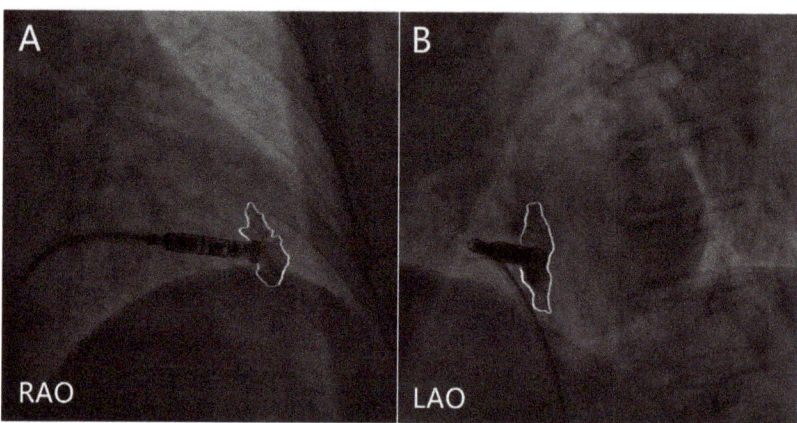

Figure 1. Contrast injection in right anterior oblique (RAO) and left anterior oblique (LAO) projections. The white lines delineate the contrast outlines. (**A**) The contrast seen both in front of and inferior to the tip of the delivery catheter in RAO projection suggests a non-apical location. (**B**) The contrast delineates the ventricular septum in LAO projection.

Device design: The tine-based fixation mechanism of the Micra permits the measurement of the electrical parameters only after deployment and active fixation into the myocardium, which inevitably increases the need for repeated attempts at deployment once the parameters are unsatisfied and there is a risk of pericardial effusion [27,35]. Different from the Micra, the contact mapping capability of the Aveir VR helps to optimally position the device before fixation [12,36], which could prevent the need for multiple attempts. Of the successful implants, 83.2% (163/196) of the Aveir VR implantation did not require repositioning in the LEADLESS II phase 2, while one deployment sufficed in only 60.0% (1583/2638) of the Micra implantations [27]. In contrast to adequate forward pressure applied to form the "goose neck" appearance of the delivery system prior to the implantation of the tine-based Micra, firm pressure is not required nor recommended and a softer touch with tissue contact is sufficient for the Aveir VR to achieve stable fixation via the slow rotation of device [36].

Rescue strategies: Unlike transvenous lead perforations, Micra perforations are often large and life-threatening. The MAUDE reports a higher rate of mortality following perforations with the Micra compared with TPMs [28]; thus, intervention that includes pericardiocentesis and surgery is required to rescue patients. In the Micra PAR, 71% (10/14) of the cardiac effusion patients required pericardiocentesis and 14% (2/14) required surgical repair [21]. Data from a real-world setting showed that 36% (82/228) of pericardial effusion patients had the need for pericardiocentesis, and 11.5% (26/228) required a thoracotomy. A higher proportion (26% (146/563)) of Micra-related perforations requiring emergency surgery was also reported in the MAUDE [37].

2.2.2. Dislodgment

Micra dislodgment was rare and limited to case reports with no dislodgment in the Micra IDE trial [20]. A total of 0.06% of the implantations resulted in dislodgment in the Micra PAR [21], and 0.51% (40/7821) of the implantations resulted in dislodgment in the real-world setting, in comparison with the relatively high rate of lead dislodgment in TPMs, which ranged between 1% and 2.55% [38]. The dislodged device could migrate to a remote location, such as the pulmonary artery, causing acute respiratory failure [39], or could produce no symptoms if the LPM is wedged in a stable manner [40], or it could be stuck in the right ventricle, causing non-sustained ventricular tachycardia [41] and damage to the TV and papillary muscles. Some types of dislodgment only manifested the loss of capture without obvious dislocation [42].

Patients' characteristics: Due to the limited amount of data, no risk factors concerning the underlying etiology for dislodgment were identified. Based on the currently available case reports, a complex heart anatomy [41,43] and myocardial fibrosis or scars in cardiac amyloidosis or ischemic cardiomyopathy might influence the engagement of the tines [41].

Procedure technique: The fixation of at least two tines is acceptable for the Micra according to the manufacturer's training recommendation; however, several dislodgment cases met the criterion of two tines [39,44,45], which indicates that the movement of two tines by the pull-and-hold test is not a guarantee against dislodgment, and that the pull-and-hold test, per se, is not an objective evaluation of the tine movement. A stable and low pacing threshold (<1 V at 0.24 ms is ideal; however, ≤2 V at 0.24 ms is considered acceptable), high sensed R wave, high impedance, and the recorded current of the injury may indicate solid fixation. Unstable impedance by the repeated measurement could suggest an insecure connection between the device and myocardium [44]. Final implant thresholds above 2 V are not recommended [33]. In situations of multiple reposition failures, it is recommended to remove and re-flush the delivery system to clean off clots, and an effective strategy is to implant LPM in the apical position and to obtain the R-wave at approximately 10 mV and the pacing threshold far below 1V in a series of three to four interrogations [46]. This strategy can be attempted by experienced operators, and is not recommended for operators at the beginning of the learning curve in consideration of the risk of cardiac perforation [46].

Rescue strategies: A Micra introducer sheath with either a delivery catheter or steerable Agilis sheath is implemented to align with the Micra with an acute rise in capture threshold, but without obvious dislocation noted, and loop snares of different sizes (range 7–10 mm) and shape (single loop or multiple loop) with integrated protective sleeves are used to capture the proximal retrieval feature or the body of LPM if the proximal retrieval feature cannot be engaged [47]. In complex situations, such as the migration of the device to the pulmonary artery or its free movement in the RV, the two-snare technique is applied as follows: one snare captures any tine that is not engaged in the endocardium to minimize the Micra movement, and a second snare captures the retrieval feature or the body of the Micra capsule [41,42,44,48]. Additionally, a gooseneck snare from the femoral venous approach can also be used to retrieve LPM, embolizing the pulmonary artery [49].

2.2.3. Vascular Complications

The Micra VR and Aveir VR are both delivered through 27F (outer diameter) introducer sheaths. Large-bore venous access for LPM implantation could induce vascular complications, such as arteriovenous fistulas (AVFs), pseudoaneurysms, bleeding and hematomas. Incidences of 0.6–1.4% for vascular complications were reported in the Micra PAR study [21] and Micra CED study [26].

Medicine preparation: The Micra VR and Aveir VR are approved for patients with AF complicated by bradycardia. The results from the Micra PAR indicated whether the intermittent interruption of anticoagulation in the perioperative setting could not significantly influence vascular-related events [50], which meant that the Micra without the interruption of anticoagulation could be performed. Although no suggestions from the guidelines are provided on the perioperative anticoagulation management in LPM procedures, continued warfarin if the international normalized ratio is <3 and the temporary interruption of new oral anticoagulants 24 h before the LPM procedure may be safe and have already been applied in clinical practice [50–52].

Procedure technique: A puncture site of the femoral vein just higher or at the level of insertion of the great saphenous vein is recommended to reduce the risk of AVF [29]. A puncture site below the common femoral artery or vein is a risk factor for pseudoaneurysm. In complex cases in which multiple arteries are inadvertently punctured, vascular ultrasound guidance or micropuncture techniques could be considered to avoid vascular complications [50]. More than half of the cases of haemostasis following LPM implantation were achieved using figure-of-eight sutures [53], and the application of pressure alone should be avoided for the 27F introducer sheath [29]. Surgical isolation of the common femoral vein for the purpose of sheath insertion in patients with severe obesity and vascular haemostasis and suture performed by vascular surgeon were effective and safe in LPM implantation [54].

Rescue strategies: Studies on AVF indicated that 38% of the cases of iatrogenic femoral AVF self-resolved at 1 year [55] and that iatrogenic AVFs should be repaired using a covered stent to seal the shunting of the AVF only when the shunting has hemodynamic consequences [56]. However, these AVFs were vascular access complications of percutaneous coronary interventions, in which sheath sizes of 7F or 8F were used. As for LPM implantation, in which a sheath of 27F is used, intervention or surgical repair may be a necessary choice. A stable pseudoaneurysm diameter of <2 cm can be conservatively managed with observation, and a pseudoaneurysm diameter of >2 cm can be managed with ultrasound-guided thrombin injection, surgical repair, or covered stent placement [57].

2.2.4. Infection

By virtue of the elimination of surgical pockets and transvenous leads, less surface area and endovascular encapsulation, LPMs have a low incidence of infection, as no infections were identified among the 3726 patients with LPMs during the 6 month follow-up in the Micra CED study [26]. A total of 33 infections out of 726 cases was recorded in the Micra IDE trial [20]; however, none of these events were associated with device- or procedure-related infections. Procedure-related infections, including abdominal wall infections, infected groin hematomas, and sepsis, occurred at 0.17% in the Micra PAR [21]; however, none of these infection cases required device removal. As for the Aveir VR, no device-related infections have been reported so far [12]. LPMs have been shown to have some unique characteristics that make them suitable for patients with high infectious risk, and in situations in which infected transvenous leads or pockets have already occurred. Suggestions according to the different scenarios are listed as follows:

Medicine preparation: Almost all the patients in an Italian clinical practice were given a prophylactic dose of antibiotics before the LPM implantation procedure without additional adverse events [36,53]; however, the specific prophylactic antibiotic usage for LPMs in the perioperative setting needs further exploration.

Application strategies: No evidence of recurrent infection was found following the LPM implantation at or after the infected TPM removal [35,58–60]. In the case of lead or pocket-related infections, the LPM implantation could even be performed before the extraction of an infected TPM for pacemaker-dependent patients, without the occurrence of reinfection [60,61]. In cases of bacteremia or endocarditis, it is recommended that the LPM not be implanted until the blood cultures turn negative, and for pacemaker-dependent patients, temporary pacing through jugular access is the interim solution after the removal of an infected TPM and prior to LPM implantation.

2.2.5. Tricuspid Valve Regurgitation

The development of tricuspid valve regurgitation (TR) after TPM implantation is primarily caused by the mechanical interference of the ventricular leads with the TV and its sub-valvular apparatus [62]. Despite the absence of leads crossing the TV, LPMs with lengths of 42 mm for the Nanostim, and with lengths of 25.9 mm for the Micra, still have the potential to interact with the valvular apparatus. The aggravation of TR was observed in 12% of patients with LPMs during the 48 month follow-up when compared with 9%

of patients with TPMs [63]. However, an age- and sex-matched analysis showed a higher increase in the TR severity in patients with TPMs than in those with LPMs [64], and the LPMs had the advantage of reducing the TR effective regurgitant orifice area, compared with conventional leads 1 month after the device implantation [65]. The TR increased 12 months after the LPM implantation; however, it was comparable to that of TPMs [66]. The conclusion concerning TR following LPM implantation is controversial, which is possibly because of the differences in the definition of TR, the follow-up period, and the proportion of the Nanostim, with a greater length than the Micra. To minimize the potential influence of LPMs on the TV, suggestions are provided for consideration.

Procedure technique: A septal implantation of the Micra is recommended to reduce the risk of cardiac perforation, which may not be a risk factor for the worsening of TR. Apical septal implantation is considered desirable to avoid the entrapment of the docking button or proximal retrieval feature within the tricuspid valve apparatus. However, a basal implantation site close to the TV annulus should be avoided to minimize mechanical interference with the valvular apparatus [66]. Despite being designed 10% shorter than its predecessor the Nanostim, the Aveir VR, which is 38.0 mm in length, is still longer than the Micra [36], and therefore the Aveir VR implantation site should maintain more of a distance from the TV and anterior interventricular groove if possible. Physicians should balance the long-term benefit of the TR severity with the short-term risk of pericardial effusion.

2.3. Gaps in Experience

Worldwide experience demonstrated that the early retrieval of Micra (median 46 days, range 1–95 days) was feasible and can be accomplished with low risk of serious complications, such as cardiac perforation, and device embolization [47]. However, the long-term experience with Micra retrieval is limited. The Micra VR was designed with 12 years of battery life, and the battery longevity was confirmed in the real-world setting [67]. As for the Micra AV, the original design of an 11.8 year battery life (1 V, 0.24 ms) with 100% pacing was reduced to 10.5 years in the real-world setting [68]. The anticipated encapsulation of LPMs during the whole battery life could further impede the extractability of LPMs. There is no recommended treatment for LPMs after battery depletion. Physicians can either retrieve the nonfunctioning LPMs and subsequently implant a new device, or abandon the nonfunctioning LPMs and implant a new adjacent one [69]. Even though the RV can host up to three Micra devices [70], this could still lead to geometric alterations of the cardiac anatomy and have a negative impact on the ventricular volume.

3. Leadless AV Synchronization

3.1. Brief Introduction of the Algorithm of the Micra AV

Four distinct segments of cardiac activity are derived from the accelerometer signal: A1, A2, A3, and A4. Their relationships to the cardiac mechanical activity, echocardiography, and ECG are displayed in Table 1. The post-ventricular atrial blanking period (PVAB) (500–550 ms by default), an interval that is used to blank the A1 and A2 signals, is followed by A3 and A4 sensing windows. The A3 window end (750–900 ms by default) is marked as "VE" annotation, denoting the end of all ventricular activity on the programmer. The A4 window starts at VE and ends with a ventricular sensed or paced event. The A3 threshold must be programmed higher than the A3 signal to blank the A3 signal, as opposed to the A4 threshold, which needs to be programmed lower than the A4 signal to sense A4. Any mechanical activity sensed during the A3/A4 window is denoted as AM. Any ventricular pacing is denoted as VP, and any ventricular activity sensed during AM-VP interval (20 ms by default) is denoted as VS. The device is programmed to accurately discern the A4 signal; that is, to accurately mark AM on the A4 signal so as to synchronize with VP [15,71–73] (Figure 2).

Table 1. Meanings of A1–A4 in relation to function, echocardiography, and electrocardiogram.

		Heart Sound	Echocardiography	Electrocardiogram
A1	Mitral/tricuspid valve closure	S1		At the end of QRS complex
A2	Aortic/pulmonic valve closure	S2		At the end of T wave
A3	Early passive ventricular filling	S3	E wave	Before the onset of the P wave
A4	Atrial contraction	S4	A wave	After the inscription of the P wave

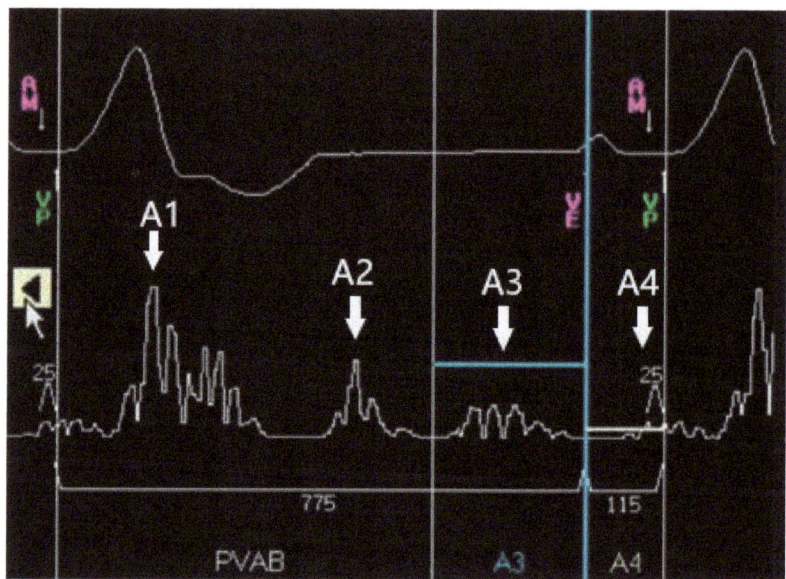

Figure 2. Schematic illustration and explanation of the key atrial sensing parameters. The top signal shows the electrocardiogram; the bottom signal shows the accelerometer signal.

3.2. Evaluation of the AV Synchrony and Recommendation of Strategies

The efficacy of the Micra AV was mainly evaluated based on the rate of AV synchrony. The median AV synchrony was 87% in the Micra Atrial TRacking using a Ventricular AccELerometer (MARVEL) study [15], and due to an enhanced algorithm, which included new features such as automated programming and mode switching, the median AV synchrony increased to 89.2% in the MARVEL2 study [16]. The average AV synchrony was 94.4% in patients with intrinsic conduction, compared with 80.0% in patients with high-degree AV blocks [15]. Patients with intrinsic conduction could have higher AV synchrony; however, the high-degree AV block with relatively low AV synchrony was the arrhythmia that the Micra AV was designed to treat. The AV synchrony in the MARVEL and MARVEL2 studies was objectively and accurately calculated with a Holter monitor; however, the processes were time-consuming. A currently published study in which the authors evaluated the relationship between AV synchrony and LPM device counters showed that the median AV synchrony of 87.1% was well correlated with a median %AM-VP of 79.1% in the MARVEL2 study [68], providing evidence for the reliability of the LPM device counters. Moreover, a linear and positive correlation between the AV synchrony determined with the Holter monitor and the LPM device counters was confirmed in another study [74]. In a real-world setting, the median %AM-VP was 74.7% among 1662 patients with %VP > 90% [68]. A highly similar ambulatory AV synchrony of 74.8%, assessed using Holter monitoring, was found in patients with complete AV blocks [75]. A theoretical AV synchrony of theoretical 100% is what clinicians and technicians expect and pursue. Factors that could influence the AV synchrony and the according strategies are listed as follows:

A. Patients' factors:
  (a) Patient characteristics: High AV synchrony was associated with a lower BMI, a lower proportion of congestive heart failure, a history of cardiac surgery, and pulmonary hypertension [71]. It is a hypothesis the A4 amplitude was negatively related to a history of coronary artery bypass grafting due to the ischemia-inducing reduced atrial contractions [76];
  (b) Electrocardiogram (ECG): Some cases of low AV synchrony could be related to sinus rates < 50/min [15], and an analysis in a real-world setting of outpatients indicated that the median AV synchrony was 91% when the patients had sinus rates of 50–80/min, and that it decreased to 33% when the patients had sinus rates of >80/min [72]. Therefore, a sinus rate of 50–80/min contributes to high AV synchrony. Several kinds of arrhythmia, such as a sinus rate variability of >5 bpm at rest [76], AF/atrial flutter [71], and a high premature atrial/ventricular complex [15], are associated with lower AV synchrony. The A4 amplitude was positively correlated with p-wave amplitude in lead aVR [76];
  (c) Echocardiography: A higher A wave in the echocardiography reflects a stronger atrial contraction and a greater possibility of being discerned by the Mica AV. In a past study, the authors demonstrated that an E/A ratio of <0.94 indicated a high AV synchrony [76], in comparison with an E/A ratio of >1.5, which is considered a contraindication to Micra AV implantation. A small-sample study indicated that an A wave velocity > 73 cm/s could predict appropriate atrial sensing [77];
  (d) Maneuver and posture: The AV synchrony ranged from 89.2% during resting to 69.8% during standing, and to 74.7% during fast walking [16]. The higher sinus rate and volatile direction of the acceleration during activity could influence the sensing of atrial mechanical contraction, as reflected by the lower ambulatory AV synchrony of 74.7% a real-world setting [68], compared with that of 80.0% in a clinical trial for patients with AV blocks [15]. Hence, the Micra AV is more suitable for patients with sedentary lifestyles.

B. Procedure technique: The Micra AV implant location has not been reported to have a significant influence on the AV synchrony [16] or A4 amplitude [76]. In terms of the implant location selection, physicians should take the electrical parameters of the RV and relevant complications into consideration; however, the AV synchrony cannot be evaluated or mediated during the procedure, which is another drawback of the Mica AV hardware design.

C. Device programming: The nominal values of the Micra AV were optimized for patients during resting. Regular postimplant device reprogramming is necessary and should be individually optimized. The manual atrial mechanical (MAM) test is to line up A1–A4 signals with the corresponding surface ECG signals (Figure 2). Firstly, the MAM test with "auto" atrial mechanical features turned-off runs in the VDI mode to allow a clear distinction of the A1–A4 signals, and subsequently, MAM test runs in the VDD mode to make adjustment based on the track of atrial activity. The systematic and stepwise approaches including MAM test and adjustments of the A4 threshold, A3 window, and A3 threshold are to accurately discern A4 [78,79].

a. The A4 threshold: In situations of low A4 amplitudes, a lower A4 threshold facilitates a reduction in the under-sensed A4 and improves the AV synchrony [72,73]; Meanwhile, in the case of low A4 amplitudes, the device's built-in 3-axis accelerometer atrial-sensing vectors can be changed from a selection of one or two vectors to a recruitment of all three vectors to improve AV synchrony at the cost of negative impact on battery longevity [78,79]. When the A4 threshold is too low, the over-sensed A4 could impair the AV synchrony which was observed in a study in which a higher A4 threshold was found to be related to a higher AV synchrony [74] (Figure 3A);
b. The A3 window end: In situations of sinus tachycardia, the A4 signal falls in the A3 window, which reduces the AV synchrony. A shorter A3 window end interval for detecting the A4 signal and improving the AV synchrony has been confirmed in multiple studies [72–74]. A rate-dependent A3 window may be promising for tracking atrial contractions at higher heart rates. However, some researchers have suggested setting the A3 window below 700 ms and deactivating the automatic adjustment to improve the AV synchrony [74] (Figure 3B);
c. The A3 threshold: In situations of sinus tachycardia, the A4 signal begins with the encroachment into the A3 window; however, as the heart rate is further elevated, the A4 signal could merge with the A3 signal and the A3 auto threshold function could result in the under-sensing of A4. Turning the A3 auto threshold function off and fixing the A3 threshold contribute to AV synchrony, and this is especially suitable for elevated sinus rates of 80–110/min [71]. A lower A3 threshold could improve the AV synchrony [74,76] (Figure 3C);
d. The PVAB: In situations of Wenckebach behavior, the progressive shortening of the RP interval means that the P wave falls in the PVAB period, which results in the intermittent loss of A4 [76]. Shortening the PVAB to minimize the p-wave blanking is recommended. Wenckebach behavior occurs in patients with intrinsic conduction for whom the AV synchrony is high; therefore, the benefit of shortening PVAB is limited (Figure 3D);
e. AV conduction mode switch: The algorithm of the Micra AV assumes intact intrinsic conduction in cases of ventricular rates of >40/min by default, and it switches to VVI-40 and VVIR pacing [16] if this function is activated. However, in situations of 2:1 AV blocks with sinus rates of ≥80/min, or complete AV blocks with ventricular escape beats of ≥40/min, such a function decreases the AV synchrony, and the recommendation is to switch it off [73,80];
f. Rate smoothing feature: This feature was delivered at a rate smoothing interval (typically 100 ms) longer than the median R-R interval if A4 was not detected and improved the AV synchrony by 9% [15]. In situations of high sinus rate variability or high/low sinus rates, the efficacy of such a feature is somewhat compromised. Some studies suggested programming the rate smoothing interval longer than 100ms in patients with high sinus rate variabilities and low sinus rates [68], and programming the interval to 50 ms in patients with sinus rates of >90/min [16];
g. Programmed lower rate: The loss of AV synchrony could be induced by sinus rates lower than the programmed lower rate [68,72]. The programmed lower rate should be set according to the sinus rate, measured using 24 h Holter monitoring.

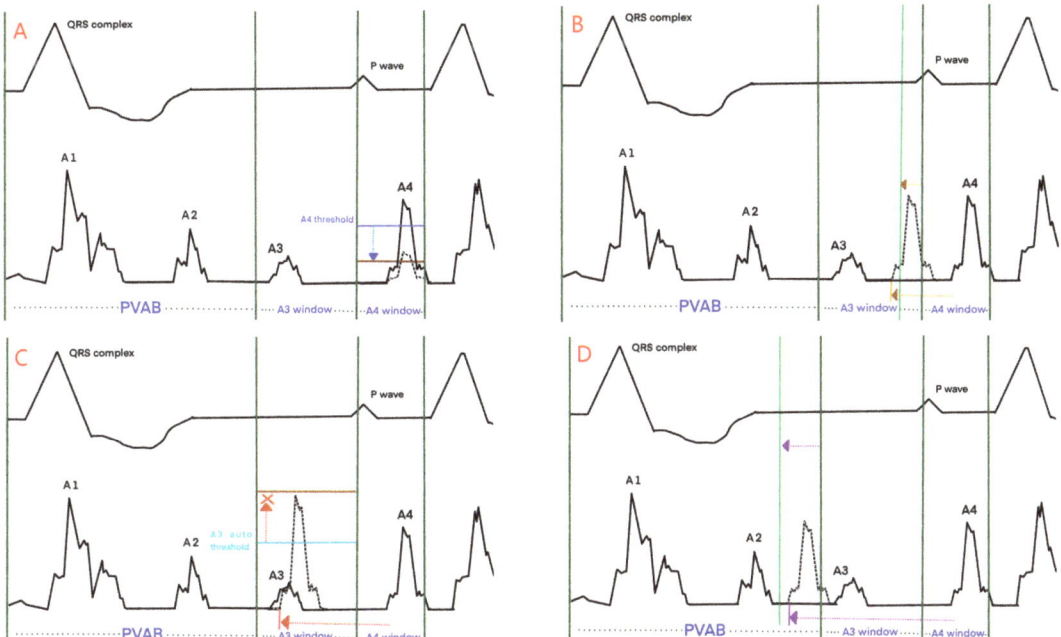

Figure 3. Schematic illustration and device programming in various situations. The blue dotted line indicates a lower A4 threshold in the situation of low A4 amplitude (**A**). The yellow dotted line indicates a shorter A3 window end interval in the situation of the A4 signal falling in the A3 window (**B**). The red dotted line indicates the deactivation of the A3 auto threshold function in the situation of the A4 signal merging with the A3 signal (**C**). The purple dotted line indicates a shorter PVAB in the situation of the A4 signal falling in the PVAB period (**D**).

4. Selection Strategy for LPMs vs. TPMs

4.1. Selection Strategy for VVI-LPMs vs. DDD-TPMs

A total of 36–38% of patients with VVI-LPMs had non-AF bradyarrhythmias [20,21], in which the absence of AV synchrony due to chronic VVI pacing could theoretically cause a decreased stroke volume and increase the incident AF and heart failure. However, only 1.1% of patients experienced heart failure and pacemaker syndrome related to the VVI pacing mode [81]. Another LPM registry from Italy found that patients without AF did not experience significantly higher rates of recurrent syncope, cardiac hospitalization, or all-cause death compared with patients with AF during a mean follow-up period of more than 600 days [82], which suggests that the effect of VVI-LPMs on patients with non-AF is reassuring. It remains to be seen whether non-AF patients will benefit more from DDD-TPMs than VVI-LPMs. A propensity-matched analysis indicated that VVI-LPMs for non-AF bradyarrhythmias significantly increased the rate of heart-failure-related rehospitalization at the 48 month follow-up compared with the use of DDD-TPMs, and a higher but not significant all-cause mortality was observed in patients with VVI-LPMs [63].

4.2. Selection Strategy for VDD-LPMs vs. DDD-TPMs

In addition to the lack of atrial pacing to treat sick sinus syndrome, the unachievable 100% AV synchrony, especially in cases of high sinus rates, is another shortcoming of the hardware design of the Micra AV. Thus, VDD-LPMs are the interim solution prior to the realization of true DDD-LPMs. Although the AV synchrony substantially decreased at sinus rates of >80/min [72], the cardiac output at higher rates has been shown to be more dependent on the heart rate than the AV synchrony [83]. A positive chronotropic response provides approximately 75% of the increment in cardiac output, whereas the maintenance of AV synchrony and increased contractility accounting for the remaining 25% [84]. Therefore, rate responsive pacing could be an adequate option for patients when exercising. As for sedentary or elderly patients with AV blocks, compared with DDD-TPMs, the Micra AV might still have the advantage, despite the less than 100% AV synchrony. However, there is an argument that the benefit of AV synchrony is not essential at rest, as the pacemaker syndrome causes symptoms, especially during exercise. Therefore, whether the added value of the Micra AV vs. Micra VR in clinical practice could be evaluated with clinical endpoints needs further exploration.

4.3. Conduction System Pacing

The RV apical pacing and RV septal pacing result in dyssynchronous activation that can impair ventricular function and have the possibility of inducing pacing-induced cardiomyopathy [85]. Conduction system pacing, including His bundle pacing and left bundle branch pacing, has gained prominence as a novel pacing modality that can activate the ventricles physiologically, correct bundle branch block, and improve cardiac function via the lead of TPMs fixed in the specific region of the His–Purkinje conduction system [86]. Improvement in the LPM hardware design, such as a more precise fixation mechanism and contact mapping capability of the Aveir VR, can perhaps provide a promise of fulfilling conduction system pacing by LPMs.

5. Leadless Atrial Pacemakers

The Atrial Micra (Medtronic) and Aveir atrial LPM (Abbott) are two kinds of LPMs that are positioned in the RA appendage and that are designed to deliver the AAI(R) mode. The two have been tested and evaluated in preclinical ovine studies. The Atrial Micra is a modified version of the Micra VR, featuring shorter and flatter tines that are adaptive for relatively thin atrial myocardium [87]. The Aveir atrial LPM is also a modified version of the Aveir VR, with a dual-helix fixation mechanism that is specific to the RA anatomy [88], and with an electrically active inner helix and mechanical fixation of the outer helix. The preliminary results indicated that both of these AAI-LPMs exhibited excellent and stable pacing performances during the 24 week follow-up for the Atrial Micra and the 12 week follow-up for the Aveir atrial LPM. Here, the Atrial Micra displayed its potential to be retrieved. As for safety concerns, one dislodgment of the Atrial Micra occurred among 17 implants and one case of hemopericardium occurred during the retrieval and implant procedure. In comparison, no dislodgments or significant myocardial perforations of the Aveir atrial LPM have been reported. Phase III clinical trials are expected to further assess the efficacy and safety of these two AAI-LPMs.

6. Dual-Chamber Leadless and Battery-Less Pacemakers

6.1. The Conception of True Dual-Chamber Leadless and Battery-Less Pacemakers

The configuration of a true DDD-LPM is conceptualized as the combination of a VVI-LPM with an AAI-LPM, and it is supported by the device–device communication technology and algorithm to coordinate the atrium and ventricle activities. An Aveir DR is under development by Abbott, which has a proprietary implant-to-implant communication technology for the regulation of AAI-LPMs and VVI-LPMs in a dual-chamber fashion [89]. Due to the limited volume of LPMs and complex environment of the beating heart, high energy efficiency, excellent interference resistance, and long-term reliability are the main requirements for the communication technology. The small form factor of the battery size constrains its long-term usage. In addition to the currently available battery technology under constant improvement, some novel energy programs are under development to address this quandary.

6.2. Communication Technology for the Realization of Dual-Chamber Leadless Pacemakers

6.2.1. Radio-Frequency (RF) Communication

Unlike communications through the air, the various tissues and organs within the body have different conductivities, dielectric constants, and impedances, which could interfere with RF communication. A frequency range of 2.4–2.5 GHz in in vivo experiments is optimal for the multi-node pacemaker technology with the least signal attenuation [90]. The RF communication is prone to electromagnetic interference and suffers from large signal leakages and the ease of eavesdropping.

6.2.2. Conductive Intracardiac Communication (CIC)

CIC, which is also known as galvanic coupled intra-body communication, is a promising novel technique for highly energy-efficient wireless communication inside the heart. The conduction of electrical signals between LPMs through the blood and myocardial tissue should be sufficient to convey information, and it is lower than the pacing threshold to avoid pacing myocardium. A frequency range of 100 kHz–1 MHz in in vivo experiments is beneficial [91]. Compared with RF communication, CIC has a lower system power consumption and electromagnetic interference, as well as higher data security, because the communication signal is confined within the human body. The trade-off for the low frequency and power consumption is the data rate; fortunately, the data rate required for the vital physiological signal transmission among implantable devices is relatively low. The dual-chamber pacing modes were tested unidirectionally, from the RA to RV and from left ventricle (LV) to the RV, through CIC, and specific algorithms have been tested in vivo in pigs [92]. The chronic preclinical feasibility of two LPMs using the novel bidirectional communication technology was evaluated in ovine subjects [93], and the stable performance of the bidirectional communication during the 13 week follow-up and the energy efficient algorithm of the communication modality were demonstrated.

6.3. Energy Programs for the Realization of Dual-Chamber Battery-Less Pacemakers

6.3.1. Acoustic Energy

The wireless Stimulation Endocardially for CRT (WiSE-CRT) system (EBR Systems, Sunnyvale, CA, USA) was developed to emit ultrasonic energy from a subcutaneous ultrasound transmitter to a wireless LV endocardial receiver electrode, which paces the LV by converting the ultrasonic energy into electrical energy [94]. Once the battery is depleted, changing the subcutaneous battery is sufficient without the need for removing the endocardial electrode. One disadvantage is that 7.7% of patients did not have an adequate acoustic window to power the receiver electrode [95], and another is the low energy efficiency of acoustic energy [96]. A narrowed ultrasound beam could increase the energy efficiency; however, it would be susceptible to the change in the beam location and posture [97]. Therefore, one subcutaneous transmitter to drive multi-site receivers is more difficult under the constraint of the acoustic window.

6.3.2. RF Energy

An intravenous cardiac pacemaker designed to be implanted in cardiac veins is a passive wireless power receiver circuit that receives bursts of power at 13.5 MHz from a subcutaneous transmitter and stimulates the tissue [98]. A novel bioresorbable leadless cardiac pacemaker for the purpose of temporary pacing is powered by a wireless inductive energy transfer at a frequency of 13.5 MHz [99]. The adoption of 13.5 MHz is because there is less absorption by biofluids or biological tissues at this frequency regime [99]. The advantage of RF energy is its potential to be extended to multi-chamber pacing by using different frequencies.

6.3.3. Kinetic Energy

The kinetic energy derived from cardiac vibrations [100,101], blood flow [102] and body motion [103] could serve as an inexhaustible source for battery-less pacemakers. A mass imbalance or oscillation weight is connected to an electrical micro generator to convert a minimal amount of the heart's kinetic energy into electric energy [100,101]. Due to the nature of kinetic energy, the selection of the implantation site should consider the direction of the cardiac contraction or blood flow. The relatively low efficiency of in vivo energy harvest is another drawback of kinetic energy. A novel coin battery-sized inertia-driven triboelectric nanogenerator that is dependent on the body motion and gravity to produce electricity demonstrated a significant power performance in preclinical settings [103].

7. Conclusions

Although LPMs have shown excellent and stable pacing performances and are associated with a low rate of complications in comparison with TPMs, some risk complications such as cardiac perforation and dislodgment, should be handled with extra caution and individualized strategies. Compared with LPMs, DDD-TPMs could bring about lower rates of heart-failure-related rehospitalizations for patients with non-AF; however, clinicians should balance the long-term benefits of the low complication rates of VVI-LPMs with the benefits of AV synchrony and/or interventricular synchrony of DDD-TPMs prior to making clinical recommendations. With the further development of AAI-LPMs, true DDD-LPMs could theoretically realize almost all the features of DDD-TPMs, except for the conduction system pacing; however, DDD-LPMs inevitably increase the risk of atrial perforation and dislodgment due to the extra AAI-LPMs. Hence, VDD-LPMs still have their own advantages for patients with sedentary lifestyles and at high risk of pericardial effusion. The prospect of LPMs is promising and encouraging. The integration of leadless pacing and conduction system pacing, more efficient and reliable communication technology, and improved battery technology or, alternatively, revolutionized energy programs, require further exploration.

Author Contributions: Conceptualization, F.T. and Z.S.; writing—original draft preparation, F.T.; writing—review and editing, Z.S.; supervision, Z.S. All authors have read and agreed to the published version of the manuscript.

Funding: This research received no external funding.

Institutional Review Board Statement: Not applicable.

Informed Consent Statement: Not applicable.

Data Availability Statement: Not applicable.

Conflicts of Interest: The authors declare no conflict of interest.

References

1. Raatikainen, M.J.P.; Arnar, D.O.; Zeppenfeld, K.; Merino, J.L.; Levya, F.; Hindriks, G.; Kuck, K.H. Statistics on the use of cardiac electronic devices and electrophysiological procedures in the European Society of Cardiology countries: 2014 report from the European Heart Rhythm Association. *Europace* **2015**, *17*, i1–i75. [PubMed]
2. Pakarinen, S.; Oikarinen, L.; Toivonen, L. Short-term implantation-related complications of cardiac rhythm management device therapy: A retrospective single-centre 1-year survey. *Europace* **2010**, *12*, 103–108. [PubMed]
3. Udo, E.O.; Zuithoff, N.P.; van Hemel, N.M.; de Cock, C.C.; Hendriks, T.; Doevendans, P.A.; Moons, K.G. Incidence and predictors of short- and long-term complications in pacemaker therapy: The FOLLOWPACE study. *Heart Rhythm* **2012**, *9*, 728–735. [CrossRef] [PubMed]
4. Kirkfeldt, R.E.; Johansen, J.B.; Nohr, E.A.; Jorgensen, O.D.; Nielsen, J.C. Complications after cardiac implantable electronic device implantations: An analysis of a complete, nationwide cohort in Denmark. *Eur. Heart J.* **2014**, *35*, 1186–1194. [PubMed]
5. Cho, M.S.; Kim, J.; Lee, J.B.; Nam, G.B.; Choi, K.J.; Kim, Y.H. Incidence and predictors of moderate to severe tricuspid regurgitation after dual-chamber pacemaker implantation. *Pacing Clin. Electrophysiol.* **2019**, *42*, 85–92.
6. Malagù, M.; Vitali, F.; Brieda, A.; Cimaglia, P.; De Raffele, M.; Tazzari, E.; Musolino, C.; Balla, C.; Serenelli, M.; Cultrera, R.; et al. Antibiotic prophylaxis based on individual infective risk stratification in cardiac implantable electronic device: The practice study. *Europace* **2022**, *24*, 413–420.
7. Cantillon, D.J.; Exner, D.V.; Badie, N.; Davis, K.; Gu, N.Y.; Nabutovsky, Y.; Doshi, R. Complications and health care costs associated with transvenous cardiac pacemakers in a nationwide assessment. *JACC Clin. Electrophysiol.* **2017**, *3*, 1296–1305.

Cantillon, D.J.; Dukkipati, S.R.; Ip, J.H.; Exner, D.V.; Niazi, I.K.; Banker, R.S.; Rashtian, M.; Plunkitt, K.; Tomassoni, G.F.; Nabutovsky, Y.; et al. Comparative study of acute and mid-term complications with leadless and transvenous cardiac pacemakers. *Heart Rhythm* **2018**, *15*, 1023–1030.

El-Chami, M.F.; Bockstedt, L.; Longacre, C.; Higuera, L.; Stromberg, K.; Crossley, G.; Kowal, R.C.; Piccini, J.P. Leadless vs. transvenous single-chamber ventricular pacing in the Micra CED study: 2-year follow-up. *Eur. Heart J.* **2022**, *43*, 1207–1215.

Sperzel, J.; Defaye, P.; Delnoy, P.P.; Garcia Guerrero, J.J.; Knops, R.E.; Tondo, C.; Deharo, J.C.; Wong, T.; Neuzil, P. Primary safety results from the LEADLESS Observational Study. *Europace* **2018**, *20*, 1491–1497.

Lakkireddy, D.; Knops, R.; Atwater, B.; Neuzil, P.; Ip, J.; Gonzalez, E.; Friedman, P.; Defaye, P.; Exner, D.; Aonuma, K.; et al. A worldwide experience of the management of battery failures and chronic device retrieval of the nanostim leadless pacemaker. *Hear Rhythm* **2017**, *14*, 1756–1763.

Reddy, V.Y.; Exner, D.V.; Doshi, R.; Tomassoni, G.; Bunch, T.J.; Estes, N.A.M.; Neužil, P.; Paulin, F.L.; Garcia Guerrero, J.J.; Cantillon, D.J.; et al. Primary results on safety and efficacy from the LEADLESS II-phase 2 worldwide clinical trial. *JACC Clin. Electrophysiol.* **2022**, *8*, 115–117. [CrossRef] [PubMed]

Piccini, J.P.; Stromberg, K.; Jackson, K.P.; Kowal, R.C.; Duray, G.Z.; El-Chami, M.F.; Crossley, G.H.; Hummel, J.D.; Narasimhan, C.; Omar, R.; et al. Patient selection, pacing indications, and subsequent outcomes with de novo leadless single-chamber VVI pacing. *Europace* **2019**, *21*, 1686–1693.

Steinwender, C.; Lercher, P.; Schukro, C.; Blessberger, H.; Prenner, G.; Andreas, M.; Kraus, J.; Ammer, M.; Stühlinger, M. State of the art: Leadless ventricular pacing: a national expert consensus of the Austrian Society of Cardiology. *J. Interv. Card. Electrophysiol.* **2020**, *57*, 27–37. [PubMed]

Chinitz, L.; Ritter, P.; Khelae, S.K.; Iacopino, S.; Garweg, C.; Grazia-Bongiorni, M.; Neuzil, P.; Johansen, J.B.; Mont, L.; Gonzalez, E.; et al. Accelerometer-based atrioventricular synchronous pacing with a ventricular leadless pacemaker: Results from the Micra atrioventricular feasibility studies. *Heart Rhythm* **2018**, *15*, 1363–1371. [PubMed]

Steinwender, C.; Khelae, S.K.; Garweg, C.; Chan, J.Y.S.; Ritter, P.; Johansen, J.B.; Sagi, V.; Epstein, L.M.; Piccini, J.P.; Pascual, M.; et al. Atrioventricular synchronous pacing using a leadless ventricular pacemaker: Results from the MARVEL 2 study. *JACC Clin. Electrophysiol.* **2020**, *6*, 94–106.

Glikson, M.; Nielsen, J.C.; Kronborg, M.B.; Michowitz, Y.; Auricchio, A.; Barbash, I.M.; Barrabés, J.A.; Boriani, G.; Braunschweig, F.; Brignole, M.; et al. 2021 ESC Guidelines on cardiac pacing and cardiac resynchronization therapy. *Eur. Heart J.* **2021**, *42*, 3427–3520.

Tonegawa-Kuji, R.; Kanaoka, K.; Mori, M.; Nakai, M.; Iwanaga, Y. Mortality and 30-day readmission rates after inpatient leadless pacemaker implantation: Insights from a nationwide readmissions database. *Can. J. Cardiol.* **2022**, *38*, 1697–1705.

Gulletta, S.; Schiavone, M.; Gasperetti, A.; Breitenstein, A.; Palmisano, P.; Mitacchione, G.; Chierchia, G.B.; Montemerlo, E.; Statuto, G.; Russo, G.; et al. Peri-procedural and mid-term follow-up age-related differences in leadless pacemaker implantation: Insights from a multicenter European registry. *Int. J. Cardiol.* **2023**, *371*, 197–203.

Reynolds, D.; Duray, G.Z.; Omar, R.; Soejima, K.; Neuzil, P.; Zhang, S.; Narasimhan, C.; Steinwender, C.; Brugada, J.; Lloyd, M.; et al. A leadless intracardiac transcatheter pacing system. *N. Engl. J. Med.* **2016**, *374*, 533–541.

El-Chami, M.F.; Al-Samadi, F.; Clementy, N.; Garweg, C.; Martinez-Sande, J.L.; Piccini, J.P.; Iacopino, S.; Lloyd, M.; Viñolas Prat, X.; Jacobsen, M.D.; et al. Updated performance of the Micra transcatheter pacemaker in the real-world setting: A comparison to the investigational study and a transvenous historical control. *Heart Rhythm* **2018**, *15*, 1800–1807. [CrossRef] [PubMed]

Darlington, D.; Brown, P.; Carvalho, V.; Bourne, H.; Mayer, J.; Jones, N.; Walker, V.; Siddiqui, S.; Patwala, A.; Kwok, C.S. Efficacy and safety of leadless pacemaker: A systematic review, pooled analysis and meta-analysis. *Indian Pacing Electrophysiol.* **2022**, *22*, 77–86.

Bertelli, M.; Toniolo, S.; Ziacchi, M.; Gasperetti, A.; Schiavone, M.; Arosio, R.; Capobianco, C.; Mitacchione, G.; Statuto, G.; Angeletti, A.; et al. Is less always more? A prospective two-centre study addressing clinical outcomes in leadless versus transvenous single-chamber pacemaker recipients. *J. Clin. Med.* **2022**, *11*, 6071. [PubMed]

Tjong, F.V.Y.; Knops, R.E.; Udo, E.O.; Brouwer, T.F.; Dukkipati, S.R.; Koruth, J.S.; Petru, J.; Sediva, L.; van Hemel, N.M.; Neuzil, P.; et al. Leadless pacemaker versus transvenous single-chamber pacemaker therapy: A propensity matched analysis. *Heart Rhythm* **2018**, *15*, 1387–1393. [CrossRef] [PubMed]

Vincent, L.; Grant, J.; Peñalver, J.; Ebner, B.; Maning, J.; Olorunfemi, O.; Goldberger, J.J.; Mitrani, R.D. Early trends in leadless pacemaker implantation: Evaluating nationwide in-hospital outcomes. *Heart Rhythm* **2022**, *19*, 1334–1342.

Piccini, J.P.; El-Chami, M.; Wherry, K.; Crossley, G.H.; Kowal, R.C.; Stromberg, K.; Longacre, C.; Hinnenthal, J.; Bockstedt, L. Contemporaneous comparison of outcomes among patients implanted with a leadless vs. transvenous single chamber ventricular pacemaker. *JAMA Cardiol.* **2021**, *6*, 1187–1195.

Piccini, J.P.; Cunnane, R.; Steffel, J.; El-Chami, M.F.; Reynolds, D.; Roberts, P.R.; Soejima, K.; Steinwender, C.; Garweg, C.; Chinitz, L.; et al. Development and validation of a risk score for predicting pericardial effusion in patients undergoing leadless pacemaker implantation: Experience with the Micra transcatheter pacemaker. *Europace* **2022**, *24*, 1119–1126.

Hauser, R.G.; Gornick, C.C.; Abdelhadi, R.H.; Tang, C.Y.; Casey, S.A.; Sengupta, J.D. Major adverse clinical events associated with implantation of a leadless intracardiac pacemaker. *Heart Rhythm* **2021**, *18*, 1132–1139. [CrossRef]

Okabe, T.; Afzal, M.R.; Houmsse, M.; Makary, M.S.; Elliot, E.D.; Daoud, E.G.; Augostini, R.S.; Hummel, J.D. Tine-based leadless pacemaker: Strategies for safe implantation in unconventional clinical scenarios. *JACC Clin. Electrophysiol.* **2020**, *6*, 1318–1331.

30. Garweg, C.; Vandenberk, B.; Foulon, S.; Haemers, P.; Ector, J.; Willems, R. Leadless pacing with Micra TPS: A comparison between right ventricular outflow tract, mid-septal, and apical implant sites. *J. Cardiovasc. Electrophysiol.* **2019**, *30*, 2002–2011. [CrossRef]
31. Chen, X.; Huang, W. Strategies to overcome complicated situations in leadless pacemaker implantation. *Pacing Clin. Electrophysiol.* **2021**, *44*, 1959–1962. [CrossRef]
32. Bhardwaj, R.; Kewcharoen, J.; Contractor, T.; Nayak, S.; Ai, S.; Kim, U.; Mandapati, R.; Garg, J. Echocardiogram-guided leadless pacemaker implantation. *JACC Clin. Electrophysiol.* **2022**, *8*, 1581–1582. [CrossRef] [PubMed]
33. Lloyd, M.S.; El-Chami, M.F.; Nilsson, K.R., Jr.; Cantillon, D.J. Transcatheter/leadless pacing. *Heart Rhythm* **2018**, *15*, 624–628. [CrossRef] [PubMed]
34. Mitacchione, G.; Arabia, G.; Schiavone, M.; Cerini, M.; Gasperetti, A.; Salghetti, F.; Bontempi, L.; Viecca, M.; Curnis, A.; Forleo G.B. Intraoperative sensing increase predicts long-term pacing threshold in leadless pacemakers. *J. Interv. Card. Electrophysiol.* **2022**, *63*, 679–686. [CrossRef]
35. Mitacchione, G.; Schiavone, M.; Gasperetti, A.; Arabia, G.; Breitenstein, A.; Cerini, M.; Palmisano, P.; Montemerlo, E.; Ziacchi, M.; Gulletta, S.; et al. Outcomes of Leadless Pacemaker implantation following transvenous lead extraction in high-volume referral centers: Real-world data from a large international registry. *Heart Rhythm* **2022**, *20*, 395–404. [CrossRef] [PubMed]
36. Laczay, B.; Aguilera, J.; Cantillon, D.J. Leadless cardiac ventricular pacing using helix fixation: Step-by-step guide to implantation. *J. Cardiovasc. Electrophysiol.* **2023**, *34*, 748–759. [CrossRef] [PubMed]
37. Hauser, R.G.; Gornick, C.C.; Abdelhadi, R.H.; Tang, C.Y.; Kapphahn-Bergs, M.; Casey, S.A.; Okeson, B.K.; Steele, E.A.; Sengupta J.D. Leadless pacemaker perforations: Clinical consequences and related device and user problems. *J. Cardiovasc. Electrophysiol.* **2022**, *33*, 154–159. [CrossRef]
38. Wang, Y.; Hou, W.; Zhou, C.; Yin, Y.; Lu, S.; Liu, G.; Duan, C.; Cao, M.; Li, M.; Toft, E.S.; et al. Meta-analysis of the incidence of lead dislodgement with conventional and leadless pacemaker systems. *Pacing Clin. Electrophysiol.* **2018**, *41*, 1365–1371. [CrossRef]
39. Terricabras, M.; Khaykin, Y. Successful leadless pacemaker retrieval from the left pulmonary artery: A case report. *Heart Rhythm Case Rep.* **2020**, *6*, 798–799. [CrossRef]
40. Sugiura, K.; Baba, Y.; Hirota, T.; Kubo, T.; Kitaoka, H. A drifting dislodged leadless pacemaker in the bilateral pulmonary arteries. *JACC Case Rep.* **2022**, *4*, 844–846. [CrossRef]
41. Fichtner, S.; Estner, H.L.; Näbauer, M.; Hausleiter, J. Percutaneous extraction of a leadless Micra pacemaker after dislocation: A case report. *Eur. Heart J. Case Rep.* **2019**, *3*, ytz113. [CrossRef]
42. Karim, S.; Abdelmessih, M.; Marieb, M.; Reiner, E.; Grubman, E. Extraction of a Micra transcatheter pacing system: First-in-human experience. *Heart Rhythm Case Rep.* **2015**, *2*, 60–62. [CrossRef] [PubMed]
43. Sterliński, M.; Demkow, M.; Plaskota, K.; Oręziak, A. Percutaneous extraction of a leadless Micra pacemaker from the pulmonary artery in a patient with complex congenital heart disease and complete heart block. *EuroIntervention* **2018**, *14*, 236–237. [CrossRef] [PubMed]
44. Hasegawa-Tamba, S.; Ikeda, Y.; Tsutsui, K.; Kato, R.; Muramatsu, T.; Matsumoto, K. Two-directional snare technique to rescue detaching leadless pacemaker. *Heart Rhythm Case Rep.* **2020**, *6*, 711–714. [CrossRef]
45. Roberts, P.R.; Clementy, N.; Al Samadi, F.; Garweg, C.; Martinez-Sande, J.L.; Iacopino, S.; Johansen, J.B.; Vinolas Prat, X.; Kowal R.C.; Klug, D.; et al. A leadless pacemaker in the real-world setting: The Micra Transcatheter Pacing System Post-Approval Registry. *Heart Rhythm* **2017**, *14*, 1375–1379. [CrossRef]
46. Sterliński, M.; Demkow, M.; Oręziak, A.; Szumowski, Ł. What is retrieved must dislocate first: Few consideration how to avoid leadless pacemaker escape. *Pacing Clin. Electrophysiol.* **2021**, *44*, 1137–1138. [CrossRef] [PubMed]
47. Afzal, M.R.; Daoud, E.G.; Cunnane, R.; Mulpuru, S.K.; Koay, A.; Hussain, A.; Omar, R.; Wei, K.K.; Amin, A.; Kidwell, G.; et al. Techniques for successful early retrieval of the Micra transcatheter pacing system: A worldwide experience. *Heart Rhythm* **2018**, *15*, 841–846. [CrossRef]
48. Romeo, E.; D'Alto, M.; Cappelli, M.; Nigro, G.; Correra, A.; Colonna, D.; Sarubbi, B.; Golino, P. Retrieval of a leadless transcatheter pacemaker from the right pulmonary artery: A case report. *Pacing Clin. Electrophysiol.* **2021**, *44*, 952–954. [CrossRef]
49. Sundaram, S.; Choe, W. The one that got away: A leadless pacemaker embolizes to the lungs. *Heart Rhythm* **2016**, *13*, 2316. [CrossRef]
50. El-Chami, M.F.; Garweg, C.; Iacopino, S.; Al-Samadi, F.; Martinez-Sande, J.L.; Tondo, C.; Johansen, J.B.; Prat, X.V.; Piccini, J.P.; Cha Y.M.; et al. Leadless pacemaker implant, anticoagulation status, and outcomes: Results from the Micra Transcatheter Pacing System Post-Approval Registry. *Heart Rhythm* **2022**, *19*, 228–234. [CrossRef]
51. Kiani, S.; Black, G.B.; Rao, B.; Thakkar, N.; Massad, C.; Patel, A.V.; Merchant, F.M.; Hoskins, M.H.; De Lurgio, D.B.; Patel, A.M.; et al. Outcomes of Micra leadless pacemaker implantation with uninterrupted anticoagulation. *J. Cardiovasc. Electrophysiol.* **2019**, *30*, 1313–1318. [CrossRef]
52. San Antonio, R.; Chipa-Ccasani, F.; Apolo, J.; Linhart, M.; Trotta, O.; Pujol-López, M.; Niebla, M.; Alarcón, F.; Trucco, E.; Arbelo, E.; et al. Management of anticoagulation in patients undergoing leadless pacemaker implantation. *Heart Rhythm.* **2019**, *16*, 1849–1854. [CrossRef] [PubMed]
53. Palmisano, P.; Iacopino, S.; De Vivo, S.; D'Agostino, C.; Tomasi, L.; Startari, U.; Ziacchi, M.; Pisanò, E.C.L.; Santobuono, V.E.; Caccavo, V.P.; et al. Leadless transcatheter pacemaker: Indications, implantation technique and peri-procedural patient management in the Italian clinical practice. *Int. J. Cardiol.* **2022**, *365*, 49–56. [CrossRef] [PubMed]

Malagù, M.; D'Aniello, E.; Vitali, F.; Balla, C.; Gasbarro, V.; Bertini, M. Leadless pacemaker implantation in superobese patient. *Rev. Cardiovasc. Med.* **2022**, *23*, 125. [CrossRef]

Kelm, M.; Perings, S.M.; Jax, T.; Lauer, T.; Schoebel, F.C.; Heintzen, M.P.; Perings, C.; Strauer, B.E. Incidence and clinical outcome of iatrogenic femoral arteriovenous fistulas: Implications for risk stratification and treatment. *J. Am. Coll. Cardiol.* **2002**, *40*, 291–297. [CrossRef]

Zilinyi, R.S.; Sethi, S.S.; Parikh, M.A.; Parikh, S.A. Iatrogenic arteriovenous fistula following femoral access precipitating high-output heart failure. *JACC Case Rep.* **2021**, *3*, 421–424. [CrossRef]

Madia, C. Management trends for postcatheterization femoral artery pseudoaneurysms. *JAAPA* **2019**, *32*, 15–18. [CrossRef]

Chang, D.; Gabriels, J.K.; Soo Kim, B.; Ismail, H.; Willner, J.; Beldner, S.J.; John, R.M.; Epstein, L.M. Concomitant leadless pacemaker implantation and lead extraction during an active infection. *J. Cardiovasc. Electrophysiol.* **2020**, *31*, 860–867. [CrossRef] [PubMed]

Beurskens, N.E.G.; Tjong, F.V.Y.; Dasselaar, K.J.; Kuijt, W.J.; Wilde, A.A.M.; Knops, R.E. Leadless pacemaker implantation after explantation of infected conventional pacemaker systems: A viable solution? *Heart Rhythm* **2019**, *16*, 66–71. [CrossRef]

Breeman, K.T.N.; Beurskens, N.E.G.; Driessen, A.H.G.; Wilde, A.A.M.; Tjong, F.V.Y.; Knops, R.E. Timing and mid-term outcomes of using leadless pacemakers as replacement for infected cardiac implantable electronic devices. *J. Interv. Card. Electrophysiol.* **2022**. [CrossRef]

Bicong, L.; Allen, J.C.; Arps, K.; Al-Khatib, S.M.; Bahnson, T.D.; Daubert, J.P.; Frazier-Mills, C.; Hegland, D.D.; Jackson, K.P.; Jackson, L.R.; et al. Leadless pacemaker implantation after lead extraction for cardiac implanted electronic device infection. *J. Cardiovasc. Electrophysiol.* **2022**, *33*, 464–470. [CrossRef] [PubMed]

Al-Mohaissen, M.A.; Chan, K.L. Prevalence and mechanism of tricuspid regurgitation following implantation of endocardial leads for pacemaker or cardioverter-defibrillator. *J. Am. Soc. Echocardiogr.* **2012**, *25*, 245–252. [CrossRef] [PubMed]

Sasaki, K.; Togashi, D.; Nakajima, I.; Suchi, T.; Nakayama, Y.; Harada, T.; Akashi, Y.J. Clinical outcomes of non-atrial fibrillation bradyarrhythmias treated with a ventricular demand leadless pacemaker compared with an atrioventricular synchronous transvenous pacemaker-a propensity score-matched analysis. *Circ. J.* **2022**, *86*, 1283–1291. [CrossRef] [PubMed]

Vaidya, V.R.; Dai, M.; Asirvatham, S.J.; Rea, R.F.; Thome, T.M.; Srivathsan, K.; Mulpuru, S.K.; Kusumoto, F.; Venkatachalam, K.L.; Ryan, J.D.; et al. Real-world experience with leadless cardiac pacing. *Pacing Clin. Electrophysiol.* **2019**, *42*, 366–373. [CrossRef]

Ohta, Y.; Goda, A.; Daimon, A.; Manabe, E.; Masai, K.; Kishima, H.; Mine, T.; Asakura, M.; Ishihara, M. The differences between conventional lead, thin lead, and leadless pacemakers regarding effects on tricuspid regurgitation in the early phase. *J. Med. Ultrason.* **2023**, *50*, 51–56. [CrossRef]

Beurskens, N.E.G.; Tjong, F.V.Y.; de Bruin-Bon, R.H.A.; Dasselaar, K.J.; Kuijt, W.J.; Wilde, A.A.M.; Knops, R.E. Impact of leadless pacemaker therapy on cardiac and atrioventricular valve function through 12 months of follow-up. *Circ. Arrhythm. Electrophysiol.* **2019**, *12*, e007124. [CrossRef]

Breeman, K.T.N.; Oosterwerff, E.F.J.; Dijkshoorn, L.A.; Salavati, A.; Beurskens, N.E.G.; Wilde, A.A.M.; Delnoy, P.H.M.; Tjong, F.V.Y.; Knops, R.E. Real-world long-term battery longevity of Micra leadless pacemakers. *J. Interv. Card. Electrophysiol.* **2022**. [CrossRef]

Garweg, C.; Piccini, J.P.; Epstein, L.M.; Frazier-Mills, C.; Chinitz, L.A.; Steinwender, C.; Stromberg, K.; Sheldon, T.; Fagan, D.H.; El-Chami, M.F. Correlation between AV synchrony and device collected AM-VP sequence counter in atrioventricular synchronous leadless pacemakers: A real-world assessment. *J. Cardiovasc. Electrophysiol.* **2023**, *34*, 197–206. [CrossRef]

Grubman, E.; Ritter, P.; Ellis, C.R.; Giocondo, M.; Augostini, R.; Neuzil, P.; Ravindran, B.; Patel, A.M.; Omdahl, P.; Pieper, K.; et al. To retrieve, or not to retrieve: System revisions with the Micra transcatheter pacemaker. *Heart Rhythm* **2017**, *14*, 1801–1806. [CrossRef]

Omdahl, P.; Eggen, M.D.; Bonner, M.D.; Iaizzo, P.A.; Wika, K. Right ventricular anatomy can accommodate multiple Micra transcatheter pacemakers. *Pacing Clin. Electrophysiol.* **2016**, *39*, 393–397. [CrossRef]

Kowlgi, G.N.; Tseng, A.S.; Tempel, N.D.; Henrich, M.J.; Venkatachalam, K.L.; Scott, L.; Shen, W.K.; Deshmukh, A.J.; Madhavan, M.; Lee, H.C.; et al. A real-world experience of atrioventricular synchronous pacing with leadless ventricular pacemakers. *J. Cardiovasc. Electrophysiol.* **2022**, *33*, 982–993. [CrossRef]

Neugebauer, F.; Noti, F.; van Gool, S.; Roten, L.; Baldinger, S.H.; Seiler, J.; Madaffari, A.; Servatius, H.; Ryser, A.; Tanner, H.; et al. Leadless atrioventricular synchronous pacing in an outpatient setting: Early lessons learned on factors affecting atrioventricular synchrony. *Heart Rhythm* **2022**, *19*, 748–756. [CrossRef]

El-Chami, M.F.; Bhatia, N.K.; Merchant, F.M. Atrio-ventricular synchronous pacing with a single chamber leadless pacemaker: Programming and trouble shooting for common clinical scenarios. *J. Cardiovasc. Electrophysiol.* **2021**, *32*, 533–539. [CrossRef] [PubMed]

Briongos-Figuero, S.; Estévez-Paniagua, Á.; Sánchez Hernández, A.; Jiménez, S.; Gómez-Mariscal, E.; Abad Motos, A.; Muñoz-Aguilera, R. Optimizing atrial sensing parameters in leadless pacemakers: Atrioventricular synchrony achievement in the real world. *Heart Rhythm* **2022**, *19*, 2011–2018. [CrossRef]

Chinitz, L.A.; El-Chami, M.F.; Sagi, V.; Garcia, H.; Hackett, F.K.; Leal, M.; Whalen, P.; Henrikson, C.A.; Greenspon, A.J.; Sheldon, T.; et al. Ambulatory atrioventricular synchronous pacing over time using a leadless ventricular pacemaker: Primary results from the AccelAV study. *Heart Rhythm* **2023**, *20*, 46–54. [CrossRef] [PubMed]

76. Garweg, C.; Khelae, S.K.; Steinwender, C.; Chan, J.Y.S.; Ritter, P.; Johansen, J.B.; Sagi, V.; Epstein, L.M.; Piccini, J.P.; Pascual, M.; et al. Predictors of atrial mechanical sensing and atrioventricular synchrony with a leadless ventricular pacemaker: Results from the MARVEL 2 Study. *Heart Rhythm* **2020**, *17*, 2037–2045. [CrossRef]
77. Pujol-López, M.; Garcia-Ribas, C.; Doltra, A.; Guasch, E.; Vazquez-Calvo, S.; Niebla, M.; Domingo, R.; Roca-Luque, I.; Tolosana, J.M.; Mont, L. Pulsed doppler A-wave as an aid in patient selection for atrioventricular synchrony through a leadless ventricular pacemaker. *J. Interv. Card. Electrophysiol.* **2023**, *66*, 261–263. [CrossRef] [PubMed]
78. Mitacchione, G.; Schiavone, M.; Gasperetti, A.; Viecca, M.; Curnis, A.; Forleo, G.B. Atrioventricular synchronous leadless pacemaker: State of art and broadened indications. *Rev. Cardiovasc. Med.* **2021**, *22*, 395–401. [CrossRef] [PubMed]
79. Mitacchione, G.; Schiavone, M.; Gasperetti, A.; Ruggiero, D.; Denora, M.; Viecca, M.; Forleo, G.B. Micra-AV leadless pacemaker and atrioventricular (dys)synchrony: A stepwise process. *Pacing Clin. Electrophysiol.* **2021**, *44*, 1738–1742. [CrossRef] [PubMed]
80. Garweg, C.; Khelae, S.K.; Chan, J.Y.S.; Chinitz, L.; Ritter, P.; Johansen, J.B.; Sagi, V.; Epstein, L.M.; Piccini, J.P.; Pascual, M.; et al. Behavior of AV synchrony pacing mode in a leadless pacemaker during variable AV conduction and arrhythmias. *J. Cardiovasc. Electrophysiol.* **2021**, *32*, 1947–1957. [CrossRef]
81. Duray, G.Z.; Ritter, P.; El-Chami, M.; Narasimhan, C.; Omar, R.; Tolosana, J.M.; Zhang, S.; Soejima, K.; Steinwender, C.; Rapallini, L.; et al. Long-term performance of a transcatheter pacing system: 12-Month results from the Micra Transcatheter Pacing Study. *Heart Rhythm* **2017**, *14*, 702–709. [CrossRef]
82. Russo, V.; D'Andrea, A.; De Vivo, S.; Rago, A.; Manzo, G.; Bocchetti, A.; Papa, A.A.; Giordano, V.; Ammendola, E.; Sarubbi, B.; et al. Single-chamber leadless cardiac pacemaker in patients without atrial fibrillation: Findings from Campania leadless registry. *Front. Cardiovasc. Med.* **2022**, *8*, 781335. [CrossRef] [PubMed]
83. Buckingham, T.A.; Janosik, D.L.; Pearson, A.C. Pacemaker hemodynamics: Clinical implications. *Prog. Cardiovasc. Dis.* **1992**, *34*, 347–366. [CrossRef]
84. Benditt, D.G.; Milstein, S.; Buetikofer, J.; Gornick, C.C.; Mianulli, M.; Fetter, J. Sensor-triggered, rate-variable cardiac pacing. Current technologies and clinical implications. *Ann. Intern. Med.* **1987**, *107*, 714–724. [CrossRef]
85. Ng, A.C.; Allman, C.; Vidaic, J.; Tie, H.; Hopkins, A.P.; Leung, D.Y. Long-term impact of right ventricular septal versus apical pacing on left ventricular synchrony and function in patients with second-or third-degree heart block. *Am. J. Cardiol.* **2009**, *103*, 1096–1101. [CrossRef]
86. Arnold, A.D.; Whinnett, Z.I.; Vijayaraman, P. His-Purkinje conduction system pacing: State of the art in 2020. *Arrhythm. Electrophysiol. Rev.* **2020**, *9*, 136–145. [PubMed]
87. Vatterott, P.J.; Eggen, M.D.; Hilpisch, K.E.; Drake, R.A.; Grubac, V.; Anderson, T.A.; Colin, B.P.; Seifert, K.R.; Mesich, M.L.; Ramor, L.C. Implant, performance, and retrieval of an atrial leadless pacemaker in sheep. *Heart Rhythm* **2021**, *18*, 288–296. [CrossRef]
88. Rashtian, M.; Banker, R.S.; Neuzil, P.; Breeman, K.; Nee, P.; Badie, N.; Victorine, K.; Ligon, D.; Rippy, M.K.; Eldadah, Z.; et al. Preclinical safety and electrical performance of novel atrial leadless pacemaker with dual-helix fixation. *Heart Rhythm* **2022**, *19*, 776–781. [CrossRef] [PubMed]
89. NCT05252702; Aveir Dual-Chamber Leadless i2i IDE Study. Abbott Medical Devices: Abbott Park, IL, USA, 2022.
90. Bose, P.; Khaleghi, A.; Albatat, M.; Bergsland, J.; Balasingham, I. RF channel modeling for implant-to-implant communication and implant to subcutaneous implant communication for future leadless cardiac pacemakers. *IEEE Trans. Biomed. Eng.* **2018**, *65*, 2798–2807. [CrossRef]
91. Bereuter, L.; Kuenzle, T.; Niederhauser, T.; Kucera, M.; Obrist, D.; Reichlin, T.; Tanner, H.; Haeberlin, A. Fundamental characterization of conductive intracardiac communication for leadless multisite pacemaker systems. *IEEE Trans. Biomed. Circuits Syst.* **2019**, *13*, 237–247. [CrossRef]
92. Bereuter, L.; Gysin, M.; Kueffer, T.; Kucera, M.; Niederhauser, T.; Fuhrer, J.; Heinisch, P.; Zurbuchen, A.; Obrist, D.; Tanner, H.; et al. Leadless Dual-chamber pacing a novel communication method for wireless pacemaker synchronization. *JACC Basic Transl. Sci.* **2018**, *3*, 813–823. [CrossRef] [PubMed]
93. Cantillon, D.J.; Gambhir, A.; Banker, R.; Rashtian, M.; Doshi, R.; Badie, N.; Booth, D.; Yang, W.; Nee, P.; Fishler, M.; et al. Wireless communication between paired leadless pacemakers for dual-chamber synchrony. *Circ. Arrhythm. Electrophysiol.* **2022**, *15*, e010909. [CrossRef] [PubMed]
94. Okabe, T.; Hummel, J.D.; Bank, A.J.; Niazi, I.K.; McGrew, F.A.; Kindsvater, S.; Oza, S.R.; Scherschel, J.A.; Walsh, M.N.; Singh, J.P. Leadless left ventricular stimulation with WiSE-CRT System-Initial experience and results from phase I of SOLVE-CRT Study (nonrandomized, roll-in phase). *Heart Rhythm* **2022**, *19*, 22–29. [CrossRef] [PubMed]
95. Reddy, V.Y.; Miller, M.A.; Neuzil, P.; Søgaard, P.; Butter, C.; Seifert, M.; Delnoy, P.P.; van Erven, L.; Schalji, M.; Boersma, L.V.A.; et al. Cardiac resynchronization therapy with wireless left ventricular endocardial pacing The SELECT-LV Study. *J. Am. Coll. Cardiol.* **2017**, *69*, 2119–2129. [CrossRef]
96. Neuzil, P.; Reddy, V.Y. Leadless cardiac pacemakers: Pacing paradigm change. *Curr. Cardiol. Rep.* **2015**, *17*, 68. [CrossRef]
97. Benditt, D.G.; Goldstein, M.; Belalcazar, A. The leadless ultrasonic pacemaker: A sound idea? *Heart Rhythm* **2009**, *6*, 749–751. [CrossRef]
98. Anwar, U.; Ajijola, O.A.; Shivkumar, K.; Markovic, D. Towards a leadless wirelessly controlled intravenous cardiac pacemaker. *IEEE Trans. Biomed. Eng.* **2022**, *69*, 3074–3086. [CrossRef]
99. Choi, Y.S.; Yin, R.T.; Pfenniger, A.; Koo, J.; Avila, R.; Benjamin Lee, K.; Chen, S.W.; Lee, G.; Li, G.; Qiao, Y.; et al. Fully implantable and bioresorbable cardiac pacemakers without leads or batteries. *Nat Biotechnol.* **2021**, *39*, 1228–1238. [CrossRef]

100. Franzina, N.; Zurbuchen, A.; Zumbrunnen, A.; Niederhauser, T.; Reichlin, T.; Burger, J.; Haeberlin, A. A miniaturized endocardial electromagnetic energy harvester for leadless cardiac pacemakers. *PLoS ONE* **2020**, *15*, e0239667. [CrossRef]
101. Zurbuchen, A.; Haeberlin, A.; Bereuter, L.; Wagner, J.; Pfenniger, A.; Omari, S.; Schaerer, J.; Jutzi, F.; Huber, C.; Fuhrer, J.; et al. The Swiss approach for a heartbeat-driven lead- and batteryless pacemaker. *Heart Rhythm* **2017**, *14*, 294–299. [CrossRef]
102. Tholl, M.V.; Haeberlin, A.; Meier, B.; Shaheen, S.; Bereuter, L.; Becsek, B.; Tanner, H.; Niederhauser, T.; Zurbuchen, A. An intracardiac flow based electromagnetic energy harvesting mechanism for cardiac pacing. *IEEE Trans. Biomed. Eng.* **2019**, *66*, 530–538. [CrossRef] [PubMed]
103. Ryu, H.; Park, H.M.; Kim, M.K.; Kim, B.; Myoung, H.S.; Kim, T.Y.; Yoon, H.J.; Kwak, S.S.; Kim, J.; Hwang, T.H.; et al. Self-rechargeable cardiac pacemaker system with triboelectric nanogenerators. *Nat. Commun.* **2021**, *12*, 4374. [CrossRef] [PubMed]

Disclaimer/Publisher's Note: The statements, opinions and data contained in all publications are solely those of the individual author(s) and contributor(s) and not of MDPI and/or the editor(s). MDPI and/or the editor(s) disclaim responsibility for any injury to people or property resulting from any ideas, methods, instructions or products referred to in the content.

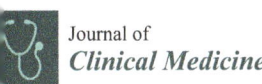

Cardiac Implantable Electronic Devices Infection Assessment, Diagnosis and Management: A Review of the Literature

Filippo Toriello [1,2,*], Massimo Saviano [2], Andrea Faggiano [1,2], Domitilla Gentile [2], Giovanni Provenzale [2], Alberto Vincenzo Pollina [2], Elisa Gherbesi [2], Lucia Barbieri [2] and Stefano Carugo [1,2]

1. Department of Clinical Sciences and Community Health, University of Milan, 20122 Milan, Italy
2. Department of Internal Medicine, Fondazione IRCCS Ca' Granda—Ospedale Maggiore Policlinico, 20122 Milan, Italy
* Correspondence: filippo.toriello@unimi.it; Tel.: +39-0255033532

Abstract: The use of increasingly complex cardiac implantable electronic devices (CIEDs) has increased exponentially in recent years. One of the most serious complications in terms of mortality, morbidity and financial burden is represented by infections involving these devices. They may affect only the generator pocket or be generalised with lead-related endocarditis. Modifiable and non-modifiable risk factors have been identified and they can be associated with patient or procedure characteristics or with the type of CIED. Pocket and systemic infections require a precise evaluation and a specialised treatment which in most cases involves the removal of all the components of the device and a personalised antimicrobial therapy. CIED retention is usually limited to cases where infection is unlikely or is limited to the skin incision site. Optimal re-implantation timing depends on the type of infection and on the results of microbiological tests. Preventive strategies, in the end, include antibiotic prophylaxis before CIED implantation, the possibility to use antibacterial envelopes and the prevention of hematomas. The aim of this review is to investigate the pathogenesis, stratification, diagnostic tools and management of CIED infections.

Keywords: cardiac implantable electronic device infection; pocket infection; antimicrobial therapy; risk factors; preventive strategies

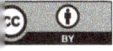

1. Introduction

Since the first pacemaker (PM) was implanted by Åke Senning in 1958, cardiac implantable electronic devices (CIEDs) have spread worldwide. More sophisticated systems such as implantable cardioverter defibrillators (ICDs) and cardiac resynchronisation therapy (CRT) devices often represent a lifesaving asset, but device-related infections (DRI), albeit infrequent, still represent a potential life-threatening complication [1]. Their clinical manifestation may be confined to the device pocket or to the leads or extended to the entire system and bloodstream [2].

DRI is a relevant clinical dilemma as it increases mortality (up to 35% at 5 years), morbidity and financial health care burden with an incremental cost of USD 16,500 per hospitalisation and an average total cost of USD 146,000 per CIED infection case [3–5].

2. Risk Factors for Cardiac Implantable Electronic Device Infections

The overall incidence of CIED infections ranges from 0.5% to 2.2% of patients according to different populations, type of device and time from implant [2]. CIED infection rate raise has surprisingly exceeded the heightened number of device implantations [6]. In the last 16 years, while the number of implanted electronic devices has almost doubled (95% more), the incidence of CIED infections recorded an increase of more than 200% [5]. This escalation of infections may be caused by the higher complexity of CIED recipients in terms of comorbidities and ageing (patient-related), as well as by more sophisticated techniques and longer procedural times (procedure-related) [7].

Risk factors for CIED infection have historically been classified into patient-related, procedure-related and additionally sub-classified into non-modifiable and modifiable [3]. According to actual evidence ICDs and CRT devices are more susceptible to infections than PMs (8.9 and 10 vs. 1.8 cases, respectively, per 1000 device/years) [8,9]. The number of implanted leads is critical in terms of risk of infections [10,11]. Whether this finding is related to the mere presence of additional hardware itself or reflects the complexity and duration of the procedure is unclear and still object of debates [12]. The end-stage renal disease brings the highest risk of infection among the non-modifiable patient-related factors showing a pooled estimate odds ratio (OR) of 8.73 [13]. Other relevant risk factors from the same category are chronic corticosteroid use, history of device infection, chronic obstructive pulmonary disease (COPD), heart failure (HF), malignancy and diabetes mellitus [2]. Although the underlying mechanism is unclear, male gender seems to be associated with an increased risk, while infections in women showed a high mortality rate [14,15]. Surprisingly, there is some evidence indicating that age is inversely related to DRI [16], probably because younger patients may have a weaker immune response against low virulence organisms and finally they go through many procedures in their lifetime [17]. Procedural time is a sizeable determinant of DRI as longer procedures are indeed independently associated with infectious complications [18]. Device replacement or upgrade, which is a non-modifiable procedure-related risk factor as well, is associated with a 2- to 5-fold risk of DRI compared with de novo implant [2]. Early re-interventions, defined as repeat procedures occurring during a single hospitalisation, are also associated with an 8.8-fold increased risk of CIED infection. Pocket hematoma, temporary pacing wires and unfamiliarity with implant techniques are all independent risk factors for DRI [19]. Modifiable factors leave room to preventive strategies to overcome the increased risk for DRI. Fever in the 24 h before implantation is certainly the most relevant (pooled estimate OR > 4). Improper trichotomy, oral anticoagulants and heparin bridging have a minor impact [3].

Ultimately, an investigation on the WRAP-IT trial population, using a machine learning analysis that considers 81 variables, identified additional non-modifiable risk factors including higher number of CIED procedures, history of atrial arrhythmia, geography (outside North America and Europe), device type (CRT vs. permanent PM/ICD) and lower body mass index. Potentially modifiable risk factors included longer procedure time, implant location (non-left pectoral subcutaneous), peri-operative glycopeptide antibiotic (vancomycin) vs. non-glycopeptide (cefazolin), anticoagulant and/or antiplatelet use and capsulectomy. Chlorhexidine skin preparation and antibiotic pocket wash have been found to be protective from early DRI [20].

3. Pathogenesis and Microbiology of Cardiac Implantable Electronic Device Infections

There are two key classes of clinical manifestations, device pocket infections and leads-related endocarditis. The most common source of contamination is the air or the hands of the operators and pocket infection is the prevalent expression of this pathway [3]. Direct lead seeding during bloodstream infections is the mechanism of late lead vegetation formation. The pathways for germs penetration are usually skin, mouth, gastrointestinal or urinary tract infections [21]. A retrograde progression of infection from the bloodstream to the pocket has been described, and device infection could represent the first clinical expression of a subclinical bacteraemia. It is commonly accepted, although controversial, that infections occurring within 1 year are probably due to contamination at the time of surgery, while those occurring later may be caused by blood-bared germs [7]. ICD infections generally occur earlier after the implant compared with PM infections (125 vs. 415 days, respectively) [8]. This finding is probably related to procedural time and higher susceptibility of ICD leads to shelter micro-organisms seeding. Data suggest that more than a half of DRI is related to procedural contamination. In 55% of patients indeed, a DRI is detected before 12 months after last procedure [22]. Similarly, it has been detected that 25% of CIED infections occur in the first month (0–28 days after device placement), 33% later (29 days to 1 year after device placement), and 42% of total DRI are delayed

(>1 year after device placement), implying that only 4 out of 10 infections are not primarily related to peri-procedural contamination [23]. A study including only patients with lead-associated endocarditis, showed that more than two-thirds of individuals developed the disease at least 1 year after the procedure, supporting the theory that late infections are mainly lead-related and secondary to bacteraemia [24]. As expected, risk factors for DRI within 6 months of implantation are different from those related to later infections. The presence of epicardial leads or immediate peri-procedural wound complications seem to be associated with early infections, while the hospitalisation span, the presence of COPD and other comorbidities are mostly associated with delayed infections. Therefore, different pathogenetic mechanisms are associated with distinct clinical presentations, both in terms of time (early versus late) and of clinical manifestation (pocket infection versus lead/systemic infection), which in turn are burdened with different prognosis. In fact, some studies have found higher mortality in lead-related CIEDs or bloodstream infections (29%) compared with isolated pocket infection (5%) [25]. The microorganisms by far most frequently involved in DRI are Gram-positive bacteria (70–90%), especially normally non-pathogenic germs such as coagulase-negative Staphylococci (CoNS, 37.6%) that usually are skin saprophytes [26]. The second most common pathogen, namely Staphylococcus aureus (StA) (30.8%), is the most lethal. It is the most common cause of bacteraemia and early pocket infections and the one that is much prone to adhere to non-biological material creating the biofilm. The biofilm is a structured community of bacterial cells enclosed in a self-produced polymeric matrix and adherent to an inert or living surface, which prevents the effective action of host defences and the penetration of antibiotics [27]. Gram-negative bacilli and other Gram-positive cocci are rarely isolated in CIED infections. Finally, a common and critical situation, ranging from 12% to 49% of situations, is that of clinical infections with negative cultures [28].

4. Pocket Infections

Uncomplicated pocket infection is defined as an infection limited to the generator pocket without systemic symptoms, clinical signs of infection or positive blood cultures [2,3]. The generator pocket is the most frequent site of CIED infection [29]; indeed, almost two-thirds of patients have a localised pocket infection [8]. Whereas later stages of pocket infection are clearly evident, with discernible features, the earliest stages of the infection may be devious and easily confused with other clinical conditions, such as pocket hematoma, post-implantation inflammation or superficial wound infection. Those complications typically occur within 30 days from the index procedure and have a different therapeutic management and prognosis (Table 1). Local signs are quite different from mild inflammation (erythema, warmth, pain and swelling), in the early stage of the disease, to the real "positive clinical pocket" in later stages. Advanced pocket infection gives raise to fluctuance (abscess) and adherence of the pocket, purulent material drainage from incision sites, fistula formation, wound dehiscence and skin erosion with externalisation of the generator or leads. In this situation, the device should be considered contaminated, independently from the results of the microbiology [2]. In this setting, diagnostic percutaneous puncture with pocket fluid aspiration should be generally avoided to prevent further inoculation with bacteria [30]. Even when performed in a sterile environment, the puncture results in a skin barrier interruption creating a gateway for microbes. The clotted blood, the warm and moist setting of the pocket, enhance bacteria proliferation. Finally, pocket infections may reach the bloodstream prompting systemic infections.

Apparently uncomplicated pocket infections should not be assumed as localised CIED infection, as germs may follow the path along leads and cause secondary blood-stream infection and endocarditis. Current data show that when a clinical pocket infection is identified, rates of lead or endocardial involvement range between 6% and 58% [31]. Precisely, complicated generator pocket infections are internationally defined as a pocket infection with evidence of lead or endocardial involvement and/or systemic signs and/or symptoms of infection or positive blood cultures. Regardless, pocket infection is uncomplicated or complicated, current International Societies Guidelines suggest CIED removal/extraction associated with a specific antibiotic regimen (Figure 1) [2,3]. The investigation of the extent of the infection, the overall management and treatment processes traditionally overlap [17]. For these reasons, some authors consider the clinical differentiation between complicated and uncomplicated pocket infection as a mere academic exercise.

Table 1. Differential diagnosis among cardiac implantable electronic device pocket complications.

Clinical Entity	Characteristics	Incidence	Time Period after Implant	Prognosis (+ Good Prognosis, − Bad Prognosis)	Management
Pocket Hematoma	Ecchymosis, mild effusion in the pocket and swelling.	1–20%	Within 2 weeks (usually <48 h)	+	Compression bandage, removal of antithrombotic therapy, specific pocket compression vest.
Post-implantation inflammation	Erythema affecting the incision site, without purulent exudate, dehiscence, fluctuance or systemic signs of infection.	1–10%	Within 30 days (usually <7 days)	+ +	Close observation. Antibiotics not mandatory.
Superficial infection of surgical wound	A small, localised area of erythema and/or purulence associated with a suture defect.	0.5–5%	Within 30 days (usually <14 days)	+/−	Removal of the suture and antimicrobial therapy, if indicated.
Uncomplicated pocket infection	From mild inflammation to deformation, fluctuance, adherence of pocket, purulent material drainage from incision sites, fistula formation, wound dehiscence and exposure of the generator or leads.	0.5–2.2%	Whenever, traditionally within 1 year	−	Cardiac implantable electronic device removal/extraction associated with a specific antibiotic regimen.

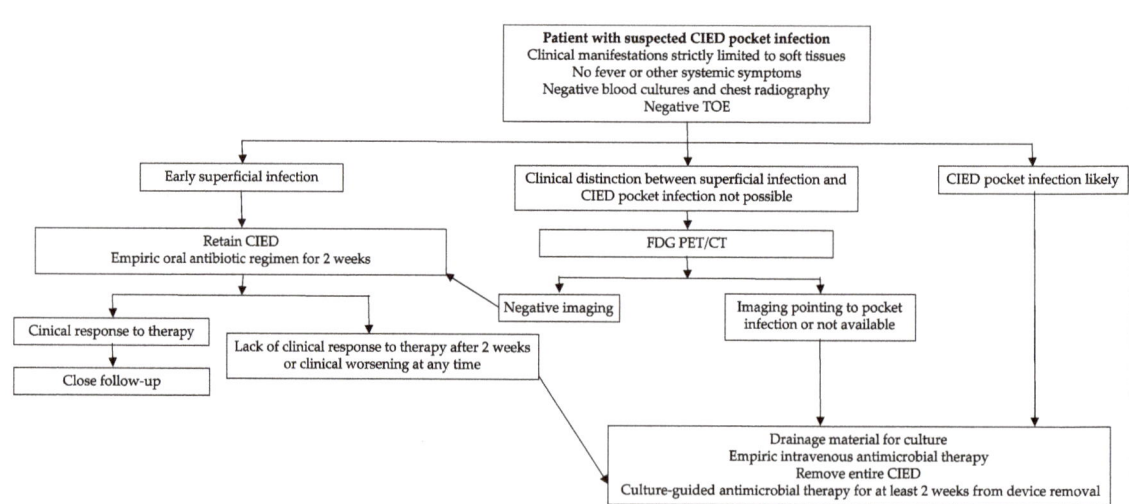

Figure 1. Proposed algorithm for the management of patients with suspected CIED pocket infection. CIED cardiovascular implantable electronic device; TOE: trans-oesophageal echocardiography; FDG PET/CT Fluorine-18-fludeoxyglucose (18F-FDG) positron emission tomography/computerised tomography.

5. Cardiac Device-Related Infective Endocarditis and Bacteriemia

Bloodstream infection usually refers to a CDRIE which is defined as the presence of lead or valvular vegetations in combination with positive blood cultures [32]. Nevertheless the clinical spectrum of systemic CIED infection includes two other conditions:

- A left-sided endocarditis in a CIED carrier: the therapeutic approach follows the current guidelines for valve endocarditis [33]. If surgery is required for left-sided endocarditis, an open-heart removal of the CIED is recommended regardless of the presence of acknowledged device involvement. If there is no indication for valve surgery, complete hardware extraction should be considered even if there is no evidence of associated device infection.
- An occult bacteraemia in a CIED carrier: in this case, there is not an alternative source of infection which resolves only after CIED extraction [34].

The diagnosis of CIED systemic infection is very challenging and it should always be suspected in case of history of fever positively responding to antibiotic therapy and relapsing after its discontinuation [35]. However, several studies have found that 20–50% of patients with CDRIE may present without systemic signs of infection, such as fever, chills, malaise or anorexia and it should spur clinicians to increase their attentiveness to CIED infections [11,23,36,37]. The most frequent complication of CDRIE is the presence of a tricuspid valve vegetation, which occurs in about one-third of the cases [38]. Tricuspid involvement can present with valve alterations (stenosis or regurgitation), pulmonary emboli or pneumonia [39,40]. Tricuspid regurgitation, which is the most prevalent, when severe may require surgical correction coupled with open-heart lead extraction. In case of small tricuspid vegetations, with mild or moderate valve insufficiency, percutaneous extraction can be performed and medical treatment continued for valve endocarditis [34]. Septic thrombophlebitis of the axillary-subclavian axis, even though it is a rare condition, can occur when multiple leads are placed through the same vessel (e.g., CRT or abandoned leads). This complication is at very high risk of pulmonary embolism and an aggressive antithrombotic therapy is recommended before the explant of the whole device [41]. The diagnosis of CDRIE is still based on the modified Duke criteria, but many studies have highlighted some criticism about their predictive value in this setting [33,42]. In order to increase the sensitivity for CIED infection diagnosis, the European Heart Rhythm Association developed the International CIED Infection Criteria in 2020; unfortunately, many limitations are still present [3]. Caution should be maintained in cases of incidental masses on leads without clinical signs of infection because they may be of thrombotic origin [43]. In this situation, four sets of blood cultures and inflammatory markers should be obtained over 2–4 days. If they are all negative, clinical and echocardiographic follow-up is warranted and anticoagulant treatment should be considered, keeping in mind that a mass on right heart CIED leads without signs of infection may also represent a malignancy [44]. Not all patients with a CIED and positive blood cultures have an underlying CIED lead infection. Individuals with positive blood cultures, but no evidence of localised CIED infection constitute a group of difficult management (Figure 2). The risk of underlying CIED lead infection in presence of bacteraemia depends on several factors including duration and source of bacteraemia, type of device, the number of device-related procedures and especially the type of microorganism isolated in blood cultures [45]. Gram-positive organisms remain the predominant pathogens associated with CIED: CoNS and StA are more prone to adhere to non-biological materials [46,47]. Moreover, StA is the most common cause of bacteraemia and early pocket infections. For this reason, many studies tried to identify the clinical predictors of underlying CDRIE in patients presenting with StA bacteraemia, but no signs of pocket infection. Uslan et al. identified different independent predictors of CIED infection such as: relapsing bacteraemia after an appropriate period of antibiotic therapy (when no other source of bacteraemia has been identified), persisting bacteraemia for more than 24 h, implanted ICD, prosthetic cardiac valve and bacteraemia within 3 months of device implantation [48].

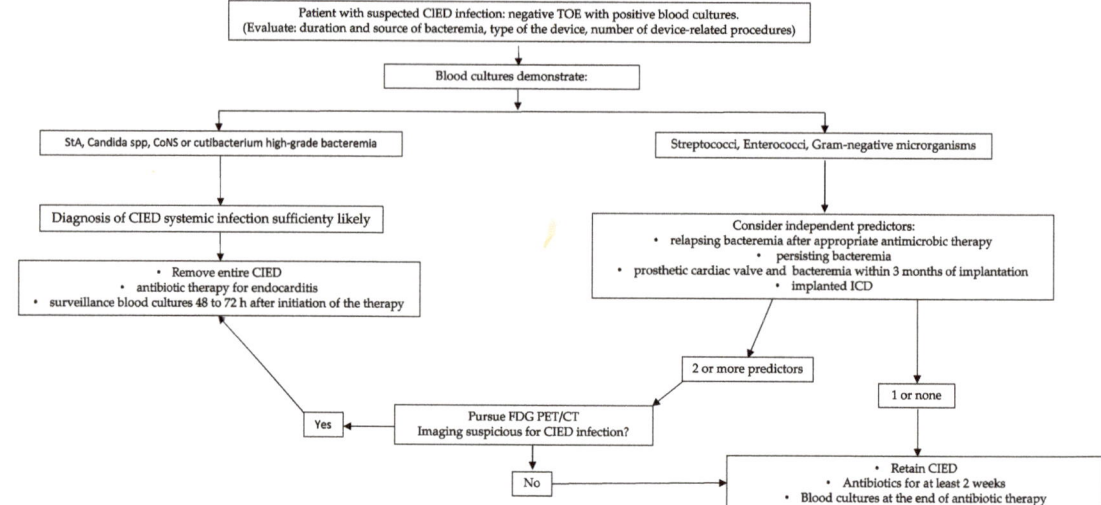

Figure 2. Proposed algorithm for the management of patients with suspected CIED infection with negative TOE and positive blood cultures. CIED: cardiovascular implantable electronic device TOE: trans-oesophageal echocardiography; StA: Staphylococcus aureus; CoNS: coagulase-negative Staphylococci; ICD: implantable cardiac defibrillator; FDG PET/CT: Fluorine-18-fludeoxyglucose (18F-FDG) positron emission tomography/computerised tomography.

6. Diagnosis of CDRIE

CDRIE is defined, according to European guidelines, as an infection extending to the electrode leads, cardiac valve leaflets or endocardial surface; however, local device infection and CDRIE are difficult to be differentiated. Clinical manifestations are the same of other forms of endocarditis, with some differences: fever is less prevalent especially in the elderly, while respiratory and rheumatological symptoms as well as local signs of infection are predominant [33]. The diagnosis should start from blood cultures, no less than two sets three or more are recommended [49]. Suspected CIED infection with negative cultural findings should consider fungal/mycobacterial blood cultures to exclude an unrecognised causative pathogen [45]. Swab samples from the device and generator pocket tissue for culture and susceptibility testing are valuable instruments [45]. Tissue cultures acquired during the surgical exploration are more sensitive than swab cultures [49]. The use of biomarkers was investigated by Lennerz et al. concluding that pro-calcitonin and high sensitivity C-reactive protein could aid in the diagnosis [50]. Recent studies have suggested that leads and generator sonification after removal may help the microbiology testing [51].

Trans-thoracic (TTE) and trans-oesophageal echocardiography (TOE) are the first essential instruments of the diagnostic workup as they help sizing and follow-up of the vegetations identifying possible valvular involvement and dysfunction. TTE can detect pericardial effusion, ventricular dysfunction and pulmonary artery pressure better than TOE, while the latter would be more accurate for the diagnosis of lead-related endocarditis and peri-valvular extension of the infection (Figure 3). TTE and TOE must be performed both when CDRIE is presumed and intracardiac echocardiography may be considered in case both tests are negative [33].

When the echocardiographic investigations are negative or doubtful and the clinical suspicion is quite reasonable, Fluorine-18-fludeoxyglucose (18F-FDG) positron emission tomography/computerised tomography (PET/CT) scanning and radiolabelled leucocyte scintigraphy have been described as a complementary tool not only in the diagnosis of CDRIE, but also in the search for complications including pulmonary septic embolism [33]

99mTc-labeled hexa-methyl-propylene-amine-oxime (HMPAO) white blood cell (WBC) scintigraphy with single-photon-emission computed tomography–computed tomography (SPECT-CT) detects and localises metabolically active cells involved in inflammation and infection. In the study by Erba et al. 99mTc-HMPAO WBC scintigraphy was 94% sensitive for both detection and localisation of CIED infection and associated complications, with a 95% negative predictive value to exclude device-associated infection during a febrile episode and sepsis [52]. 18F-FDG-PET/CT (Figure 4), conversely, performs better for pocket infections than for lead infections: for pocket infections, pooled sensitivity and specificity were 93% and 98%, respectively, while for lead infections sensitivity was 65% although specificity was still high (88%) [53]. Aside from that, delayed image acquisition could increase 18F-FDG-PET/CT diagnostic accuracy in suspected CDRIE [54]. Previous antibiotic therapy may yield false-negative PET/CT imaging despite CDRIE being present [55].

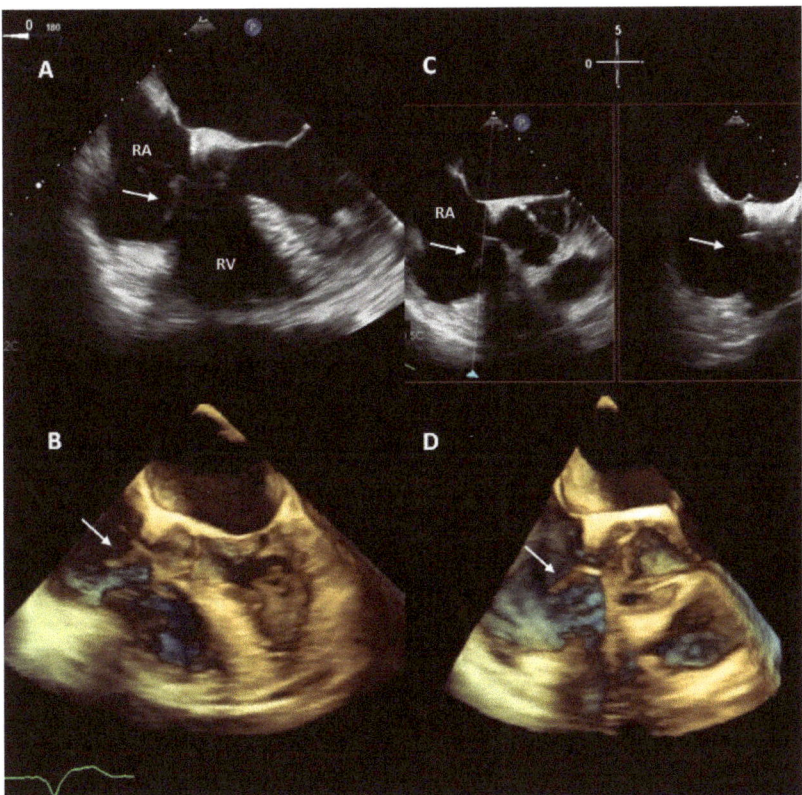

Figure 3. Transesophageal echocardiogram, 5 chamber view, showing a vegetation (19 × 6 mm) adherent to pacemaker's ventricular lead in 2D (panel (**A**), white arrow) and 3D (panel (**B**)). The same vegetation is also shown in right ventricular inflow-outflow view (and its orthogonal plane-bicaval view) in 2D (panel (**C**)) and in 3D (panel (**D**)). RV: right ventricle; RA: right atrium.

No validated clinical tools are available to date, EHRA has proposed to combine modified Duke and ESC 2015 criteria [33]. Positive lead-culture is the major criterion to establish CDRIE among those proposed in the modified Duke [36]. Nevertheless, the use of positive lead cultures can be misleading as the lead tip could be contaminated during the extraction passing through the infected pocket. In addition, previous antibiotics administration and biofilm protection could affect culture sensitivity preventing colony formation [56].

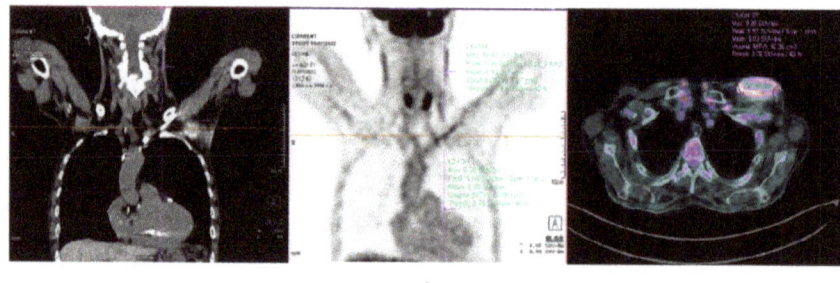

Figure 4. Fluorodeoxyglucose (FDG)-positron emission tomography (PET)/computed tomography (CT) of CIED pocket infection. Coronal slices of CT (panel (**A**)) and of PET (panel (**B**)) showing FDG uptake of the proximal part of the lead; fused PET/CT with abnormal FDG uptake at the pocket (panel (**C**)).

7. Device Removal Versus Device Retention

Key aspects in the management of CIED infections are rapid diagnosis and timely treatment. Early intervention, performed within three days of diagnosis, conducts to a significant reduction in in-hospital mortality [57]. A large-population cohort study reported high short- and medium-term complication rates related to CIED removal. However, at the multivariate analysis, the use of initial antimicrobial therapy as unique strategy was associated with a 7-fold increase in 30-day mortality, while immediate device removal showed a 3-fold decrease in 1-year mortality compared to delayed extraction [58].

International position and consensus documents highlight how effective treatments require complete removal of the system and any transvenous or subcutaneous component as well as any residual non-functional lead. A significant cause of relapses is represented, in fact, by retained hardware.

Complete device extraction should be performed when a valve is replaced or repaired for infective endocarditis since CIEDs could serve as a pabulum for pathogen's persistence and multiplication [59].

Lead vegetation recorded through TOE, after having ruled out the presence of a non-infected fibrin stranding (a very common finding in long-duration leads) is an absolute indication for device extraction [3].

Device removal outcomes for CDRIE does not differ in elderly and younger population [60]. The laser excimers devices appear to be more incline to vascular damage particularly involving the superior vena cava [61].

The therapeutic strategy to be adopted in presence of positive blood cultures varies depending on the microorganism that is found. A single positive test for StA (especially within three months of CIED manipulation or in case of recurrences despite specific antimicrobial therapy) or Candida species is enough to suggest the extraction of the system. On the other hand, in presence of CoNS, Cutibacterium or other pathogens commonly causing endocarditis, high-grade bacteraemia (two or more separate blood cultures positive for the same organism) is required to have a specific diagnosis. A single positive blood culture for one of the last listed pathogens may represent skin contamination. However, if the clinical suspicion persists, it may be reasonable to perform other diagnostic imaging tests such as 18F-FDG PET/CT and to discuss the subsequent management with an infectious disease expert [3,62]. In the aforementioned cases, the procedural risks related to CIED removal are significantly lower than the rate of mortality or recurrence of infection even if alternative strategies are adopted, such as antibiotic therapy or generator extraction with retention of the leads [63].

Signs and symptoms of pocket infection including oedema, erythema, purulent drainage, skin erosion with exposure of the generator or leads and pain, are a warning of the need to remove the device, even in absence of a positive culture of the drainage of the wound or bacteriemia [64]. Superficial incision infections, especially if they occur in the first weeks after implantation, with the involvement of the skin and the subcutaneous tissue without the participation of the fascia and the muscle, provide for close monitoring for one to two weeks to rule out the progression to deeper tissues which would require extraction. A similar approach should be adopted in presence of pocket hematoma. Some authors suggest the opportunity to start an empiric antibiotic therapy with activity against staphylococcus spp. [49].

Where indicated, transvenous removal of all leads, including the abandoned ones, is the most recommended technique with low rates of mortality and major complications [2]. Usually, leads implanted at least two years earlier are technically more difficult to extract and the procedure should be performed by experienced operators. Different types of leads involve different challenges during the removal: ICD leads, with the presence of one or two coils steering to the formation of more extensive adherences, are more prone to procedural complication, especially when a caval coil is present; the same applies to those with passive fixing compared to those with active fixing.

The evaluation of the balance between the surgical risk of removal and the benefits in terms of eradication of the infection is mandatory in presence of epicardial leads or patches connected to pectoral or abdominal generators. When the contamination is isolated to the pocket, an option is to perform a separate incision away from the pocket, adjacent to the thoracic entrance of the epicardial leads or patches, and to cut their connection with the generator. Their proximal end can then be removed from the pocket [65].

Large vegetations should be carefully assessed in terms of risk for pulmonary embolism with the transvenous method and the risk-benefit balance of a surgical procedure. The surgical threshold, in fact, has still to be defined and this approach is associated with greater morbidity [57]. Observational studies with small sample sizes, on the other hand, showed low rates of hemodynamically relevant pulmonary embolism with transvenous removal independently from vegetative mass dimensions [66,67]. Percutaneous removal of such vegetations, with a suction and debulking technique, before lead transvenous extraction, has been reported [68]. Filtering of vegetations using an in-line filtered veno-venous extracorporeal circulation has been described for very large masses. This technique shows beneficial effects reducing post-operative sepsis or pneumonia related to small vegetations embolisation [69].

Pocket management is likewise a crucial aspect of device removal. It requires an accurate debridement with complete excision of the fibrotic capsule and of the non-adsorbable suture material and following plenty sterile saline irrigation [70].

Sometimes the removal of the CIED is desirable, but not feasible. It is the case of patients with relevant comorbidities, limited life-expectancy, with devices implanted for a long time and with PM dependency. Evidence is limited in this setting. Current recommendations are that such individuals should undergo full targeted antibiotic therapy for at least six weeks as last resort. In most cases they experience limited survival rates and high likelihood of relapses [71].

CIED retention strategy is limited to few instances where the infection of the system is unlikely. For example, when the established pathogen in the blood stream is not a StA, the definition of CIED or valvular vegetation matters. With this kind of setting, imaging techniques should identify the vegetations location, pocket infection should be excluded, and the device should not have been manipulated for less than three months.

CIED retention may also be considered in case of skin incision site infections with superficial cellulitis or stitch abscess, without the involvement of the pocket. Such a diagnosis is often difficult, and these patients should be carefully followed up. The surgical technique used for superficial infection should include wide excision of healthy skin around the infected area and must be performed in a proper sterile environment. The first manoeuvre, crucial in the analysis of the infected wound, must be the verification of a possible communication between the pocket of the device and the outside. If the integrity of the pocket is compromised, total removal of the system deserves to be considered [49].

The definition of optimal re-implantation timing requires further analysis (Figure 5). About one third of patients who undergo CIED extraction do not require a new device. A temporary system, when the need to place a cardiac pacing device is not deferrable, could be implanted, considering that this increases the infectious risk. Individuals who showed valve vegetations on TOE should be implanted after at least 14 days from last negative blood cultures. In case of isolated lead involvement or in case of bacteraemia without demonstration of vegetations on TOE, waiting 72 h from last negative blood cultures could be enough [3]. Finally, as soon as an isolated pocket infection has completely healed, new CIED positioning is possible. In the case of PM-dependent patients, local pocket infection may be managed with device extraction and, once specific antibiotic regimen has been started, contralateral device implant may be considered.

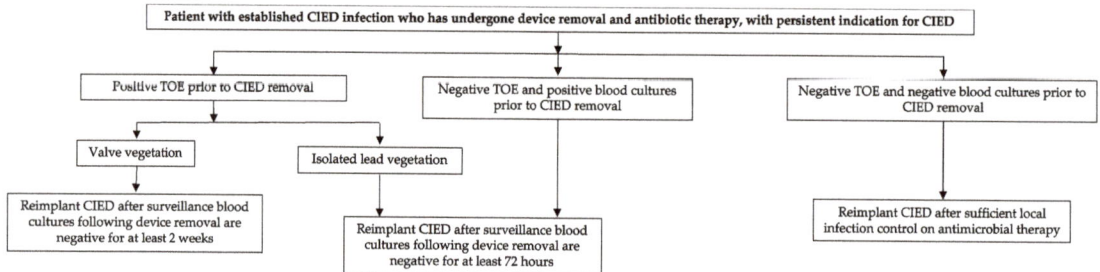

Figure 5. Proposed algorithm for optimal re-implantation timing in patients with persistent indication to CIED. CIED: cardiovascular implantable electronic device; TOE: trans-oesophageal echocardiography.

Different devices as subcutaneous ICDs (S-ICDs) or leadless PMs may also be taken into account to reduce the risk of relapses [49].

Due to their recent introduction into clinical practice, little data is available on the risk of infection for leadless PMs. However, when compared with conventional permanent pacing, they showed lower rates and a lower predisposition to hematogenous infections even when implanted in the presence of active bacteraemia [72,73]. The reason could be related to the specific coating system of the devices, the small surface area and the progressive fibrous encapsulation in the right ventricle which make them more resistant to bacterial seeding. Furthermore, the absence of the generator pocket and the use of a delivery system avoids physical handling of the device during implantation [73].

8. Antimicrobial Therapy

Although randomised studies are currently lacking, resolutive treatment of CIED infections requires early and complementary association between complete system removal and antimicrobial therapy [2,33,49,74].

Multiple antimicrobial regimens may be considered, depending on several different clinical scenarios. The available data are mostly based on in vitro susceptibility, observational studies, pharmacokinetic/pharmacodynamic data and clinical experience. Antimicrobial choice for CIED infection depends on multiple factors such as severity of clinical presentation, plans for device management, cardiac involvement, extra-cardiac foci of infection, allergy, concurrent medications and renal impairment. An appropriate treatment should therefore be discussed by a multidisciplinary team with expertise in CIED infections (i.e., "Endocarditis Team") [2].

Even though empirical treatments (before the pathogen identification) cover a broad spectrum of bacilli, sometimes requiring complex and potentially toxic antimicrobial associations, they are usually less effective than "targeted" approaches. Potential life-threatening conditions as severe sepsis/septic shock require an empirical treatment urgently after sampling for blood cultures to minimise the prognostic impact of systemic involvement. On the other hand, many CIED-related infections show indolent clinical course enabling, whenever possible, to await cultures report and susceptibility testing to set up a "targeted" strategy

Antimicrobial regimens should be kept as simple as possible until microbiological results and CIED system management are defined. Antibiotic treatment recommendations are summarised in (Table 2), as listed in the 2020 EHRA international consensus document [2].

Table 2. Antibiotic treatment recommendation.

Surgical Incision Infection	
Empirical Treatment	
Oral antibiotic covering StA:	flucloxacillin 1 gr (every 6–8 h)
If high MRSA prevalence:	trimethoprim-sulfamethoxazole, clyndamicin, doxyciclin, linezolid
	Targeted after culture results
	Duration: 7–10 days
Isolated Pocket Infection	
Empirical Treatment	
Intravenous treatment covering StA and multi-resistant CoNS	vancomycin 30–60 mg/kg/day i.v. in 2–3 doses daptomycin 8–10 mg/kg i.v. o.d.)
	If systemic symptoms
For additional Gram-negative coverage, combine with 3rd generation cephalosporin (or broader beta-lactam) or gentamicin	cephalosporins standard dose or gentamicin 5–7 mg/kg i.v. o.d.
	Targeted after culture results
If sensitive Staphylococci:	flucloxacillin 8 g/day i.v. in 4 doses or 1st generation cephalosporins (standard dose)
	Targeted after culture results
	Duration post-extraction: 10–14 days
Systemic Infections	
Without Vegetation on Leads or Valves ± Pocket Infection	
Empirical combination treatment covering multi-resistant Staphylococci and Gram-negative bacteria	vancomycin 30–60 mg/kg/day i.v. in 2–3 doses (alternative: daptomycin 8–10 mg/kg i.v. o.d.) plus 3rd generation cephalosporins standard dose i.v (or broader beta-lactam) or gentamicin 5–7 mg/kg i.v. o.d.
	Targeted after culture results
If sensitive Staphylococci	flucloxacillin 8 g/day i.v. in 4 doses 1st generation cephalosporin (standard dose)
	Targeted after culture results
	Duration post-extraction: 4 weeks (2 weeks if negative blood cultures)
CIED endocarditis with vegetation on leads and/or valves ± embolism	
Empirical treatment	vancomycin 30–60 mg/kg/day i.v. in 2–3 doses (alternative: daptomycin 8–10 mg/kg i.v. o.d.) plus 3rd generation cephalosporins standard dose i.v (or broader beta-lactam) or gentamicin 5–7 mg/kg i.v. o.d.
If prosthetic valve and staphylococcal infection	add rifampicin after 5–7 days, 900–1200 mg/day in two doses (orally or i.v.)
	Adjust to culture results according to ESC Endocarditis Guidelines

Duration:
- for native valve infective endocarditis: 4 weeks post-extraction
- for prosthetic valve endocarditis: 4 to 6 weeks
- for isolated lead vegetation: 2 weeks after extraction may be sufficient (4 weeks in total) except for StA infection

Bacteraemia in a CIED patient without signs of pocket infection or echocardiographic evidence of lead or valve involvement	
According to pathogen-specific treatment guidelines	
Attempted Salvage Therapy and Long-Term Suppressive Therapy	
I.v. antibiotics as in prosthetic valve endocarditis for 4–6 weeks	
Stop antibiotic therapy under close follow-up or continue individualised long-term suppressive oral therapy	

Adapted from Blomstrom-Lundqvist C. et al. European Heart Journal (2020) 41, 2012–2032. CIED: cardiovascular implantable electronic device; StA: Staphylococcus aureus; MRSA: methicillin-resistant Staphylococcus aureus; CoNS: coagulase-negative Staphylococci; i.v.: intravenous; o.d.: once daily.

Successful antibiotic rescue therapy and long-term suppressive antibiotic therapy have been used in selected cases when device removal is considered contraindicated, but there is only limited clinical experience reinforcing the need of multidisciplinary "Endocarditis Team" management [71,74].

Finally, yeasts are a rare cause of CIED infections and routine empirical antifungal therapy is generally not recommended. Candida species are the most frequently involved (ranging from C. albicans to C. parapsilosis). When clinical features suggest fungal aetiology and require urgent treatment initiation, empirical approach should include amphotericin B with/without 5-flucytosine or an echinocandin agent such as micafungin as primary therapy. In stable patients with documented susceptible microorganism and negative blood cultures, step-down therapy with fluconazole 400–800 mg daily could be a reasonable choice [75].

Administration of antimicrobial treatment should be managed orally or intravenously according to patients' clinical features and needs. Although no clinical trial is available on this topic, there is a wide consensus advising that IV therapy is the best choice for CDRIE and attempted CIED salvage, while oral treatment could be more appropriate in localised pocket infections and after system removal. Central venous catheterisation is preferably to be avoided, except when requested for clinical instability or difficult peripheral access. The peripheral venous cannula has the lowest infection potential (with 72h replacement) and reduces the risk of damaging future sites for CIED implantation. When long-term IV therapy is planned, peripherally inserted central catheter (PICC) or 'midline' (MID) is preferable [3]. Vascular accesses-related risk of infections shows a direct correlation with the permanence of the cannula, and periodic switches between peripheral cannula and PICC/MID should be planned by nursing professionals in order to manage this risk [2].

9. Prevention of CDRIE

Even if there are no large, controlled studies on this topic, antibiotic prophylaxis is recommended before implantation of CIEDs. A first-generation cephalosporin, such as cefazolin, is usually used as prophylaxis and should be parenterally administered one hour before the procedure. Vancomycin, teicoplanin and daptomycin may be considered instead of cefazolin in centres where oxacillin resistance among staphylococci is high, in high-risk patients or in patients with contraindications to cephalosporins. They should be started before the procedure according to the drug pharmacokinetics [33]. In patients who are allergic to both cephalosporins and vancomycin, daptomycin and linezolid represent an option [49]. Potential sources of sepsis should be eliminated at least two weeks before implantation in deferrable procedures [33].

Antibiotic prophylaxis before invasive procedures that are not directly related to CIEDs manipulation is not recommended based on limited evidence. Furthermore, the predominant pathogens in CDRIE are staphylococci, which are different from the expected pathogen associated with translocation during dental, gastrointestinal, or genitourinary procedures. Post-procedural antibiotics are not recommended given the lack of evidence in terms of benefits and potential risks.

According to the PADIT trial, incremental administration of antibiotics on the basis of the clinical risk of CDRIE does not significantly impact the prevalence of infections [76].

An interesting role could be played by antimicrobial eluting antibacterial envelopes. The TYRX™ (MEDTRONIC TYRX™ Inc. New Jersey USA) antibacterial envelope (the last available type) is a monofilament polypropylene mesh that holds the cardiac implantable electronic device in place and emits rifampin and minocycline slowly over time [51]. More recently, two prospective cohort studies were conducted to evaluate the use of antibacterial envelope among high-risk patients receiving ICD and CRT. These studies showed a very low infection rate of 0.4%, which was significantly lower than the 12-month benchmark rate of 2.2% [77]. Moreover, a large randomised clinical trial enrolling patients from multiple sites across the world reported a 40% reduction in major CDRIE within 12 months after the procedure with the use of antibacterial envelopes [78].

Pocket hematoma that complicates CIEDs placement or invasive manipulation has been identified as a risk factor for infection [79]. Prevention of hematoma during the procedure is desirable: meticulous cautery of bleeding sites, application of topical thrombin, irrigation of the pocket, the use of monofilament suture for sub-cuticular layer, a pressure dressing applied for 12 to 24 h after skin closure may decrease the risk of hematoma formation [49]. The "bridging approach" with anticoagulation increases the risk of hematoma and should be avoided in CIEDs-related procedures [80]. For patients undergoing device implantation, prospective and randomised data in vitamin K antagonists (VKA)-treated patients indicated lower thromboembolic and bleeding rates if the VKA is continued, without any bridging [81]. For Direct Oral Anticoagulant (DOAC)- treated patients, the BRUISE-CONTROL 2 trial demonstrated similar bleeding and embolic rates in patients with a last intake two days before the implantation compared to those who continued DOAC until the morning of the procedure [82]. A balance between thrombotic and bleeding risks must be pursued: to stop DOAC the day before the procedure seems reasonable in most cases, especially when bleeding risk exceeds stroke risk. Resumption of DOAC regimen on the first postoperative day is usually feasible [83].

Patients on dual antiplatelet therapy carry an increased risk of post-operative pocket hematoma compared to patients treated with aspirin alone or without antiplatelet therapy. In such cases, European guidelines recommend P2Y12 receptor-inhibitors discontinuation for 3–7 days (according to the specific drug) before the procedure, where possible, accordingly to an individualised risk assessment [80].

Needle aspiration should be avoided because of the risk of introducing skin flora into the pocket with the subsequent development of infection [49].

In elective procedures, StA colonisation can be detected by nasal swabs. Nasal treatment with mupirocin and chlorhexidine skin washing reduce colonisation and should be preferred to iodine solution [20,76].

AHA/ACC/HRS guidelines suggest a S-ICD in patients who are at high risk for infection and in whom pacing is neither needed nor anticipated [84]. Even if the CIED infection rate for S-ICDs is still not demonstrated to be lower than transvenous ICDs, the absence of the possibility for infective endocarditis with S-ICDs is the reason for this recommendation [85]. When available and according to the clinical indication, leadless PMs carry a lower incidence of CDRIE [86].

A summary of possible strategies to prevent CDRIE is available in Table 3.

Table 3. Preventive strategies for cardiac device-related infective endocarditis.

Strategy	Description
Antibiotic prophylaxis before CIED implantation	A first-generation cephalosporin. Vancomycin, teicoplanin and daptomycin in patients with contraindications to cephalosporins.
Antibiotic prophylaxis before other procedures	It is not recommended based on limited evidence
Antibacterial envelope	Reduces the rate of CDRIE
Hematoma pocket prevention	It is a risk factor for infection. Needle aspiration should be avoided.
Nasal swab	No studies for patients with CIED

CIED: cardiovascular implantable electronic device; CDRIE: cardiac device-related infective endocarditis.

10. Conclusions

Infections represent one of the main factors of mortality and morbidity that afflict patients with CIEDs. Their correct definition and an appropriate diagnosis allow a precise treatment in terms of removal or retention of the device, antimicrobial therapy and optimal timing of re-implantation. Nowadays, however, there are alternative strategies and prevention mechanisms that must be employed and implemented to reduce the burden of this problem.

Author Contributions: Conceptualization, F.T. and M.S.; methodology, F.T.; validation, F.T. and M.S.; writing—original draft preparation, F.T., M.S., A.F., D.G., G.P., A.V.P., E.G. and L.B.; writing—review and editing, F.T., M.S. and S.C; supervision, S.C. All authors have read and agreed to the published version of the manuscript.

Funding: This study was partially funded by Italian Ministry of Health, Current research IRCCS.

Institutional Review Board Statement: Not applicable.

Informed Consent Statement: Not applicable.

Data Availability Statement: Not applicable.

Conflicts of Interest: The authors declare no conflict of interest.

References

1. Senning, Ä. Cardiac Pacing in Retrospect. *Am. J. Surg.* **1983**, *145*, 733–739. [CrossRef]
2. Sandoe, J.A.T.; Barlow, G.; Chambers, J.B.; Gammage, M.; Guleri, A.; Howard, P.; Olson, E.; Perry, J.D.; Prendergast, B.D.; Spry, M.J.; et al. Guidelines for the Diagnosis, Prevention and Management of Implantable Cardiac Electronic Device Infection. Report of a Joint Working Party Project on Behalf of the British Society for Antimicrobial Chemotherapy (BSAC, Host Organization), British Heart Rh. *J. Antimicrob. Chemother.* **2015**, *70*, 325–359. [CrossRef]
3. Blomströ M-Lundqvist, C.; Erba, P.A.; Burri, H.; Nielsen, J.C.; Bongiorni, M.G.; Poole, J. European Heart Rhythm Association (EHRA) International Consensus Document on How to Prevent, Diagnose, and Treat Cardiac Implantable Electronic Device Infections. *Eur. Heart J.* **2020**, *12*, 515–549.
4. Sohail, M.R.; Henrikson, C.A.; Braid-Forbes, M.J.; Forbes, K.F.; Lerner, D.J. Mortality and Cost Associated with Cardiovascular Implantable Electronic Device Infections. *Arch. Intern. Med.* **2011**, *171*, 1821–1828. [CrossRef]
5. Greenspon, A.J.; Patel, J.D.; Lau, E.; Ochoa, J.A.; Frisch, D.R.; Ho, R.T.; Pavri, B.B.; Kurtz, S.M. 16-Year Trends in the Infection Burden for Pacemakers and Implantable Cardioverter-Defibrillators in the United States: 1993 to 2008. *J. Am. Coll. Cardiol.* **2011**, *58*, 1001–1006. [CrossRef] [PubMed]
6. Voigt, A.; Shalaby, A.; Saba, S. Continued Rise in Rates of Cardiovascular Implantable Electronic Device Infections in the United States: Temporal Trends and Causative Insights. *PACE-Pacing Clin. Electrophysiol.* **2010**, *33*, 414–419. [CrossRef]
7. Korantzopoulos, P.; Sideris, S.; Dilaveris, P.; Gatzoulis, K.; Goudevenos, J.A. Infection Control in Implantation of Cardiac Implantable Electronic Devices: Current Evidence, Controversial Points, and Unresolved Issues. *Europace* **2016**, *18*, 473–478. [CrossRef] [PubMed]
8. Sohail, M.R.; Uslan, D.Z.; Khan, A.H.; Friedman, P.A.; Hayes, D.L.; Wilson, W.R.; Steckelberg, J.M.; Stoner, S.; Baddour, L.M. Management and Outcome of Permanent Pacemaker and Implantable Cardioverter-Defibrillator Infections. *J. Am. Coll. Cardiol.* **2007**, *49*, 1851–1859. [CrossRef] [PubMed]
9. Landolina, M.; Gasparini, M.; Lunati, M.; Iacopino, S.; Boriani, G.; Bonanno, C.; Vado, A.; Proclemer, A.; Capucci, A.; Zucchiatti, C.; et al. Long-Term Complications Related to Biventricular Defibrillator Implantation: Rate of Surgical Revisions and Impact on Survival: Insights from the Italian Clinicalservice Database. *Circulation* **2011**, *123*, 2526–2535. [CrossRef] [PubMed]
10. Chauhan, A.; Grace, A.A.; Newell, S.A.; Stone, D.L.; Shapiro, L.M.; Schofield, P.M.; Petch, M.C. Early Complications After Dual Chamber Versus Single Chamber Pacemaker Implantation. *Pacing Clin. Electrophysiol.* **1994**, *17*, 2012–2015. [CrossRef]
11. Sohail, M.R.; Uslan, D.Z.; Khan, A.H.; Friedman, P.A.; Hayes, D.L.; Wilson, W.R.; Steckelberg, J.M.; Stoner, S.M.; Baddour, L.M. Risk Factor Analysis of Permanent Pacemaker Infection. *Clin. Infect. Dis.* **2007**, *45*, 166–173. [CrossRef]
12. Barbar, T.; Patel, R.; Thomas, G.; Cheung, J. Strategies to Prevent Cardiac Implantable Electronic Device Infection. *J. Innov. Card. Rhythm Manag.* **2020**, *11*, 3949. [CrossRef]
13. Polyzos, K.A.; Konstantelias, A.A.; Falagas, M.E. Risk Factors for Cardiac Implantable Electronic Device Infection: A Systematic Review and Meta-Analysis. *Europace* **2015**, *17*, 767–777. [CrossRef]
14. Catanchin, A.; Murdock, C.J.; Athan, E. Pacemaker Infections: A 10-Year Experience. *Heart Lung Circ.* **2007**, *16*, 434–439. [CrossRef]
15. Sohail, M.R.; Henrikson, C.A.; Braid-Forbes, M.J.; Forbes, K.F.; Lerner, D.J. Comparison of Mortality in Women versus Men with Infections Involving Cardiovascular Implantable Electronic Device. *Am. J. Cardiol.* **2013**, *112*, 1403–1409. [CrossRef] [PubMed]
16. Johansen, J.B.; Jørgensen, O.D.; Møller, M.; Arnsbo, P.; Mortensen, P.T.; Nielsen, J.C. Infection after Pacemaker Implantation: Infection Rates and Risk Factors Associated with Infection in a Population-Based Cohort Study of 46299 Consecutive Patients. *Eur. Heart J.* **2011**, *32*, 991–998. [CrossRef]
17. Leung, S.; Danik, S. Prevention, Diagnosis, and Treatment of Cardiac Implantable Electronic Device Infections. *Curr. Cardiol. Rep.* **2016**, *18*, 58. [CrossRef]
18. Romeyer-Bouchard, C.; Da Costa, A.; Dauphinot, V.; Messier, M.; Bisch, L.; Samuel, B.; Lafond, P.; Ricci, P.; Isaaz, K. Prevalence and Risk Factors Related to Infections of Cardiac Resynchronization Therapy Devices. *Eur. Heart J.* **2010**, *31*, 203–210. [CrossRef]
19. Sadeghi, H.; Alizadehdiz, A.; Fazelifar, A.; Emkanjoo, Z.; Haghjoo, M. New Insights into Predictors of Cardiac Implantable Electronic Device Infection. *Texas Heart Inst. J.* **2018**, *45*, 128–135. [CrossRef]

10. Tarakji, K.G.; Krahn, A.D.; Poole, J.E.; Mittal, S.; Kennergren, C.; Biffi, M.; Korantzopoulos, P.; Dallaglio, P.D.; Lexcen, D.R.; Lande, J.D.; et al. Risk Factors for CIED Infection after Secondary Procedures: Insights from the WRAP-IT Trial. *JACC Clin. Electrophysiol.* **2022**, *8*, 101–111. [CrossRef]
11. Uslan, D.Z.; Sohail, M.R.; St Sauver, J.L.; Friedman, P.A.; Hayes, D.L.; Stoner, S.M.; Wilson, W.R.; Steckelberg, J.M.; Baddour, L.M. Permanent Pacemaker and Implantable Cardioverter Defibrillator Infection: A Population-Based Study. *Arch. Intern. Med.* **2007**, *167*, 669–675. [CrossRef] [PubMed]
12. Welch, M.; Uslan, D.Z.; Greenspon, A.J.; Sohail, M.R.; Baddour, L.M.; Blank, E.; Carrillo, R.G.; Danik, S.B.; Del Rio, A.; Hellinger, W.; et al. Variability in Clinical Features of Early versus Late Cardiovascular Implantable Electronic Device Pocket Infections. *PACE-Pacing Clin. Electrophysiol.* **2014**, *37*, 955–962. [CrossRef] [PubMed]
13. Chua, J.D.; Wilkoff, B.L.; Lee, I.; Juratli, N.; Longworth, D.L.; Gordon, S.M. Diagnosis and Management of Infections Involving Implantable Electrophysiologic Cardiac Devices. *Ann. Intern. Med.* **2000**, *133*, 604–608. [CrossRef] [PubMed]
14. Del Río, A.; Anguera, I.; Miró, J.M.; Mont, L.; Fowler, V.G.; Azqueta, M.; Mestres, C.A. Surgical Treatment of Pacemaker and Defibrillator Lead Endocarditis: The Impact of Electrode Lead Extraction on Outcome. *Chest* **2003**, *124*, 1451–1459. [CrossRef] [PubMed]
15. Viganego, F.; O'Donoghue, S.; Eldadah, Z.; Shah, M.H.; Rastogi, M.; Mazel, J.A.; Platia, E.V. Effect of Early Diagnosis and Treatment with Percutaneous Lead Extraction on Survival in Patients with Cardiac Device Infections. *Am. J. Cardiol.* **2012**, *109*, 1466–1471. [CrossRef]
16. Priori, S.G.; Blomstrom-Lundqvist, C.; Mazzanti, A.; Bloma, N.; Borggrefe, M.; Camm, J.; Elliott, P.M.; Fitzsimons, D.; Hatala, R.; Hindricks, G.; et al. 2015 ESC Guidelines for the Management of Patients with Ventricular Arrhythmias and the Prevention of Sudden Cardiac Death the Task Force for the Management of Patients with Ventricular Arrhythmias and the Prevention of Sudden Cardiac Death of the Europea. *Eur. Heart J.* **2015**, *17*, 1601–1687. [CrossRef]
17. Del Pozo, J.L.; Patel, R. The Challenge of Treating Biofilm-Associated Bacterial Infections. *Clin. Pharmacol. Ther.* **2007**, *82*, 204–209. [CrossRef] [PubMed]
18. Jan, E.; Camou, F.; Texier-Maugein, J.; Whinnett, Z.; Caubet, O.; Ploux, S.; Pellegrin, J.L.; Ritter, P.; Metayer, P.L.; Roudaut, R.; et al. Microbiologic Characteristics and in Vitro Susceptibility to Antimicrobials in a Large Population of Patients with Cardiovascular Implantable Electronic Device Infection. *J. Cardiovasc. Electrophysiol.* **2012**, *23*, 375–381. [CrossRef]
19. Palmisano, P.; Accogli, M.; Zaccaria, M.; Luzzi, G.; Nacci, F.; Anaclerio, M.; Favale, S. Rate, Causes, and Impact on Patient Outcome of Implantable Device Complications Requiring Surgical Revision: Large Population Survey from Two Centres in Italy. *Europace* **2013**, *15*, 531–540. [CrossRef] [PubMed]
20. Nielsen, J.C.; Gerdes, J.C.; Varma, N. Infected Cardiac-Implantable Electronic Devices: Prevention, Diagnosis, and Treatment. *Eur. Heart J.* **2015**, *36*, 2484–2490. [CrossRef]
21. Martinelli, M.; D'Orio Nishioka, S.A.; Varejão, T.; Uipe, D.; Pedrosa, A.A.A.; Costa, R.; Danik, S.B.; De Oliveira, J.C. Efficacy of Antibiotic Prophylaxis before the Implantation of Pacemakers and Cardioverter-Defibrillators: Results of a Large, Prospective, Randomized, Double-Blinded, Placebo-Controlled Trial. *Circ. Arrhythmia Electrophysiol.* **2009**, *2*, 29–34. [CrossRef]
22. Li, J.S.; Sexton, D.J.; Mick, N.; Nettles, R.; Fowler, V.G.; Ryan, T.; Bashore, T.; Corey, G.R. Proposed Modifications to the Duke Criteria for the Diagnosis of Infective Endocarditis. *Clin. Infect. Dis.* **2000**, *30*, 633–638. [CrossRef] [PubMed]
23. Habib, G.; Lancellotti, P.; Antunes, M.J.; Bongiorni, M.G.; Casalta, J.P.; Del Zotti, F.; Dulgheru, R.; El Khoury, G.; Erba, P.A.; Iung, B.; et al. The Task Force for the Management of infective Endocarditis of the European Society of Cardiology (ESC) Endorsed by European Association for Cardio-Thoracic Surgery (EACTS), the European Association of Nuclear Medicine (EANM). 2015 ESC Guidelines for the management of infective endocarditis. *Eur. Heart J.* **2015**, *36*, 3075–3123. [CrossRef] [PubMed]
24. Durante-Mangoni, E.; Mattucci, I.; Agrusta, F.; Tripodi, M.F.; Utili, R. Current Trends in the Management of Cardiac Implantable Electronic Device (CIED) Infections. *Intern. Emerg. Med.* **2013**, *8*, 465–476. [CrossRef]
25. Gould, P.A.; Gula, L.J.; Yee, R.; Skanes, A.C.; Klein, G.J.; Krahn, A.D. Cardiovascular Implantable Electrophysiological Device-Related Infections: A Review. *Curr. Opin. Cardiol.* **2011**, *26*, 6–11. [CrossRef] [PubMed]
26. Massoure, P.L.; Reuter, S.; Lafitte, S.; Laborderie, J.; Bordachard, P.; Clementy, J.; Roudaut, R. Pacemaker Endocarditis: Clinical Features and Management of 60 Consecutive Cases. *Pacing Clin. Electrophysiol.* **2007**, *30*, 12–19. [CrossRef] [PubMed]
27. Cengiz, M.; Okutucu, S.; Ascioglu, S.; Şahin, A.; Aksoy, H.; Deveci, O.S.; Kaya, E.B.; Aytemir, K.; Kabakci, G.; Tokgozoglu, L.; et al. Permanent Pacemaker and Implantable Cardioverter Defibrillator Infections: Seven Years of Diagnostic and Therapeutic Experience of a Single Center. *Clin. Cardiol.* **2010**, *33*, 406–411. [CrossRef]
28. Leone, S.; Ravasio, V.; Durante-Mangoni, E.; Crapis, M.; Carosi, G.; Scotton, P.G.; Barzaghi, N.; Falcone, M.; Chinello, P.; Pasticci, M.B.; et al. Epidemiology, Characteristics, and Outcome of Infective Endocarditis in Italy: The Italian Study on Endocarditis. *Infection* **2012**, *40*, 527–535. [CrossRef]
29. Sohail, M.R.; Palraj, B.R.; Khalid, S.; Uslan, D.Z.; Al-Saffar, F.; Friedman, P.A.; Hayes, D.L.; Lohse, C.M.; Wilson, W.R.; Steckelberg, J.M.; et al. Predicting Risk of Endovascular Device Infection in Patients with Staphylococcus Aureus Bacteremia (PREDICT-SAB). *Circ. Arrhythmia Electrophysiol.* **2015**, *8*, 137–144. [CrossRef]
30. Voet, J.G.; Vandekerckhove, Y.R.; Muyldermans, L.L.; Missault, L.H.; Matthys, L.J. Pacemaker Lead Infection: Report of Three Cases and Review of the Literature. *Heart* **1999**, *81*, 88–91. [CrossRef]

41. Santangelo, L.; Russo, V.; Ammendola, E.; De Crescenzo, I.; Pagano, C.; Savarese, C.; Caruso, A.; Utili, R.; Calabrò, R. Superior Vena Cava Thrombosis after Intravascular AICD Lead Extraction: A Case Report. *J. Vasc. Access* **2006**, *7*, 90–93. [CrossRef] [PubMed]
42. Polewczyk, A.; Janion, M.; Kutarski, A. Cardiac Device Infections: Definition, Classification, Differential Diagnosis, and Management. *Pol. Arch. Med. Wewn.* **2016**, *126*, 275–283. [CrossRef] [PubMed]
43. Downey, B.C.; Juselius, W.E.; Pandian, N.G.; Estes, N.A.M.; Link, M.S. Incidence and Significance of Pacemaker and Implantable Cardioverter-Defibrillator Lead Masses Discovered during Transesophageal Echocardiography. *PACE-Pacing Clin. Electrophysiol.* **2011**, *34*, 679–683. [CrossRef] [PubMed]
44. Kojodjojo, P.; John, R.M.; Epstein, L.M. Disseminated Malignancies Masquerading as Cardiovascular Implantable Electronic Devices Infections. *Europace* **2011**, *13*, 821–824. [CrossRef]
45. DeSimone, D.C.; Sohail, M.R. Infection Management. *Card. Electrophysiol. Clin.* **2018**, *10*, 601–607. [CrossRef]
46. Veloso, T.R.; Amiguet, M.; Rousson, V.; Giddey, M.; Vouillamoz, J.; Moreillon, P.; Entenza, J.M. Induction of Experimental Endocarditis by Continuous Low-Grade Bacteremia Mimicking Spontaneous Bacteremia in Humans. *Infect. Immun.* **2011**, *79*, 2006–2011. [CrossRef]
47. Morgan, S.R. Original Articles. *Except. Child* **1984**, *31*, 74–79. [CrossRef]
48. Uslan, D.Z.; Dowsley, T.F.; Sohail, M.R.; Hayes, D.L.; Friedman, P.A.; Wilson, W.R.; Steckelberg, J.M.; Baddour, L.M. Cardiovascular Implantable Electronic Device Infection in Patients with Staphylococcus Aureus Bacteremia. *PACE-Pacing Clin. Electrophysiol.* **2010**, *33*, 407–413. [CrossRef]
49. Baddour, L.M.; Epstein, A.E.; Erickson, C.C.; Knight, B.P.; Levison, M.E.; Lockhart, P.B.; Masoudi, F.A.; Okum, E.J.; Wilson, W.R.; Beerman, L.B.; et al. Update on Cardiovascular Implantable Electronic Device Infections and Their Management: A Scientific Statement from the American Heart Association. *Circulation* **2010**, *121*, 458–477. [CrossRef]
50. Lennerz, C.; Vrazic, H.; Haller, B.; Braun, S.; Petzold, T.; Ott, I.; Lennerz, A.; Michel, J.; Blažek, P.; Deisenhofer, I.; et al. Biomarker-Based Diagnosis of Pacemaker and Implantable Cardioverter Defibrillator Pocket Infections: A Prospective, Multicentre, Case-Control Evaluation. *PLoS ONE* **2017**, *12*, e0172384. [CrossRef]
51. Arnold, C.J.; Chu, V.H. Cardiovascular Implantable Electronic Device Infections. *Infect. Dis. Clin. N. Am.* **2018**, *32*, 811–825. [CrossRef] [PubMed]
52. Erba, P.A.; Sollini, M.; Conti, U.; Bandera, F.; Tascini, C.; De Tommasi, S.M.; Zucchelli, G.; Doria, R.; Menichetti, F.; Bongiorni, M.G.; et al. Radiolabeled WBC Scintigraphy in the Diagnostic Workup of Patients with Suspected Device-Related Infections. *JACC Cardiovasc. Imaging* **2013**, *6*, 1075–1086. [CrossRef] [PubMed]
53. Ten Hove, D.; Slart, R.H.J.A.; Sinha, B.; Glaudemans, A.W.J.M.; Budde, R.P.J. 18 F-FDG PET/CT in Infective Endocarditis. Indications and Approaches for Standardization. *Curr. Cardiol. Rep.* **2021**, *23*, 130. [CrossRef] [PubMed]
54. Juneau, D.; Golfam, M.; Hazra, S.; Zuckier, L.S.; Garas, S.; Redpath, C.; Bernick, J.; Leung, E.; Chih, S.; Wells, G.; et al. Positron Emission Tomography and Single-Photon Emission Computed Tomography Imaging in the Diagnosis of Cardiac Implantable Electronic Device Infection: A Systematic Review and Meta-Analysis. *Circ. Cardiovasc. Imaging* **2017**, *10*, e005772. [CrossRef] [PubMed]
55. Cautela, J.; Alessandrini, S.; Cammilleri, S.; Giorgi, R.; Richet, H.; Casalta, J.P.; Habib, G.; Raoult, D.; Mundler, O.; Deharo, J.C. Diagnostic Yield of FDG Positron-Emission Tomography/Computed Tomography in Patients with CEID Infection: A Pilot Study. *Europace* **2013**, *15*, 252–257. [CrossRef]
56. Sohail, M.R.; Uslan, D.Z.; Khan, A.H.; Friedman, P.A.; Hayes, D.L.; Wilson, W.R.; Steckelberg, J.M.; Jenkins, S.M.; Baddour, L.M. Infective Endocarditis Complicating Permanent Pacemaker and Implantable Cardioverter-Defibrillator Infection. *Mayo Clin. Proc.* **2008**, *83*, 46–53. [CrossRef]
57. Mulpuru, S.K.; Pretorius, V.G.; Birgersdotter-Green, U.M. Device Infections: Management and Indications for Lead Extraction. *Circulation* **2013**, *128*, 1031–1038. [CrossRef]
58. Le, K.Y.; Sohail, M.R.; Friedman, P.A.; Uslan, D.Z.; Cha, S.S.; Hayes, D.L.; Wilson, W.R.; Steckelberg, J.M.; Baddour, L.M. Impact of Timing of Device Removal on Mortality in Patients with Cardiovascular Implantable Electronic Device Infections. *Heart Rhythm* **2011**, *8*, 1678–1685. [CrossRef]
59. Huang, X.M.; Fu, H.X.; Zhong, L.; Cao, J.; Asirvatham, S.J.; Baddour, L.M.; Sohail, M.R.; Nkomo, V.T.; Nishimura, R.A.; Greason, K.L.; et al. Outcomes of Transvenous Lead Extraction for Cardiovascular Implantable Electronic Device Infections in Patients with Prosthetic Heart Valves. *Circ. Arrhythmia Electrophysiol.* **2016**, *9*, e004188. [CrossRef]
60. Okada, A.; Tabata, H.; Shoda, M.; Shoin, W.; Kobayashi, H.; Okano, T.; Yoshie, K.; Kato, K.; Saigusa, T.; Ebisawa, S.; et al. Safe and Effective Transvenous Lead Extraction for Elderly Patients Utilizing Non-Laser and Laser Tools: A Single-Center Experience in Japan. *Heart Vessels* **2021**, *36*, 882–889. [CrossRef]
61. Starck, C.T.; Gonzalez, E.; Al-Razzo, O.; Mazzone, P.; Delnoy, P.P.; Breitenstein, A.; Steffel, J.; Eulert-Grehn, J.; Lanmüller, P.; Melillo, F.; et al. Results of the Patient-Related Outcomes of Mechanical Lead Extraction Techniques (PROMET) Study: A Multicentre Retrospective Study on Advanced Mechanical Lead Extraction Techniques. *Europace* **2020**, *22*, 1103–1110. [CrossRef] [PubMed]
62. Kusumoto, F.M.; Schoenfeld, M.H.; Wilkoff, B.L.; Berul, C.I.; Birgersdotter-Green, U.M.; Carrillo, R.; Cha, Y.M.; Clancy, J.; Deharo, J.C.; Ellenbogen, K.A.; et al. 2017 HRS Expert Consensus Statement on Cardiovascular Implantable Electronic Device Lead Management and Extraction. *Heart Rhythm* **2017**, *14*, e503–e551. [CrossRef] [PubMed]

1. Athan, E.; Chu, V.H.; Tattevin, P.; Selton-Suty, C.; Jones, P.; Naber, C.; Miró, J.M.; Ninot, S.; Fernández-Hidalgo, N.; Durante-Mangoni, E.; et al. Clinical Characteristics and Outcome of Infective Endocarditis Involving Implantable Cardiac Devices. *JAMA* **2012**, *307*, 1727–1735. [CrossRef]
2. Blomström-Lundqvist, C.; Traykov, V.; Erba, P.A.; Burri, H.; Nielsen, J.C.; Bongiorni, M.G.; Poole, J.; Boriani, G.; Costa, R.; Deharo, J.C.; et al. European Heart Rhythm Association (EHRA) International Consensus Document on How to Prevent, Diagnose, and Treat Cardiac Implantable Electronic Device Infections-Endorsed by the Heart Rhythm Society (HRS), the Asia Pacific Heart Rhythm Society (APHRS), The Latin American Heart Rhythm Society (LAHRS), International Society for Cardiovascular Infectious Diseases (ISCVID) and the European Society of Clinical Microbiology and Infectious Diseases (ESCMID) in collaboration with the European Association for Cardio-Thoracic Surgery (EACTS). *Eur. Heart J.* **2020**, *41*, 2012–2032. [CrossRef] [PubMed]
3. Riaz, T.; Nienaber, J.J.C.; Baddour, L.M.; Walker, R.C.; Park, S.J.; Sohail, M.R. Cardiovascular Implantable Electronic Device Infections in Left Ventricular Assist Device Recipients. *Pacing Clin. Electrophysiol.* **2014**, *37*, 225–230. [CrossRef] [PubMed]
4. Grammes, J.A.; Schulze, C.M.; Al-Bataineh, M.; Yesenosky, G.A.; Saari, C.S.; Vrabel, M.J.; Horrow, J.; Chowdhury, M.; Fontaine, J.M.; Kutalek, S.P. Percutaneous Pacemaker and Implantable Cardioverter-Defibrillator Lead Extraction in 100 Patients with Intracardiac Vegetations Defined by Transesophageal Echocardiogram. *J. Am. Coll. Cardiol.* **2010**, *55*, 886–894. [CrossRef] [PubMed]
5. Pérez Baztarrica, G.; Gariglio, L.; Salvaggio, F.; Reolón, E.; Blanco, N.; Mazzetti, H.; Villecco, S.; Botbol, A.; Porcile, R. Transvenous Extraction of Pacemaker Leads in Infective Endocarditis with Vegetations ≥20 Mm: Our Experience. *Clin. Cardiol.* **2012**, *35*, 244–249. [CrossRef] [PubMed]
6. Starck, C.T.; Schaerf, R.H.M.; Breitenstein, A.; Najibi, S.; Conrad, J.; Berendt, J.; Esmailian, F.; Eulert-Grehn, J.; Dreizler, T.; Falk, V. Transcatheter Aspiration of Large Pacemaker and Implantable Cardioverter-Defibrillator Lead Vegetations Facilitating Safe Transvenous Lead Extraction. *Europace* **2020**, *22*, 133–138. [CrossRef] [PubMed]
7. Schaerf, R.H.M.; Najibi, S.; Conrad, J. Percutaneous Vacuum-Assisted Thrombectomy Device Used for Removal of Large Vegetations on Infected Pacemaker and Defibrillator Leads as an Adjunct to Lead Extraction. *J. Atr. Fibrillation* **2016**, *9*, 1455. [CrossRef] [PubMed]
8. Nakajima, I.; Narui, R.; Tokutake, K.; Norton, C.A.; Stevenson, W.G.; Richardson, T.D.; Ellis, C.R.; Crossley, G.H.; Montgomery, J.A. Staphylococcus Bacteremia without Evidence of Cardiac Implantable Electronic Device Infection. *Heart Rhythm* **2021**, *18*, 752–759. [CrossRef] [PubMed]
9. Tan, E.M.; Desimone, D.C.; Sohail, M.R.; Baddour, L.M.; Wilson, W.R.; Steckelberg, J.M.; Virk, A. Outcomes in Patients With Cardiovascular Implantable Electronic Device Infection Managed with Chronic Antibiotic Suppression. *Clin. Infect. Dis.* **2017**, *64*, 1516–1521. [CrossRef]
10. El-Chami, M.F.; Al-Samadi, F.; Clementy, N.; Garweg, C.; Martinez-Sande, J.L.; Piccini, J.P.; Iacopino, S.; Lloyd, M.; Viñolas Prat, X.; Jacobsen, M.D.; et al. Updated Performance of the Micra Transcatheter Pacemaker in the Real-World Setting: A Comparison to the Investigational Study and a Transvenous Historical Control. *Heart Rhythm* **2018**, *15*, 1800–1807. [CrossRef] [PubMed]
11. Garweg, C.; Vandenberk, B.; Jentjens, S.; Foulon, S.; Hermans, P.; Poels, P.; Haemers, P.; Ector, J.; Willems, R. Bacteraemia after Leadless Pacemaker Implantation. *J. Cardiovasc. Electrophysiol.* **2020**, *31*, 2440–2447. [CrossRef] [PubMed]
12. Peacock, J.E.; Stafford, J.M.; Le, K.; Sohail, M.R.; Baddour, L.M.; Prutkin, J.M.; Danik, S.B.; Vikram, H.R.; Hernandez-Meneses, M.; Miró, J.M.; et al. Attempted Salvage of Infected Cardiovascular Implantable Electronic Devices: Are There Clinical Factors That Predict Success? *Pacing Clin. Electrophysiol.* **2018**, *41*, 524–531. [CrossRef] [PubMed]
13. Halawa, A.; Henry, P.D.; Sarubbi, F.A. Candida Endocarditis Associated with Cardiac Rhythm Management Devices: Review with Current Treatment Guidelines. *Mycoses* **2011**, *54*, e168–e174. [CrossRef]
14. Krahn, A.D.; Longtin, Y.; Philippon, F.; Birnie, D.H.; Manlucu, J.; Angaran, P.; Rinne, C.; Coutu, B.; Low, R.A.; Essebag, V.; et al. Prevention of Arrhythmia Device Infection Trial: The PADIT Trial. *J. Am. Coll. Cardiol.* **2018**, *72*, 3098–3109. [CrossRef]
15. Henrikson, C.A.; Sohail, M.R.; Acosta, H.; Johnson, E.E.; Rosenthal, L.; Pachulski, R.; Dan, D.; Paladino, W.; Khairallah, F.S.; Gleed, K.; et al. Antibacterial Envelope Is Associated with Low Infection Rates after Implantable Cardioverter-Defibrillator and Cardiac Resynchronization Therapy Device Replacement: Results of the Citadel and Centurion Studies. *JACC Clin. Electrophysiol.* **2017**, *3*, 1158–1167. [CrossRef] [PubMed]
16. Mittal, S.; Wilkoff, B.L.; Kennergren, C.; Poole, J.E.; Corey, R.; Bracke, F.A.; Curnis, A.; Addo, K.; Martinez-Arraras, J.; Issa, Z.F.; et al. The World-Wide Randomized Antibiotic Envelope Infection Prevention (WRAP-IT) Trial: Long-Term Follow-Up. *Heart Rhythm* **2020**, *17*, 1115–1122. [CrossRef]
17. Kewcharoen, J.; Kanitsoraphan, C.; Thangjui, S.; Leesutipornchai, T.; Saowapa, S.; Pokawattana, A.; Navaravong, L. Postimplantation Pocket Hematoma Increases Risk of Cardiac Implantable Electronic Device Infection: A Meta-Analysis. *J. Arrhythmia* **2021**, *37*, 635–644. [CrossRef]
18. Glikson, M.; Nielsen, J.C.; Kronborg, M.B.; Michowitz, Y.; Auricchio, A.; Barbash, I.M.; Barrabés, J.A.; Boriani, G.; Braunschweig, F.; Brignole, M.; et al. 2021 ESC Guidelines on Cardiac Pacing and Cardiac Resynchronization TherapyDeveloped by the Task Force on Cardiac Pacing and Cardiac Resynchronization Therapy of the European Society of Cardiology (ESC) With the Special Contribution of the European Heart Rhythm Association (EHRA). *Eur. Heart J.* **2021**, *42*, 3427–3520. [CrossRef]

81. Birnie, D.H.; Healey, J.S.; Wells, G.A.; Verma, A.; Tang, A.S.; Krahn, A.D.; Simpson, C.S.; Ayala-Paredes, F.; Coutu, B.; Leiria, T.L.L.; et al. Pacemaker or Defibrillator Surgery without Interruption of Anticoagulation. *N. Engl. J. Med.* **2013**, *368*, 2084–2093. [CrossRef] [PubMed]
82. Birnie, D.H.; Healey, J.S.; Wells, G.A.; Ayala-Paredes, F.; Coutu, B.; Sumner, G.L.; Becker, G.; Verma, A.; Philippon, F.; Kalfon, E.; et al. Continued vs. Interrupted Direct Oral Anticoagulants at the Time of Device Surgery, in Patients with Moderate to High Risk of Arterial Thrombo-Embolic Events (BRUISE CONTROL-2). *Eur. Heart J.* **2018**, *39*, 3973–3979. [CrossRef] [PubMed]
83. Steffel, J.; Collins, R.; Antz, M.; Cornu, P.; Desteghe, L.; Haeusler, K.G.; Oldgren, J.; Reinecke, H.; Roldan-Schilling, V.; Rowell, N.; et al. 2021 European Heart Rhythm Association Practical Guide on the Use of Non-Vitamin K Antagonist Oral Anticoagulants in Patients with Atrial Fibrillation. *Europace* **2021**, *23*, 1612–1676. [CrossRef]
84. Al-Khatib, S.M.; Stevenson, W.G.; Ackerman, M.J.; Bryant, W.J.; Callans, D.J.; Curtis, A.B.; Deal, B.J.; Dickfeld, T.; Field, M.E.; Fonarow, G.C.; et al. 2017 AHA/ACC/HRS Guideline for Management of Patients With Ventricular Arrhythmias and the Prevention of Sudden Cardiac Death: Executive Summary: A Report of the American College of Cardiology/American Heart Association Task Force on Clinical Practice Gui. *J. Am. Coll. Cardiol.* **2018**, *72*, 1677–1749. [CrossRef] [PubMed]
85. Baddour, L.M.; Weiss, R.; Mark, G.E.; El-Chami, M.F.; Biffi, M.; Probst, V.; Lambiase, P.D.; Miller, M.A.; McClernon, T.; Hansen, L.K.; et al. Diagnosis and Management of Subcutaneous Implantable Cardioverter-Defibrillator Infections Based on Process Mapping. *Pacing Clin. Electrophysiol.* **2020**, *43*, 958–965. [CrossRef]
86. El-Chami, M.F.; Bonner, M.; Holbrook, R.; Stromberg, K.; Mayotte, J.; Molan, A.; Sohail, M.R.; Epstein, L.M. Leadless Pacemakers Reduce Risk of Device-Related Infection: Review of the Potential Mechanisms. *Heart Rhythm* **2020**, *17*, 1393–1397. [CrossRef] [PubMed]

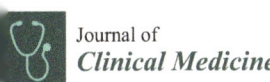

Review

Stereotactic Radiotherapy: An Alternative Option for Refractory Ventricular Tachycardia to Drug and Ablation Therapy

Wenfeng Shangguan [1,†], Gang Xu [1,†], Xin Wang [1], Nan Zhang [1], Xingpeng Liu [2], Guangping Li [1], Gary Tse [1,3,4,*] and Tong Liu [1,*]

1. Tianjin Key Laboratory of Ionic-Molecular Function of Cardiovascular Disease, Department of Cardiology, Tianjin Institute of Cardiology, Second Hospital of Tianjin Medical University, Tianjin 300211, China; sgwf@163.com (W.S.); xugang_163com@163.com (G.X.); 13502076469@163.com (X.W.); zhangnancardiac@126.com (N.Z.); tjcardiol@126.com (G.L.)
2. Department of Heart Center, Beijing Chaoyang Hospital, Capital Medical University, 8th Gongtinanlu Rd., Chaoyang District, Beijing 100020, China; xpliu71@hotmail.com
3. Faculty of Health and Medical Sciences, University of Surrey, Guildford GU2 7XH, UK
4. Kent and Medway Medical School, Canterbury CT2 7FS, UK
* Correspondence: garytse86@gmail.com (G.T.); liutongdoc@126.com (T.L.)
† These authors contributed equally to this work.

Abstract: Refractory ventricular tachycardia (VT) often occurs in the context of organic heart disease. It is associated with significantly high mortality and morbidity rates. Antiarrhythmic drugs and catheter ablation represent the two main treatment options for refractory VT, but their use can be associated with inadequate therapeutic responses and procedure-related complications. Stereotactic body radiotherapy (SBRT) is extensively applied in the precision treatment of solid tumors, with excellent therapeutic responses. Recently, this highly precise technology has been applied for radioablation of VT, and its early results demonstrate a favorable safety profile. This review presents the potential value of SBRT in refractory VT.

Keywords: stereotactic body radiotherapy; refractory ventricular tachycardia; treatment

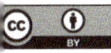

1. Background

Refractory ventricular tachycardia (VT) is characterized by recurrent sustained VT despite medical or interventional treatment. Antiarrhythmic drugs have been used to treat VT for many years [1], but they are ineffective in some cases, and their use can be associated with side effects [2,3]. Catheter ablation utilizes radiofrequency or cryo-energy to destroy the scarred cardiac tissue and its surrounding tissue, effectively disrupting the re-entrant VT substrate [4,5]. Catheter ablation can be more effective than antiarrhythmic drugs [4] but may fail due to its inability to reach the arrhythmogenic target tissue or deliver adequate energy to the deep target myocardium-tissue from which the VT originates. Catheter ablation application is also limited by the occurrence of transmural injury. The recurrence rate after VT catheter ablation is as high as 50% [6]. Catheter ablation may also be associated with procedural risks and mortality [7]. An implantable cardioverter-defibrillator (ICD) can effectively terminate VT or ventricular fibrillation, reducing the risk of sudden death [8]. However, recurrent ICD shocks are painful, contribute to impaired quality of life [9,10], and are associated with higher mortality and worsening of heart failure [11,12].

2. Stereotactic Body Radiotherapy

Stereotactic body radiotherapy (SBRT) is mostly used to treat solid tumors [13]. Unlike traditional radioablation, SBRT employs radiation delivered to a 3D target volume created by various imaging technologies, accurately ablating the target volume while avoiding damage to the surrounding tissue, with up to submillimeter accuracy. Early findings reported that this noninvasive technology could effectively treat refractory VT. Unlike radiofrequency or cryo-energy ablation, SBRT is noninvasive and painless. SBRT targeting of the VT substrate of origin is an alternative for patients with refractory VT after several failed catheter ablations.

3. Mechanisms of SBRT

The exact mechanisms through which radioablation injures the target myocardium during refractory VT treatment have not been fully characterized. Some proposed radiotherapy injury mechanisms include double-strand DNA breaks that lead to cell apoptosis, vascular injury that induces tissue hypoxia, and ischemia-related cell death. Kiani [14] described the cellular effects of radiotherapy on the human myocardium. Histopathologic features were indicative of cell injury, death, and fibrosis; electron microscopy demonstrated features consistent with disruption of the cardiomyocyte architecture and cellular machinery. Indirect radiotherapy mechanisms related to tissue vasculature damage, cell hypoxia, and necrosis induce myocardial fibrosis and conduction block that may prevent further arrhythmic events [15,16].

Previous studies speculated that radioablation induced transmural fibrosis and a homogeneous myocardium, which might account for the reduced VT after SBRT. Heart radioablation with a dose of 25 Gy or higher in animal studies produced target myocardial tissue degeneration and fibrosis and full transmural heart-injury months after the treatment [17]. Sharma et al. [18] found that radiotherapy with a single dose of at least 25 Gy could produce cavotricuspid isthmus and atrioventricular (AV) nodal blocks, and alter the electrophysiological properties at the pulmonary vein–left atrial junction. Blanck et al. [19] reported that a radioablation dose above 32.5 Gy to a healthy pig heart can induce transmural heart injury six months after treatment. Refaat et al. [20] reported that AV conduction block was induced by radioablation at a dose of 35–40 Gy, showing myocardial fibrosis in the AV node radioablation target area using immunostaining. Patients treated with a single radioablation dose of 25 Gy showed a reduced VT burden within days [21] or weeks after treatment [19,22]. Therefore, radiotherapy-induced myocardial fibrosis cannot fully explain the early effect of radioablation. An animal study found no apparent myocardial necrosis and apoptosis one month after a high-dose cardiac radioablation, further supporting the notion that fibrosis cannot explain the early antiarrhythmic effects of such a treatment [23].

Zhang et al. [24] presented evidence in an animal model and in patients that cardiac radioablation induced electrical conduction reprogramming rather than causing transmural fibrosis during the early period after treatment. Six weeks after a 25-Gy radioablation was delivered to murine hearts, no significant myocardial fibrosis or increased collagen content was detected. However, cardiac-electrophysiology remolding was found, with a significantly shortened QRS interval and increased ventricular conduction velocity. These results showed that 25-Gy radioablation induced cardiac-electrophysiology remolding without transmural fibrosis. This explains why the SBRT effect was observed within days to weeks. Western blots showed a significant increase in the expression of NaV1.5 (the cardiac voltage-gated sodium channel subunit that plays a key role in phase-0 depolarization of the action potential) and connexin 43 (a major subunit of the ventricular gap junction that helps pulse diffusion) after radioablation in murine hearts. The high expression of NaV1.5 and connexin 43 was present even 42 weeks after radioablation, achieving persistent cardiac electrical reprogramming. The Notch signaling pathway plays an important role in radioablation-induced cardiac electrophysiology reprogramming. Kim et al. [25] explored the immediate effect of radioablation on myocardial cells, showing that high-dose radioablation regulated cardiomyocyte electrophysiological activities immediately, possibly accounting for the immediate antiarrhythmic effect of SBRT on refractory VT. Additionally, animal experiments showed that radiation increased connexin 43 expression, improved the myocardial conduction velocity, reduced repolarization spatial heterogeneity, and decreased the risk of ventricular arrhythmias after myocardial infarction [26]. We can see from the above studies that radioablation-induced myocardial electrophysiology remolding, rather than fibrosis, accounted for the early effect of VT radiotherapy. The exact effects of radiation on the biology and electrophysiologic properties of the myocardium need further research.

4. SBRT Planning and Implementation

Unlike radiotherapy for tumors, the radioablation target in VT is defined by electrical properties and cannot be accurately displayed by imaging alone. Therefore, SBRT requires a multi-disciplinary team that includes oncologists, medical physicians, and cardiac electrophysiologists. Cardiac electrophysiologists can identify potential candidates and localize the re-entrant substrate using electroanatomic or other noninvasive mapping techniques. These details could assist medical physicians and oncologists to create an accurate 3D target volume, transferring these data into the SBRT system, and formulating and implementing VT radiotherapy plans.

The first VT radioablation step is to precisely identify the substrate causing the VT, often related to the underlying structural heart disease. In scar-related VT, the arrhythmia often originates from ventricular scar border zones [27]. In cases with non-ischemic causes such as dilated cardiomyopathy, the arrhythmogenic substrate often involves fibrotic areas in the myocardium and has a dispersed distribution. However, only part of the scar volume contributes to VT generation. Some surviving cardiac fibers within and around the scar tissue create slow conduction pathways and form the basis for the re-entrant VT-generating substrate. Therefore, an extensive substrate ablation that homogenizes the scar would improve the ablation success rate [28]. The myocardial scar tissue can be identified using delayed-enhanced magnetic resonance imaging (MRI), positron emission tomography–computed tomography (PET-CT), nuclear perfusion imaging, or echocardiography. Most patients with refractory VT have undergone 3D electroanatomic mapping and an unsuccessful catheter ablation procedure before cardiac SBRT. Noninvasive arrhythmia substrate mapping before SBRT would help define and localize the ablation targets [29].

Precise targeting of the arrhythmogenic substrate is crucial in VT radioablation, as it could help reduce off-target ablation of surrounding healthy myocardium, organs, and implantable electronic devices. Accurately transforming the substrate information to target volume planning is a difficult task. Multimodal integration of the electroanatomic mapping with computed tomography (CT) planning could help accurately localize the target on the CT images [30]. High-quality endocardial-surface and -chamber mapping could help to precisely merge the information with cardiac CT [31]. The RAVENTA trial found remarkable differences between the electroanatomic mapping outcomes and target volume planning during VT radioablation [32]. Therefore, highly effective and uniform standards or guidelines are required to transfer the electroanatomic mapping information to the CT planning.

The heart is a moving target due to its intrinsic spontaneous mechanical activity and motions caused by respiration. Initially, SBRT was thought to be unsuitable for cardiac arrhythmia treatment due to difficulties in localizing a moving target. However, with the great progress in imaging technologies such as the gating and tracking systems, the scope of SBRT has been expanded to include VT treatment [22]. Imaging strategies are used to differentiate the target tissue volume from the surrounding healthy tissue. Motion compensation strategies include dampening or inhibition to restrain respiratory motion, gating to release radiation at a specific time of the respiratory cycle, and tracking to make the radiation beam follow the moving target [33]. Ho et al. [34] reported that computational ECG mapping and a protocol-guided respiratory gating system could improve target volume planning precision, helping with SBRT planning and implementation. Cha et al. [35] proposed a new method, using deep-inspiration breath-hold to separate the target from the stomach, reducing the dose delivered to the gastrointestinal tract during cardiac SBRT. Real-time cardiorespiratory-motion-mitigated MRI could help compensate for cardiac and respiratory motions simultaneously [36]. Although many techniques have been used to minimize injury to the surrounding tissues, it is impossible to fully avoid the off-target delivery of radiation beams due to the respiratory and cardiac motions.

SBRT duration ranges between 10 and 90 min, depending on the radiation dose, the machines used, and the target tissue volume, location, and size (Table 1). Another key issue in SBRT for VT ablation is the radiation dose. Blanck et al. [19] showed, in a pig model, that a dose of 17.5 Gy did not induce any significant fibrosis in pulmonary veins, a dose of 25 Gy induced mild fibrosis, and a dose above 32.5 Gy might lead to transmural fibrosis. Animal study outcomes supported 25 Gy as the radioablation threshold dosage to create target myocardial-tissue fibrosis, but higher radiation dosages (35–40 Gy) increased the risks of radiation-related complications [18,19,37]. Based on preclinical results and experience in oncology SBRT, most clinical studies used 25 Gy as the basic treatment dose. The currently prescribed 25-Gy dose might be insufficient to form a homogenous transmural scar. Zhang et al. [24] proposed that the radioablation mechanism was mediated by electrophysiologic reprogramming rather than myocardial fibrosis. Using a dose de-escalation method, they found that a dose of 5–10 Gy did not induce significant electrophysiologic reprogramming, while a dose higher than 15 Gy increased the ventricular conduction velocity and shortened the QRS interval. The largest electrophysiologic effects were detected at a dose of 25 Gy. Elucidation of the optimal dose regimen needs further study.

Table 1. Summary of the different studies on stereotactic radiotherapy for ventricular arrhythmia.

Study Year	Patient Number	Sex	Mean Age (Years)	Type of CMP	LVEF (Mean, %)	Dose (Gy)	PTV (Mean, mL)	Treatment Time (Mean, Min)	Delay for Efficacy	Follow-Up (Months)	Complications
Loo et al. [36] 2015	1	M	71	ICMP	24	25	-	90	After 2 months	9	Died from COPD exacerbation at month 9
Cuculich et al. [22] 2017	5	4 M; 1 F	66	2 ICMP; 3 NICMP	23	25	49	14	Progressive effect after ablation, but maximum effect after 6 weeks	12	One fatal stroke 3 weeks after treatment
Jumeau et al. [21] 2018	1	M	75	NICMP	30	25	21	45	Immediate	4	None
Neuwirth et al. [39] 2019	10	9 M; 1 F	66	8 ICMP; 2 NICMP	27	25	22.2	68	Progressive effect	28	Three died of non-arrhythmic causes; progression of mitral valve regurgitation at 17 months
Robinson et al. [40] 2019	19	17 M; 2 F	66	11 ICMP; 5 NICMP; 3 others	25	25	98.9	15	Within the first 6 weeks	13	Pericarditis; heart failure exacerbation at 2 months
Lloyd et al. [41] 2020	10	7 M; 3 F	62	4 ICMP; 4 NICMP; 2 others	-	25	81.4	-	Within the first 2 weeks	6	Mild pneumonitis responsive to corticosteroids in two patients
Gianni et al. [42] 2020	5	5 M	63	4 ICMP; 1 NICMP	34	25	143	82	Four patients had marked reduction in VT burden during first 6 months	12	Two died of heart failure
Chin et al. [43] 2021	8	8 M	75	4 ICMP; 4 NICMP	21	22.2	121.4	18.2	3 months	7.8	No acute complications, three patient deaths in the follow-up period, unrelated to SBRT.
Carbucicchio C [44] 2021	7	8 M	70	3 ICMP; 4 NICMP	27	25	183	31	3 months	8	three patient deaths in the follow-up period, unrelated to SBRT.
Qian et al. [45] 2021	6	6 M	72	6 ICMP	20	25	319	-	6 months	7.7	3 patients died of heart failure; 3 of 6 patients had possible adverse events
Ho et al. [34] 2021	6	6 M	74	2 ICMP; 4 NICMP	29	25	120.3	21.1	-	6	1 patient Pericardial effusion 12 months after therapy
Haskova et al. [46] 2018	1	-	34	NICMP	-	25	-	-	8 months	8	-

Table 1. Cont.

Study Year	Patient Number	Sex	Mean Age (Years)	Type of CMP	LVEF (Mean, %)	Dose (Gy)	PTV (Mean, mL)	Treatment Time (Mean, Min)	Delay for Efficacy	Follow-Up (Months)	Complications
Marti Almor et al. [47] 2020	1	M	64	NICMP	-	25	-	4	Immediate	4	None
Scholz et al. [48] 2019	1	M	53	ICMP	-	30	82.4	5/30	2 weeks	2	None
Zeng et al. [49] 2019	1	M	29	NICMP	-	24	71	-	1 month	4	None
Krug et al. [50] 2019	1	M	78	NICMP	15	25	42.2	15	Days	-	Died 57 days after ablation due to sepsis-associated cardiac circulatory failure
Mayinger et al. [51] 2020	1	M	71	NICMP	25	25	115.1	24	48 h	3	None

CMP—cardiomyopathy; COPD—chronic obstructive pulmonary disease; F—female; PTV—planning target volume; ICMP—ischemic cardiomyopathy; LVEF—left ventricular ejection fraction; M—male; NICMP—non-ischemic cardiomyopathy; VT—ventricular tachycardia.

5. SBRT for VT Ablation: Clinical Experience

To date, a limited number of prospective and retrospective studies or case series focusing on the clinical evidence of SBRT for VT have been published. Loo et al. [38] delivered the first in-human cardiac arrhythmia treatment in 2012 using stereotactic radioablation with a radiation dose of 25 Gy. After a 2-month blanking period, the number of VT episodes remained low for seven months, with no acute or late complications. However, refractory VT occurred nine months after the procedure in the context of an exacerbation of chronic obstructive pulmonary disease, culminating in the patient's death.

In a case series reported by Cuculich et al. [22], five patients at high risk of refractory VT underwent SBRT with a single delivery dose of 25 Gy and a 14-min mean radioablation duration. The pre-procedural VT burden of these patients was 6577 episodes over a 3-month time period. During the 6-week post-ablation blanking period, the VT episodes decreased to 680 and declined to 4 over the next 46 patient-months. All five patients presented with a significant reduction in VT burden from the baseline. The mean left-ventricular-ejection fraction was preserved throughout the follow-up.

In 2019, Robinson et al. [40] published a phase I-II prospective trial of VT radioablation. Nineteen patients with treatment-refractory VT or premature-ventricular-contraction (PVC) cardiomyopathy were enrolled and received noninvasive electrophysiology-guided cardiac radioablation with a single delivery of 25 Gy. The number of VT episodes decreased from 119 to 3 in 18 patients after the ablation, 17 of which (94%) presented with reduced VT or PVC burden. The overall 6- and 12-month survival rates were 89% and 72%, respectively; the dual antiarrhythmic drug use declined from 59 to 12%; and the quality of life at six months improved in five of the nine Short Form-36 domains. Evidently, noninvasive electrophysiology-guided cardiac radioablation could bring favorable clinical benefits to patients with VT or PVC-related cardiomyopathy.

Neuwirth et al. [39] reported a case series of ten patients with structural heart disease and refractory VT. They delivered 25 Gy to the planning target volumes using CyberKnife. Compared to the baseline, the VT burden significantly decreased by 87.5% during the 28-month follow-up. Three patients died of non-arrhythmic causes. After a blanking period of 90 days, eight of the patients experienced a recurrence of VT. The mean times from treatment to the first antitachycardia pacing and ICD shock were 6.5 and 21 months, respectively. The follow-up results showed that SBRT failed in two patients, and two patients showed a delayed response of three and six months, respectively. One patient with previously known mitral regurgitation showed progression of the regurgitation and valvular morphology changes 17 months after the radioablation procedure. This study showed that SBRT was a safe and effective long-term treatment for refractory VT and could improve the survival rate of these patients.

Gianni et al. [42] described five patients with structural heart disease and refractory VT. A single-fraction radiation dose of 25 Gy was delivered to the target volume using

CyberKnife at a mean treatment duration of 82 min. Four of the five patients presented with significant reductions in the number of VT episodes and in the use of antiarrhythmic drugs during the first six months after the ablation. All five patients experienced VT recurrence during the 12-month follow-up, of which two died from heart failure worsening. Those researchers found no evidence that the radioablation injured the cardiac tissue around the target volume. Despite the initial promising results, SBRT did not show long-term effectiveness in patients with refractory VT. No radiation-related complications were noted during follow-up, suggesting an acceptable safety profile for SBRT. Further studies are needed to elucidate the mechanisms associated with the lack of long-term efficacy.

Lloyd et al. [41] reported ten patients with advanced heart failure (four with ischemic and six with non-ischemic cardiomyopathy) and refractory VT who underwent SBRT. The mean patient age was 61 years. The results showed that the number of VT episodes decreased by 69%, antitachycardia pacing sequences decreased by 48%, and ICD shocks decreased by 68% after the SBRT. One patient in this study did not respond to the SBRT. After excluding this patient, a significant decrease in the VT burden was observed after treatment.

Chin et al. [43] retrospectively analyzed eight consecutive patients with refractory VT who underwent SBRT, with an average age of 75 years and a mean ejection fraction of 21%. All patients were male, half with ischemic and half with non-ischemic cardiomyopathy. A mean dose of 22.2 Gy was delivered to the planning target volume during a single radioablation treatment session. During the 7.8-month follow-up, the number of ICD shocks decreased from 69.5 to 13.3. No acute complications or definite peripheral organ toxicities occurred during follow-up. Three patients died during follow-up, of causes unrelated to the SBRT. This patient group experienced VT burden reduction after the SBRT, but, unlike previous reports, they showed no immediate effects.

Carbucicchio et al. [44] presented the preliminary results of their spontaneous, prospective, single-arm, phase Ib/II single-center STRA-MI-VT Study. The study investigated the safety and efficacy of SBRT in eight patients with intractable VT. Of the seven patients who underwent SBRT (mean age, 70 ± 7 years; ejection fraction, 27 ± 11%), three had ischemic and four had non-ischemic cardiomyopathy. No treatment-related serious adverse events occurred at a median follow-up of eight months. Three patients died from non-SBRT-related causes, while four completed the 6-month follow-up. The number of VT episodes decreased from 29 to 11 and 2, three and six months post-treatment, respectively. The respective number of ICD shocks decreased from 11 to 0 and 2. All patients showed a significant reduction in the number of VT episodes and no electrical storm recurrence six months after treatment. The STRA-MI-VT Study showed excellent short-term VT radioablation treatment outcomes but showed no long-term effects.

The study by Qian et al. [45] aimed to determine the feasibility of using radioablation on the arrhythmogenic substrate of myocardial scars in patients with ischemic cardiomyopathy. Six male patients with ischemic cardiomyopathy and refractory VT underwent SBRT targeting of the extensive scar substrate. The median planning target volume was 319 mL, and the radioablation dose was 25 Gy. ICD-treated or sustained VT episodes did not decrease significantly after SBRT, but ICD shocks decreased significantly from 12 to 0. Three patients died of heart failure during the 7.7-month follow-up period, and three experienced complications, including heart failure exacerbation, pneumonia, and asymptomatic pericardial effusion. Repeat catheter ablation was performed in four patients at 32, 167, 288, and 396 days post-SBRT. This study suggested that SBRT-induced substrate modifications did not significantly reduce the VT burden in patients with ischemic cardiomyopathy, similar to a recent report demonstrating that radioablation did not have long-term effectiveness in patients with serious ischemic cardiomyopathy [38]. Further study is warranted to evaluate the radiobiology of myocardial scars, optimal radiation dose, target location, and the effectiveness and safety of refractory VT radioablation in patients with ischemic cardiomyopathy.

Ho et al. [34] enrolled six consecutive patients with refractory VT managed by SBRT. The VT origin sites were identified noninvasively by a 3D computational electrocardiogram

(ECG) algorithm and compared to available electroanatomic maps. A 25-Gy radioablation was delivered to the target at the end of expiration. Respiratory gating facilitated small planning target volumes and prevented gastrointestinal complications. ICD shocks decreased from 23 to 0.67 per patient six months post-SRBT. This study showed that a workflow that combined computational ECG mapping and protocol-guided respiratory gating was effective and safe, and could improve SRBT planning.

However, long-term follow-ups indicate a high VT recurrence rate in patients with refractory VT after SRBT, the reasons for which remain unknown. Gianni et al. [42] described three patients with recurrent VT after radioablation. Voltage mapping during repeated radiofrequency catheter ablation showed remaining low voltage, fractionated electrograms within the radioablation target regions. Some surviving cardiomyocytes in the scar suggested incomplete homogenization. Therefore, the 25-Gy radiation dose used in previous studies might be insufficient to destroy the entire target tissue. The uniform delivery of a 25-Gy radiation dose, regardless of the planning target volume, size, and characteristics, needs further exploration and study. Another possibility is that the identified substrate might not be very accurate, as location discrepancies were introduced when the data were transferred to the CT imaging system [32]. Furthermore, aggravation of the myocardial ischemia or exacerbation of the heart failure might produce a new VT substrate, especially in patients with severe ischemic cardiomyopathy. The findings of the many ongoing clinical trials will be able to address some of these issues.

6. Safety and Complications

Several studies have reported that the VT radioablation treatment was safe during short-to-medium follow-ups, with only a few complications reported. These included pericarditis ($n = 1$), the progression of valvular disease ($n = 1$), self-resolving pneumonitis ($n = 2$), and delayed pericardial effusion ($n = 5$) [39,40]. There have been no reports of VT radioablation treatment as the direct cause of death (Table 1). Longer-term results from the Phase I/II ENCORE-VT Study showed one serious Grade 4 complication (gastropericardial fistula) at 2.4 years requiring surgical repair [52]. Haskova et al. [53] reported a refractory VT patient who died because of a bleeding esophago-pericardial fistula six months after a 25-Gy radioablation. To date, not many patients have undergone SBRT, so two fistula cases suggest that this fatal complication is not uncommon. Nevertheless, we may gain some insights from cancer radiotherapy. Several studies showed a significant relationship between the delivered cardiac radiation doses and the long-term (several years or even decades) cumulative incidence of cardiac events in the coronary arteries, conduction system, valvular structures, myocardium, and pericardium [54]. We need to be alert to late complications such as esophago-pericardial fistula. Long-term follow-up is needed to fully identify potential late complications.

7. Limitations

The following limitations of SBRT should be taken into consideration. First, it requires accurate identification and localization of the substrate. Second, an optimal radiation dosing regimen is still lacking and should be further elucidated. Third, the long-term safety and efficacy of SBRT remain unknown. Therefore, SBRT should be reserved for patients with refractory VT following failed medical therapy and ablation.

8. Conclusions

SBRT represents a noninvasive option for cases of refractory VT with failed antiarrhythmic therapy and ablation. Further clinical trials and registry studies are needed to better inform and optimize its treatment parameters and characterize its long-term safety.

Author Contributions: Conceptualization, G.X., T.L.; writing—original draft preparation, W.S., G.X. and X.W.; writing—review and editing, W.S., N.Z., X.L. and G.T.; supervision, G.L. and T.L. All authors have read and agreed to the published version of the manuscript.

Funding: This study was supported by grants from the National Natural Science Foundation of China (No. 82000313 to W.S., No. 81970270 to T.L.), Tianjin Natural Science Foundation (No. 18JCYBJC92700 to G.X), and Tianjin Key Medical Discipline (Specialty) Construction Project.

Conflicts of Interest: The authors declare that they have no conflicts of interest.

References

1. Bazoukis, G.; Tse, G.; Letsas, K.P.; Thomopoulos, C.; Naka, K.K.; Korantzopoulos, P.; Bazoukis, X.; Michelongona, P.; Papadatos, S.S.; Vlachos, K.; et al. Impact of ranolazine on ventricular arrhythmias—A systematic review. *J. Arrhythmia* **2018**, *34*, 124–128. [CrossRef] [PubMed]
2. Antiarrhythmics versus Implantable Defibrillators Investigators. A comparison of antiarrhythmic-drug therapy with implantable defibrillators in patients resuscitated from near-fatal ventricular arrhythmias. *N. Engl. J. Med.* **1997**, *337*, 1576–1583. [CrossRef] [PubMed]
3. Connolly, S.J.; Dorian, P.; Roberts, R.S.; Gent, M.; Bailin, S.; Fain, E.S.; Thorpe, K.; Champagne, J.; Talajic, M.; Coutu, B.; et al. Comparison of beta-blockers, amiodarone plus beta-blockers, or sotalol for prevention of shocks from implantable cardioverter defibrillators: The optic study: A randomized trial. *JAMA* **2006**, *295*, 165–171. [CrossRef] [PubMed]
4. Sapp, J.L.; Wells, G.A.; Parkash, R.; Stevenson, W.G.; Blier, L.; Sarrazin, J.F.; Thibault, B.; Rivard, L.; Gula, L.; Leong-Sit, P.; et al. Ventricular tachycardia ablation versus escalation of antiarrhythmic drugs. *N. Engl. J. Med.* **2016**, *375*, 111–121. [CrossRef]
5. Rivera, S.; Ricapito, M.D.; Tomas, L.; Parodi, J.; Bardera Molina, G.; Banega, R.; Bueti, P.; Orosco, A.; Reinoso, M.; Caro, M.; et al. Results of cryoenergy and radiofrequency-based catheter ablation for treating ventricular arrhythmias arising from the papillary muscles of the left ventricle, guided by intracardiac echocardiography and image integration. *Circ. Arrhythmia Electrophysiol.* **2016**, *9*, e003874. [CrossRef]
6. Piers, S.R.; Leong, D.P.; van Taxis, C.F.; Tayyebi, M.; Trines, S.A.; Pijnappels, D.A.; Delgado, V.; Schalij, M.J.; Zeppenfeld, K. Outcome of ventricular tachycardia ablation in patients with nonischemic cardiomyopathy: The impact of noninducibility. *Circ. Arrhythmia Electrophysiol.* **2013**, *6*, 513–521. [CrossRef]
7. Santangeli, P.; Muser, D.; Maeda, S.; Filtz, A.; Zado, E.S.; Frankel, D.S.; Dixit, S.; Epstein, A.E.; Callans, D.J.; Marchlinski, F.E. Comparative effectiveness of antiarrhythmic drugs and catheter ablation for the prevention of recurrent ventricular tachycardia in patients with implantable cardioverter-defibrillators: A systematic review and meta-analysis of randomized controlled trials. *Heart Rhythm* **2016**, *13*, 1552–1559. [CrossRef]
8. Al-Khatib, S.M.; Stevenson, W.G.; Ackerman, M.J.; Bryant, W.J.; Callans, D.J.; Curtis, A.B.; Deal, B.J.; Dickfeld, T.; Field, M.E.; Fonarow, G.C.; et al. 2017 aha/acc/hrs guideline for management of patients with ventricular arrhythmias and the prevention of sudden cardiac death: Executive summary: A report of the american college of cardiology/american heart association task force on clinical practice guidelines and the heart rhythm society. *Heart Rhythm* **2018**, *15*, e190–e252.
9. Schron, E.B.; Exner, D.V.; Yao, Q.; Jenkins, L.S.; Steinberg, J.S.; Cook, J.R.; Kutalek, S.P.; Friedman, P.L.; Bubien, R.S.; Page, R.L.; et al. Quality of life in the antiarrhythmics versus implantable defibrillators trial: Impact of therapy and influence of adverse symptoms and defibrillator shocks. *Circulation* **2002**, *105*, 589–594. [CrossRef]
10. Perini, A.P.; Kutyifa, V.; Veazie, P.; Daubert, J.P.; Schuger, C.; Zareba, W.; McNitt, S.; Rosero, S.; Tompkins, C.; Padeletti, L.; et al. Effects of implantable cardioverter/defibrillator shock and antitachycardia pacing on anxiety and quality of life: A madit-rit substudy. *Am. Heart J.* **2017**, *189*, 75–84. [CrossRef]
11. Bazoukis, G.; Tse, G.; Korantzopoulos, P.; Liu, T.; Letsas, K.P.; Stavrakis, S.; Naka, K.K. Impact of implantable cardioverter defibrillator interventions on all-cause mortality in heart failure patients: A meta-analysis. *Cardiol. Rev.* **2019**, *27*, 160–166. [CrossRef] [PubMed]
12. Poole, J.E.; Johnson, G.W.; Hellkamp, A.S.; Anderson, J.; Callans, D.J.; Raitt, M.H.; Reddy, R.K.; Marchlinski, F.E.; Yee, R.; Guarnieri, T.; et al. Prognostic importance of defibrillator shocks in patients with heart failure. *N. Engl. J. Med.* **2008**, *359*, 1009–1017. [CrossRef] [PubMed]
13. Potters, L.; Kavanagh, B.; Galvin, J.M.; Hevezi, J.M.; Janjan, N.A.; Larson, D.A.; Mehta, M.P.; Ryu, S.; Steinberg, M.; Timmerman, R.; et al. American society for therapeutic radiology and oncology (astro) and american college of radiology (acr) practice guideline for the performance of stereotactic body radiation therapy. *Int. J. Radiat. Oncol. Biol. Phys.* **2010**, *76*, 326–332. [CrossRef] [PubMed]
14. Kiani, S.; Kutob, L.; Schneider, F.; Higgins, K.A.; Lloyd, M.S. Histopathologic and ultrastructural findings in human myocardium after stereotactic body radiation therapy for recalcitrant ventricular tachycardia. *Circ. Arrhythmia Electrophysiol.* **2020**, *13*, e008753. [CrossRef] [PubMed]
15. Song, C.W.; Lee, Y.J.; Griffin, R.J.; Park, I.; Koonce, N.A.; Hui, S.; Kim, M.S.; Dusenbery, K.E.; Sperduto, P.W.; Cho, L.C. Indirect tumor cell death after high-dose hypofractionated irradiation: Implications for stereotactic body radiation therapy and stereotactic radiation surgery. *Int. J. Radiat. Oncol. Biol. Phys.* **2015**, *93*, 166–172. [CrossRef] [PubMed]
16. Song, C.W.; Glatstein, E.; Marks, L.B.; Emami, B.; Grimm, J.; Sperduto, P.W.; Kim, M.S.; Hui, S.; Dusenbery, K.E.; Cho, L.C. Biological principles of stereotactic body radiation therapy (sbrt) and stereotactic radiation surgery (srs): Indirect cell death. *Int. J. Radiat. Oncol. Biol. Phys.* **2021**, *110*, 21–34. [CrossRef]

7. Lehmann, H.I.; Deisher, A.J.; Takami, M.; Kruse, J.J.; Song, L.; Anderson, S.E.; Cusma, J.T.; Parker, K.D.; Johnson, S.B.; Asirvatham, S.J.; et al. External Arrhythmia Ablation Using Photon Beams: Ablation of the Atrioventricular Junction in an Intact Animal Model. *Circ. Arrhythmia Electrophysiol.* **2017**, *10*, e004304. [CrossRef]
8. Sharma, A.; Wong, D.; Weidlich, G.; Fogarty, T.; Jack, A.; Sumanaweera, T.; Maguire, P. Noninvasive stereotactic radiosurgery (cyberheart) for creation of ablation lesions in the atrium. *Heart Rhythm* **2010**, *7*, 802–810. [CrossRef]
9. Blanck, O.; Bode, F.; Gebhard, M.; Hunold, P.; Brandt, S.; Bruder, R.; Grossherr, M.; Vonthein, R.; Rades, D.; Dunst, J. Dose-escalation study for cardiac radiosurgery in a porcine model. *Int. J. Radiat. Oncol. Biol. Phys.* **2014**, *89*, 590–598. [CrossRef]
10. Refaat, M.M.; Ballout, J.A.; Zakka, P.; Hotait, M.; Al Feghali, K.A.; Gheida, I.A.; Saade, C.; Hourani, M.; Geara, F.; Tabbal, M.; et al. Swine atrioventricular node ablation using stereotactic radiosurgery: Methods and in vivo feasibility investigation for catheter-free ablation of cardiac arrhythmias. *J. Am. Heart Assoc.* **2017**, *6*, e007193. [CrossRef]
11. Jumeau, R.; Ozsahin, M.; Schwitter, J.; Vallet, V.; Duclos, F.; Zeverino, M.; Moeckli, R.; Pruvot, E.; Bourhis, J. Rescue procedure for an electrical storm using robotic non-invasive cardiac radio-ablation. *Radiother. Oncol.* **2018**, *128*, 189–191. [CrossRef] [PubMed]
12. Cuculich, P.S.; Schill, M.R.; Kashani, R.; Mutic, S.; Lang, A.; Cooper, D.; Faddis, M.; Gleva, M.; Noheria, A.; Smith, T.W.; et al. Noninvasive cardiac radiation for ablation of ventricular tachycardia. *N. Engl. J. Med.* **2017**, *377*, 2325–2336. [CrossRef] [PubMed]
13. Cha, M.J.; Seo, J.W.; Kim, H.J.; Kim, M.K.; Yoon, H.S.; Jo, S.W.; Oh, S.; Chang, J.H. Early Changes in Rat Heart After High-Dose Irradiation: Implications for Antiarrhythmic Effects of Cardiac Radioablation. *J. Am. Heart Assoc.* **2021**, *10*, e019072. [CrossRef] [PubMed]
14. Zhang, D.M.; Navara, R.; Yin, T.; Szymanski, J.; Goldsztejn, U.; Kenkel, C.; Lang, A.; Mpoy, C.; Lipovsky, C.E.; Qiao, Y.; et al. Cardiac radiotherapy induces electrical conduction reprogramming in the absence of transmural fibrosis. *Nat. Commun.* **2021**, *12*, 5558. [CrossRef]
15. Kim, J.S.; Choi, S.W.; Park, Y.G.; Kim, S.J.; Choi, C.H.; Cha, M.J.; Chang, J.H. Impact of High-Dose Irradiation on Human iPSC-Derived Cardiomyocytes Using Multi-Electrode Arrays: Implications for the Antiarrhythmic Effects of Cardiac Radioablation. *Int. J. Mol. Sci.* **2021**, *23*, 351. [CrossRef]
16. Amino, M.; Yoshioka, K.; Tanabe, T.; Tanaka, E.; Mori, H.; Furusawa, Y.; Zareba, W.; Yamazaki, M.; Nakagawa, H.; Honjo, H.; et al. Heavy ion radiation up-regulates Cx43 and ameliorates arrhythmogenic substrates in hearts after myocardial infarction. *Cardiovasc. Res.* **2006**, *7*, 412–421. [CrossRef]
17. Aliot, E.M.; Stevenson, W.G.; Almendral-Garrote, J.M.; Bogun, F.; Calkins, C.H.; Delacretaz, E.; Bella, P.D.; Hindricks, G.; Jaïs, P.; Josephson, M.E.; et al. EHRA/HRS expert consensus on catheter ablation of ventricular arrhythmias: Developed in a partnership with the European heart rhythm association (EHRA), a registered branch of the European society of cardiology (ESC), and the heart rhythm society (HRS); in collaboration with the American college of cardiology (ACC) and the American heart association (AHA). *Heart Rhythm* **2009**, *6*, 886–933.
18. Di Biase, L.; Burkhardt, J.D.; Lakkireddy, D.; Carbucicchio, C.; Mohanty, S.; Mohanty, P.; Trivedi, C.; Santangeli, P.; Bai, R.; Forleo, G.; et al. Ablation of stable VTs versus substrate ablation in ischemic cardiomyopathy: The vista randomized multicenter trial. *J. Am. Coll. Cardiol.* **2015**, *66*, 2872–2882. [CrossRef]
19. Kim, E.J.; Davogustto, G.; Stevenson, W.G.; John, R.M. Non-invasive cardiac radiation for ablation of ventricular tachycardia: A new therapeutic paradigm in electrophysiology. *Arrhythmia Electrophysiol. Rev.* **2018**, *7*, 8–10. [CrossRef]
20. Hohmann, S.; Henkenberens, C.; Zormpas, C.; Christiansen, H.; Bauersachs, J.; Duncker, D.; Veltmann, C. A novel open-source software-based high-precision workflow for target definition in cardiac radioablation. *J. Cardiovasc. Electrophysiol.* **2020**, *31*, 2689–2695. [CrossRef]
21. Abdel-Kafi, S.; Sramko, M.; Omara, S.; de Riva, M.; Cvek, J.; Peichl, P.; Kautzner, J.; Zeppenfeld, K. Accuracy of electroanatomical mapping-guided cardiac radiotherapy for ventricular tachycardia: Pitfalls and solutions. *Europace* **2021**, *23*, 1989–1997. [CrossRef] [PubMed]
22. Boda-Heggemann, J.; Blanck, O.; Mehrhof, F.; Ernst, F.; Buergy, D.; Fleckenstein, J.; Tülümen, E.; Krug, D.; Siebert, F.A.; Zaman, A.; et al. Interdisciplinary clinical target volume generation for cardiac radioablation: Multicenter benchmarking for the radiosurgery for ventricular tachycardia (raventa) trial. *Int. J. Radiat. Oncol. Biol. Phys.* **2021**, *110*, 745–756. [CrossRef]
23. Timmerman, R.D.; Kavanagh, B.D.; Cho, L.C.; Papiez, L.; Xing, L. Stereotactic body radiation therapy in multiple organ sites. *J. Clin. Oncol.* **2007**, *25*, 947–952. [CrossRef] [PubMed]
24. Ho, G.; Atwood, T.F.; Bruggeman, A.R.; Moore, K.L.; McVeigh, E.; Villongco, C.T.; Han, F.T.; Hsu, J.C.; Hoffmayer, K.S.; Raissi, F.; et al. Computational ECG mapping and respiratory gating to optimize stereotactic ablative radiotherapy workflow for refractory ventricular tachycardia. *Heart Rhythm O2* **2021**, *2*, 511–520. [CrossRef] [PubMed]
25. Cha, M.J.; Cuculich, P.S.; Robinson, C.G.; Chang, J.H. Tailored stereotactic radiotherapy technique using deep inspiration breath-hold to reduce stomach dose for cardiac radioablation. *Radiat. Oncol. J.* **2021**, *39*, 167–173. [CrossRef]
26. Akdag, O.; Borman, P.T.; Woodhead, P.; Uijtewaal, P.; Mandija, S.; Van Asselen, B.; Verhoeff, J.J.; Raaymakers, B.W.; Fast, M.F. First experimental exploration of real-time cardiorespiratory motion management for future stereotactic arrhythmia radioablation treatments on the MR-linac. *Phys. Med. Biol.* **2022**, *67*, 065003. [CrossRef]
27. Zei, P.C.; Wong, D.; Gardner, E.; Fogarty, T.; Maguire, P. Safety and efficacy of stereotactic radioablation targeting pulmonary vein tissues in an experimental model. *Heart Rhythm* **2018**, *15*, 1420–1427. [CrossRef]

38. Loo, B.W., Jr.; Soltys, S.G.; Wang, L.; Lo, A.; Fahimian, B.P.; Iagaru, A.; Norton, L.; Shan, X.; Gardner, E.; Fogarty, T.; et al. Stereotactic ablative radiotherapy for the treatment of refractory cardiac ventricular arrhythmia. *Circ. Arrhythmia Electrophysiol.* **2015**, *8*, 748–750. [CrossRef]
39. Neuwirth, R.; Cvek, J.; Knybel, L.; Jiravsky, O.; Molenda, L.; Kodaj, M.; Fiala, M.; Peichl, P.; Feltl, D.; Januška, J.; et al. Stereotactic radiosurgery for ablation of ventricular tachycardia. *Europace* **2019**, *21*, 1088–1095. [CrossRef]
40. Robinson, C.G.; Samson, P.P.; Moore, K.M.; Hugo, G.D.; Knutson, N.; Mutic, S.; Goddu, S.M.; Lang, A.; Cooper, D.H.; Faddis, M.; et al. Phase i/ii trial of electrophysiology-guided noninvasive cardiac radioablation for ventricular tachycardia. *Circulation* **2019**, *139*, 313–321. [CrossRef]
41. Lloyd, M.S.; Wight, J.; Schneider, F.; Hoskins, M.; Attia, T.; Escott, C.; Lerakis, S.; Higgins, K.A. Clinical experience of stereotactic body radiation for refractory ventricular tachycardia in advanced heart failure patients. *Heart Rhythm* **2020**, *17*, 415–422. [CrossRef]
42. Gianni, C.; Rivera, D.; Burkhardt, J.D.; Pollard, B.; Gardner, E.; Maguire, P.; Zei, P.C.; Natale, A.; Al-Ahmad, A. Stereotactic arrhythmia radioablation for refractory scar-related ventricular tachycardia. *Heart Rhythm* **2020**, *17*, 1241–1248. [CrossRef]
43. Chin, R.; Hayase, J.; Hu, P.; Cao, M.; Deng, J.; Ajijola, O.; Do, D.; Vaseghi, M.; Buch, E.; Khakpour, H.; et al. Non-invasive stereotactic body radiation therapy for refractory ventricular arrhythmias: An institutional experience. *J. Interv. Cardiol. Electrophysiol.* **2021**, *61*, 535–543. [CrossRef]
44. Carbucicchio, C.; Andreini, D.; Piperno, G.; Catto, V.; Conte, E.; Cattani, F.; Bonomi, A.; Rondi, E.; Piccolo, C.; Vigorito, S.; et al. Stereotactic radioablation for the treatment of ventricular tachycardia: Preliminary data and insights from the STRA-MI-VT phase Ib/II study. *J. Interv. Cardiol. Electrophysiol.* **2021**, *62*, 427–439. [CrossRef]
45. Qian, P.C.; Quadros, K.; Aguilar, M.; Wei, C.; Boeck, M.; Bredfeldt, J.; Cochet, H.; Blankstein, R.; Mak, R.; Sauer, W.H.; et al. Substrate Modification Using Stereotactic Radioablation to Treat Refractory Ventricular Tachycardia in Patients With Ischemic Cardiomyopathy. *JACC Clin. Electrophysiol.* **2022**, *8*, 49–58. [CrossRef]
46. Haskova, J.; Peichl, P.; Pirk, J.; Cvek, J.; Neuwirth, R.; Kautzner, J. Stereotactic radiosurgery as a treatment for recurrent ventricular tachycardia associated with cardiac fibroma. *HeartRhythm Case Rep.* **2019**, *5*, 44–47. [CrossRef]
47. Marti-Almor, J.; Jimenez-Lopez, J.; Rodriguez de Dios, N.; Tizon, H.; Valles, E.; Algara, M. Noninvasive ablation of ventricular tachycardia with stereotactic radiotherapy in a patient with arrhythmogenic right ventricular cardiomyopathy. *Rev. Esp. Cardiol. (Engl. Ed).* **2020**, *73*, 97–99. [CrossRef]
48. Scholz, E.P.; Seidensaal, K.; Naumann, P.; Andre, F.; Katus, H.A.; Debus, J. Risen from the dead: Cardiac stereotactic ablative radiotherapy as last rescue in a patient with refractory ventricular fibrillation storm. *HeartRhythm Case Rep.* **2019**, *5*, 329–332. [CrossRef]
49. Zeng, L.J.; Huang, L.H.; Tan, H.; Zhang, H.C.; Mei, J.; Shi, H.F.; Jiang, C.Y.; Tan, C.; Zheng, J.W.; Liu, X.P. Stereotactic body radiation therapy for refractory ventricular tachycardia secondary to cardiac lipoma: A case report. *Pacing Clin. Electrophysiol.* **2019**, *42*, 1276–1279. [CrossRef]
50. Krug, D.; Blanck, O.; Demming, T.; Dottermusch, M.; Koch, K.; Hirt, M.; Kotzott, L.; Zaman, A.; Eidinger, L.; Siebert, F.A.; et al. Stereotactic body radiotherapy for ventricular tachycardia (cardiac radiosurgery): First-in-patient treatment in Germany. *Strahlenther. Onkol.* **2020**, *196*, 23–30. [CrossRef]
51. Mayinger, M.; Kovacs, B.; Tanadini-Lang, S.; Ehrbar, S.; Wilke, L.; Chamberlain, M.; Moreira, A.; Weitkamp, N.; Brunckhorst, C.; Duru, F.; et al. First magnetic resonance imaging-guided cardiac radioablation of sustained ventricular tachycardia. *Radiother. Oncol.* **2020**, *152*, 203–207. [CrossRef] [PubMed]
52. Robinson, C.G.; Samson, P.; Moore, K.M.S.; Hugo, G.D.; Knutson, N.; Mutic, S. Longer Term Results from a Phase I/II Study of EP-guided Noninvasive Cardiac Radioablation for Treatment of Ventricular Tachycardia (ENCORE-VT). *Int. J. Radiat. Oncol. Biol. Phys.* **2019**, *105*, 682. [CrossRef]
53. Haskova, J.; Jedlickova, K.; Cvek, J.; Knybel, L.; Neuwirth, R.; Kautzner, J. Oesophagopericardial fistula as a late complication of stereotactic radiotherapy for recurrent ventricular tachycardia. *Europace* **2022**, euab326. [CrossRef]
54. Bergom, C.; Bradley, J.A.; Ng, A.K.; Samson, P.; Robinson, C.; Lopez-Mattei, J.; Mitchell, J.D. Past, Present, and Future of Radiation-Induced Cardiotoxicity: Refinements in Targeting, Surveillance, and Risk Stratification. *JACC CardioOncol.* **2021**, *3*, 343–359. [CrossRef] [PubMed]

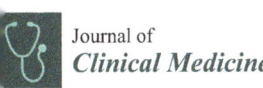

Systematic Review

Do Elderly Patients with Atrial Fibrillation Have Comparable Ablation Outcomes Compared to Younger Ones? Evidence from Pooled Clinical Studies

Feng Li [†], Lei Zhang [†], Li-Da Wu, Zhi-Yuan Zhang, Huan-Huan Liu, Zhen-Ye Zhang, Jie Zhang, Ling-Ling Qian and Ru-Xing Wang *

Department of Cardiology, Wuxi People's Hospital Affiliated to Nanjing Medical University, Wuxi 214023, China; lifeng212910@njmu.edu.cn (F.L.); leizhanglz@163.com (L.Z.); lidawunjmu@outlook.com (L.-D.W.); zzy18862935193@163.com (Z.-Y.Z.); hhliu1224@163.com (H.-H.L.); zhangzhenye@njmu.edu.cn (Z.-Y.Z.); jiezhang980216@163.com (J.Z.); qll900@sina.com (L.-L.Q.)
* Correspondence: ruxingw@njmu.edu.cn; Tel.: +86-510-85351593
† These authors contributed equally to this work.

Abstract: **Background:** Age is an independent risk factor of the progress and prognosis of atrial fibrillation (AF). However, ablation outcomes between elderly and younger patients with AF remain elusive. **Methods:** Cochrane Library, Embase, PubMed, and Web of Science were systematically searched up to 1 April 2022. Studies comparing AF ablation outcomes between elderly and younger patients and comprising outcomes of AF ablation for elderly patients were included. Trial sequential analysis (TSA) was performed to adjust for random error and lower statistical power in our meta-analysis. Subgroup analysis identified possible determinants of outcome impact for elderly patients after ablation. Moreover, linear and quadratic prediction fit plots with confidence intervals were performed, as appropriate. **Results:** A total of 27 studies with 113,106 AF patients were eligible. Compared with the younger group, the elderly group was significantly associated with a lower rate of freedom from AF (risk ratio [RR], 0.95; $p = 0.008$), as well as a higher incidence of safety outcomes (cerebrovascular events: RR, 1.64; $p = 0.000$; serious hemorrhage complications: RR, 1.50; $p = 0.035$; all-cause death: RR, 2.61; $p = 0.003$). Subgroup analysis and quadratic prediction fit analysis revealed the follow-up time was the potential determinant of freedom from AF for elderly patients after AF ablation. **Conclusions:** Our meta-analysis suggests that elderly patients may have inferior efficacy and safety outcomes to younger patients with AF ablation. Moreover, the follow-up time may be a potential determinant of outcome impact on freedom from AF for elderly patients after AF ablation.

Keywords: ablation; atrial fibrillation; elderly patients; younger patients; outcomes

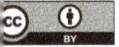

1. Introduction

Atrial fibrillation (AF) has become the most common sustained cardiac arrhythmia worldwide, with an estimated prevalence ranging from 2% to 4% in adults. Approximately 12 million individuals will experience AF in the US by 2050 and nearly 18 million in Europe by 2060. Remarkably, the prevalence could increase to as high as 5–10% among those aged 65 years and older [1,2]. Meanwhile, accumulated studies have reported that the elderly population with AF has a high risk of arrhythmic burden, stroke, bleeding, and heart failure, ultimately leading to longer hospitalization and increased mortality. Additionally, old age is an independent risk factor of AF progression and prognosis [3]. Therefore, the prevention and management of AF in elderly individuals have been hotpots in the cardiac electrophysiology field.

Ablation has been demonstrated as an effective strategy for rhythm control and life-quality improvement in symptomatic and drug-refractory AF patients [4,5]. The latest AF guidelines emphasized that catheter ablation for selected elderly AF patients might be a safe and effective option with comparable success rates and acceptable complication incidence in younger AF patients [3]. However, recommendations to date have not been made in either the European Society of Cardiology or American Heart Association guidelines, which indicates a potentially unresolved controversy in AF ablation therapy for the elderly. Alternatively, a recent retrospective study on the efficacy of second-generation cryoballoon ablation for elderly patients with persistent AF reported that old individuals ($\geq$75 years) were significantly associated with a higher AF recurrence than younger individuals (63.9 vs. 53.0%, $p = 0.03$) with the median follow-up of 24 months [6].

The results comparing ablation outcomes between elderly and younger patients with AF remain elusive and are thus vigorously debated. Accordingly, we aimed to perform a meta-analysis of a relatively large sample to comprehensively evaluate ablation outcomes between elderly and younger patients with AF.

2. Methods

2.1. Study Design

This systematic review was performed based on the PRISMA guidelines. The registered protocol for our study is available in the PROSPERO database (https://www.crd.york.ac.uk/prospero/display_record.php?ID=CRD42022325471, accessed on 10 May 2022).

2.2. Search Strategy

Two independent reviewers (F. Li and L. Zhang) comprehensively searched four online databases—the Cochrane Library, Embase, PubMed, and Web of Science—from their establishment to 1 April 2022. Search keywords were "elderly", "older", "septuagenarians", "octogenarians", "nonagenarians", "centenarians", "younger", "atrial fibrillation", and "ablation". Trials on the outcomes of AF ablation for elderly patients or comparing ablation outcomes between elderly patients and younger patients with AF were included. A manual search of reference lists of review literature and retrieved eligible literature was performed for potential publications not identified previously. In addition, we also contacted the relevant corresponding authors for missing outcome data in their publications.

2.3. Search Design

Two independent reviewers (L.-D. Wu and Z.-Y. Zhang) searched and reviewed the titles, abstracts, and full texts to select the eligible studies. A study was eligible if meeting the following inclusion criteria: randomized controlled trials and cohort, observational studies, and single-arm studies; studies comparing AF ablation outcomes between elderly patients and younger patients, including efficacy outcome (e.g., freedom from AF) and safety outcomes (e.g., cerebrovascular events, serious hemorrhage complications, phrenic nerve injury, and all-cause death); studies on outcomes of AF ablation for elderly patients; and studies with full text published in peer-reviewed journals; and studies containing the most data for multiple publications of the same study. Studies without original data, case reports, editorials, review articles, letters, and animal studies were all excluded. Meanwhile, a third reviewer (R.-X. Wang) resolved any disagreements about eligibility.

2.4. Data Extraction and Quality Assessment

Two independent researchers (F. Li and L. Zhang) extracted the data for each eligible study, and any disagreements were settled by a third researcher (R.-X. Wang). First, we documented study characteristics: first author, publication year, study design, country, sample size in the elderly and younger groups, and follow-up time. Then, patients' demographic and clinical characteristics and procedure-related indices were also recorded.

Study quality was evaluated using two appraisal tools by two independent researchers (L. Zhang and L.-D. Wu). For two-arm observational studies, the Newcastle–Ottawa Quality Assessment Scale was used, which has three domains with nine points [7]. The quality levels of studies were divided into moderate-to-high quality (score $\geq$ 6) and low quality (score < 6). For the single-arm study, the Institute of Health Economics checklist with a total of 20 items was used, and scores ranged from 0 (poor) to 20 (excellent) [8]. Any disagreements were discussed and resolved by consulting a third researcher (R.-X. Wang).

2.5. Statistical Analysis

Continuous variables are displayed as means ± standard deviations or medians with interquartile ranges, and categorical variables are displayed as frequencies and percentages. Relative risk (RR) and corresponding 95% confidence intervals (CIs) were calculated for each outcome for observational studies with two arms, whereas in terms of single-arm analysis, pooled results are presented as incidence of the events (event numbers divided by patient numbers) and 95% CI. Stata version 12.0 (http://www.stata.com, accessed on 10 May 2022) was used for statistical analyses. $p < 0.05$ was considered statistically significant.

We used the chi-squared test and I-squared (I^2) to quantify and assess statistical heterogeneity among studies. If the I^2 value was more than 50% and/or $p < 0.05$ for the chi-squared test, we considered the between-study heterogeneity to be substantial, and a random-effect model was used. Otherwise, a fixed-effect model was used. Sensitivity analysis was performed to assess the effect of a single study on the overall risk by sequentially omitting one study at a time, and potential publication bias was also evaluated via Egger's and Begg's tests. Importantly, trial sequential analysis (TSA), a useful method providing the required information size (RIS), was performed by TSA viewer (version 0.9.5.10 beta; Copenhagen Trial Unit) to adjust the random error and lower statistical power caused by the limited number of trials in a meta-analysis [9]. Type I and type II errors were set to 5% and 20% (80% power), respectively.

In addition, subgroup analysis was performed to screen sources of heterogeneity and potential determinants of AF ablation outcomes between elderly and younger patients. According to the characteristics of eligible studies, some potential factors, and previously reported factors, 13 subgroup factors were identified: study design, publication date, elderly age cutoff, elderly group sample size, AF type, female proportion, hypertension proportion, diabetes mellitus (DM) proportion, LAD (left atrial diameter), AF history duration, ablation strategy, ablation energy, and follow-up time. If the study design included only one center, it was defined as a single-center subgroup; otherwise, it was defined as a multicenter subgroup. If the publication date was within nearly 3 years (2020–2022), it was defined as the "recently" subgroup; otherwise, it was defined as the "not recently" subgroup. According to cutoff values of 75 and 100, the elderly age cutoff and the elderly group sample size were divided into two subgroups, respectively. If the AF types of the eligible patients were all paroxysmal AF (PAF) in the elderly group, it was assigned to the PAF subgroup; otherwise, it was assigned to the non-PAF subgroup. If the female proportion was significantly higher (elderly group versus younger group), it was defined as a "higher" subgroup; if the female proportion was equal, it was defined as an "equal" subgroup. Similarly, hypertension, DM proportion, LAD, and AF history duration with "higher" and "equal" subgroup also were defined, respectively. If the ablation strategy included only PVI, it was assigned to the PVI subgroup, and if PVI plus linear and/or substrate ablation had been performed, it was assigned to the "PVI-plus" subgroup. Based on the energy source of radiofrequency ablation (RF) and cryoablation (Cryo), RF and Cryo subgroups were defined. Follow-up time was divided into two subgroups (≥24 months and <24 months).

Additionally, linear and quadratic prediction fit plots with confidence intervals were constructed as appropriate to assess the correlation between the follow-up time and the rate of freedom from AF for elderly and younger patients.

3. Results

3.1. Study Selection and Quality Assessment

A total of 27 studies with 113,106 AF patients (8686 elderly patients and 104,420 younger patients) were eligible, including 23 observational two-arm studies [6,10–31] (8133 elderly AF patients and 104,420 younger AF patients) and four single-arm studies [32–35] (553 elderly AF patients). The selection flowchart is displayed in Figure 1. Two studies (Romero et al. [18] and

Hao et al. [28]) reported only the safety outcomes without the rate of freedom from AF. A total of five studies contained multiple age-based subgroups: four subgroups in Sciarra et al. [11], six subgroups in Hartl et al. [17], five subgroups in Bunch et al. [25], three subgroups in Kusumoto et al. [30], and three subgroups in Bhargava et al. [31]. Therefore, for these five studies, multiple subgroups were integrated into two groups (elderly group and younger group) based on the elderly age cutoff value in each study. The baseline characteristics and procedure-related indices of the eligible studies are presented in Table 1. In this meta-analysis, all two-arm studies had a moderate-to-high quality, as presented in Supplementary Table S1. Four single-arm studies all had a score higher than 15, and are presented in Supplementary Table S2.

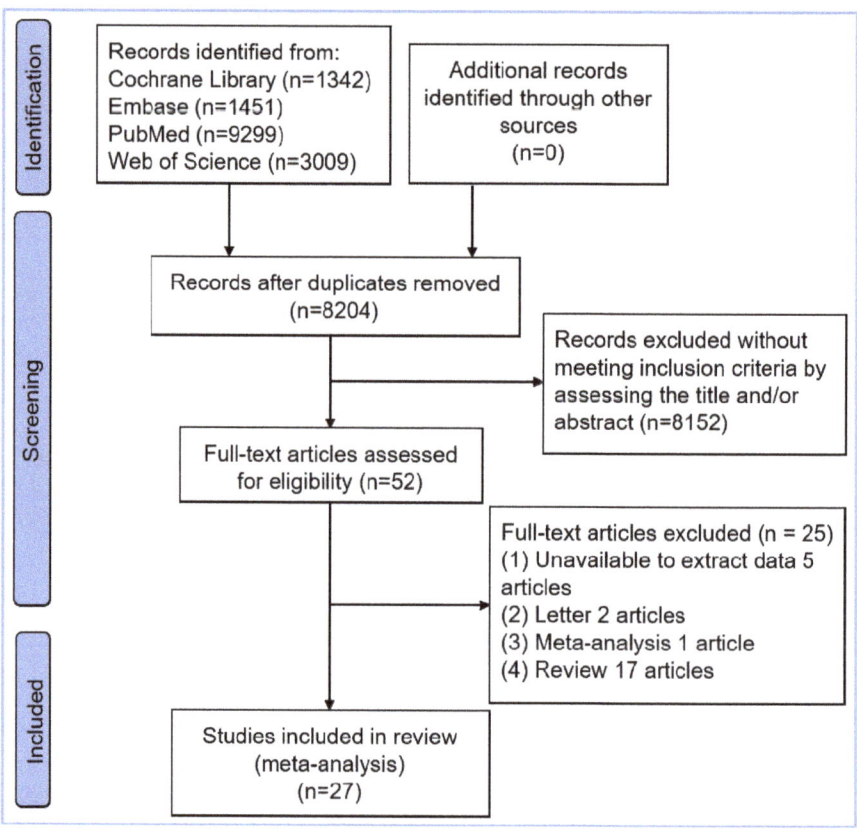

Figure 1. Flowchart of study selection.

Table 1. Baseline characteristics and procedure-related indices of eligible studies.

First Author	Year	Study Design	Country	Sample Size		Elderly Age Cutoff (Years)	Gender (Female, %)		AF Type (PAF, %)		Hypertension (%)		DM (%)	
				Elderly Group	Younger Group		Elderly Group	Younger Group	Elderly Group	Younger Group	Elderly Group	Younger Group	Elderly Group	Younger Group
Natale [10]	2021	Observational single-center	America	221	352	75	100.0	100.0	10.9	14.8	69.7 $	53.4	10.9	14.8
Vermeersch [6]	2021	Retrospective single-center	Belgium	83	166	75	41.0	39.2	0	0	73.5 $	55.4	14.5	13.9
Sciarra [11]	2021	Prospective multicenter	Italy	726	1808	67	37.5 #	23.4	73.6	75.5	62.8 $	41.3	7.2 &	4.7
Hartl [12]	2021	Observational single-center	Germany	299	487	70	44.5 #	41.9	49.2	70.0	73.6 $	60.0	NA	NA
Zhou [13]	2020	Observational single-center	China	89	244	80	55.1	59.4	64.0	62.7	75.3	64.8	36.0 &	22.1
Kanda [14]	2019	Retrospective single-center	Japan	49	241	80	51.0	40	100.0	100.0	63.0	56.0	14.0	16.0
Fink [15]	2019	Prospective multicenter	Germany	108	630	70	38.0 #	27.6	55.6	63.0	NA	NA	9.3	6.3
Zhang-1 [16]	2019	Retrospective single-center	China	127	550	75	55.1 #	40.5	92.9	88.2	67.2 $	59.8	18.1	15.1
Heeger [17]	2019	Prospective multicenter	Germany	104	104	75	50.0	48.1	57.7	56.7	77.9	78.9	15.4	14.4
Romero [18]	2019	Retrospective multicenter	America	3482	82,637	80	61.0	31.1	NA	NA	65.7	55.3	19.6	14.9
Abdin [19]	2019	Retrospective single-center	Germany	55	183	75	54.6 #	34.5	31.0	40.5	85.4 $	69.3	20.0 &	8.7
Zhang-2 [20]	2018	Retrospective single-center	China	308	360	60	41.5 #	21.4	71.4	75.0	55.0 $	37.0	12.6	9.9
Tscholl [21]	2018	Retrospective single-center	Germany	40	40	75	50.0	35	45.0	47.5	80.0	60.0	10.0	12.5
Moser [22]	2017	Retrospective multicenter	Germany	227	4222	75	48.0 #	31.1	59.9	63.3	NA	NA	8.8	7.6
Abugattas [23]	2017	Retrospective single-center	Belgium	53	106	75	54.7	41.5	100.0	100.0	79.2 $	41.3	11.3	8.7
Kautzner [24]	2017	Retrospective single-center	Czech Republic	394	2803	70	49.0 #	29.4	66.5	68.2	79.2 $	56.7	15.7 &	11.2
Bunch-2 [25]	2016	Observational multicenter	America	46	877	80	58.7 #	40.2	52.2	54.7	82.6	70.0	17.4	22.1
Lioni [26]	2014	Retrospective single-center	Greece	95	221	65	49.5	41.2	100.0	100.0	41.1	33.5	20.0 &	6.8

Table 1. Cont.

First Author	Year	Study Design	Country	Sample Size		Elderly Age Cutoff (Years)	Gender (Female, %)		AF Type (PAF, %)		Hypertension (%)		DM (%)	
				Elderly Group	Younger Group		Elderly Group	Younger Group	Elderly Group	Younger Group	Elderly Group	Younger Group	Elderly Group	Younger Group
Santangeli [27]	2012	Retrospective single-center	America	103	2651	80	41.0 #	28.0	25.0	27.0	48.0 $	37.0	15.0	11.0
Hao [28]	2012	Retrospective multicenter	America	1325	4622	65	41.0 #	23.0	NA	NA	68.0	57.0	21.0	16.0
Bunch-1 [29]	2010	Retrospective single-center	America	35	717	80	54.3	40.7	45.7	54.1	57.1	49.2	8.6	12.4
Kusumoto [30]	2009	Retrospective single-center	America	61	179	75	39.3 #	24.1	34.0	70.9	NA	NA	NA	NA
Bhargava [31]	2004	Retrospective single-center	America	103	220	60	23.3	18.2	52.4	54.5	35.0 $	20.9	NA	NA
Liu [32]	2022	Multicenter single-arm	China	270	-	80	42.6	-	65.6	-	73.7	-	29.3	-
Akhtar [33]	2020	Single-center single-arm	America	15	-	80	40.0	-	87.0	-	80.0	-	20.0	-
Metzner [34]	2016	Single-center single-arm	Germany	94	-	75	41.5	-	58.5	-	88.3	-	4.3	-
Corrado [35]	2008	Single-center single-arm	America	174	-	75	36.8	-	55.0	-	56.0	-	13.0	-

First Author	LVEF		CHA$_2$DS$_2$-VASc Score		LAD (mm)		AF History Duration		AADs Usage (Elderly vs. Younger)
	Elderly Group	Younger Group	Elderly Group	Younger Group	Elderly Group	Younger Group	Elderly Group	Younger Group	
Natale [10]	58.2 ± 9.6	57.8 ± 9.4	NA	NA	42.6 ± 7.8	41.9 ± 7.6	NA	NA	NA
Vermeersch [6]	53.2 ± 9.4	54.4 ± 9.0	NA	NA	45.8 ± 7.8	45.6 ± 7.0	45.7 ± 46.2 M	52.4 ± 61.1 M	NA
Sciarra [11]	58.8 ± 7.2	59.3 ± 6.9	2.4 ± 0.7	1.1 ± 0.9	22.9 ± 6.2 cm² *	21.8 ± 6.0 cm²	62.0 ± 107.1 M ‡	52.0 ± 105.8 M	Failed ≥ 2 AADs (higher)
Hartl [12]	56.2 ± 5.9	56.8 ± 6.5	NA	NA	46.1 ± 7.0 *	43.5 ± 6.9	NA	NA	The proportion of AADs at baseline (equal)
Zhou [13]	62.7 ± 5.4	63.1 ± 5.7	4.3 ± 1.3	3.3 ± 1.4	41.2 ± 4.8	41.5 ± 6.2	12.0 (2.5–36.0) M	24.0 (5.0–48.0) M	NA
Kanda [14]	NA	NA	3.8 ± 0.9	2.2 ± 1.4	40.0 ± 6.0	38.0 ± 6.0	NA	NA	The proportion of AADs at baseline: Class I (lower), other classes (equal)
Fink [15]	NA	NA	NA	NA	NA	NA	NA	NA	NA
Zhang-1 [16]	58.7 ± 9.0	61.5 ± 6.5	4.8 ± 1.6	2.6 ± 1.7	41.0 ± 5.3	41.3 ± 5.6	NA	NA	The proportion of AADs at baseline, Class I, I and III (equal)
Heeger [17]	NA	NA	3.8 ± 1.1	2.1 ± 1.3	44.5 ± 5.6	44.5 ± 5.6	NA	NA	NA
Romero [18]	NA	NA	NA	NA	40.8 ± 5.5	40.8 ± 6.6	24.6 ± 34.1 M	21.9 ± 34.6 M	NA
Abdin [19]	51.6 ± 8.3	52.5 ± 8.0	4.0 ± 1.3	2.0 ± 1.3	49.2 ± 5.8	38.6 ± 6.1	NA	NA	NA

Table 1. *Cont.*

First Author	LVEF Elderly Group	LVEF Younger Group	CHA$_2$DS$_2$-VASc Score Elderly Group	CHA$_2$DS$_2$-VASc Score Younger Group	LAD (mm) Elderly Group	LAD (mm) Younger Group	AF History Duration Elderly Group	AF History Duration Younger Group	AADs Usage (Elderly vs. Younger)
Zhang-2 [20]	66.3 ± 5.7	69.1 ± 8.9	NA	NA	NA	NA	NA	NA	NA
Tscholl [21]	63.0 (60.0, 66.0)	65.0 (60.0, 70.0)	4.0 (4.0, 5.0)	2.0 (1.0, 3.0)	NA	NA	NA	NA	NA
Moser [22]	NA	NA	3.7 ± 1.0	1.7 ± 1.2	41.4 ± 7.2	40.9 ± 6.6	NA	NA	NA
Abugattas [23]	59.2 ± 5.2	59.9 ± 6.4	4.0 ± 1.3	1.3 ± 1.2	42.5 ± 5.4	42.3 ± 5.7	NA	NA	NA
Kautzner [24]	55.8 ± 8.8	56.4 ± 7.6	3.1 ± 1.3	1.5 ± 1.2	41.2 ± 4.8	41.5 ± 6.2	NA	NA	The proportion of AADs at baseline (equal)
Bunch-2 [25]	53.8 ± 13.3	52.5 ± 11.4	NA	NA	NA	NA	12.0 (2.5–36) M	24.0 (5.0–48.0) M	NA
Lioni [26]	60.0 ± 3.8	61.1 ± 4.0	NA	NA	42.6 ± 4.5 *	39.5 ± 4.3	5.9 ± 5.1 Y ¢	4.7 ± 4.4 Y	The proportion of AADs after ablation, Class I and III (equal)
Santangeli [27]	55.0 ± 12.0	57.0 ± 9.0	NA	NA	46.0 ± 5.0	45.0 ± 8.0	52.0 (24.0–78.0) M	58.0 (31.0–96.0) M	Failed AADs (equal)
Hao [28]	NA	NA	NA	NA	24.8 ± 9.1 cm^2	28.7 ± 9.5 cm^2	NA	NA	NA
Bunch-1 [29]	52.7 ± 13.2	51.3 ± 13.1	NA	NA	NA	NA	NA	NA	NA
Kusumoto [30]	NA	NA	NA	NA	42.6 ± 4.5	39.1 ± 4.3	5.9 ± 5.1 Y	4.7 ± 4.4 Y	The proportion of AADs after ablation, Class I and III (equal)
Bhargava [31]	51.4 ± 9.8	53.4 ± 7.6	NA	NA	43.4 ± 6.5	43.3 ± 13.2	6.5 ± 3.7 Y	6.0 ± 4.8 Y	Failed AADs (equal)
Liu [32]	63.7 ± 7.2	-	3.9 ± 1.2	-	39.9 ± 6.3	-	2.9 ± 5.2 Y	-	-
Akhtar [33]	63.7 ± 3.5	-	4.2 ± 1.7	-	45.0 ± 1.2	-	8.9 ± 8.2 Y	-	-
Metzner [34]	NA	-	4.0 ± 1.0	-	44.8 ± 6.2	-	75.0 M Median	-	-
Corrado [35]	53.0 ± 7.0	-	NA	-	46.0 ± 6.0	-	7.0 ± 4.0 Y	-	-

First Author	Key Points of Ablation Procedure						Ablation Strategy	Ablation Energy	Follow-Up (Months)
Natale [10]	Isolation of pulmonary veins, posterior wall and superior vena cava was performed in all patients. Non-pulmonary vein triggers from other areas were ablated based on operator's discretion						PVI-plus	RF	48.0
Vermeersch [6]	PVI only						PVI	Cryo	24.0 (18.4–25.5)
Sciarra [11]	PVI only						PVI	Cryo	12.0
Hartl [12]	PVI with or without additional linear ablation based on decision						PVI-plus	Cryo	36.0
Zhou [13]	After PVI, additional linear ablation was performed when necessary						PVI-plus	RF	24.4 ± 9.6
Kanda [14]	PVI with or without additional linear ablation based on decision						PVI-plus	Cryo	12.0
Fink [15]	PVI first, and then additional ablation strategies including the creation of right atrial and left atrial linear lesions including block of the cavo-tricuspid isthmus, or ablation of complex fractionated atrial electrograms were at the discretion of the operator						PVI-plus	RF	14.9
Zhang-1 [16]	PVI only						PVI	Cryo	12.0
Heeger [17]	PVI only						PVI	Cryo	36.0
Romero [18]	NA						NA	NA	NA

Table 1. *Cont.*

First Author	Key Points of Ablation Procedure	Ablation Strategy	Ablation Energy	Follow-Up (Months)
Abdin [19]	PVI only	PVI	Cryo	11.8 ± 5.4
Zhang-2 [20]	PVI with linear ablation	PVI-plus	RF	6.0
Tscholl [21]	PVI only	PVI	Cryo	12.0 (6.0, 18.0)
Moser [22]	PVI first, and then ablation of fragmented signals and/or lines in the left atrial (mitral isthmus line, roof line, anterior line) were performed in order to achieve termination to sinus rhythm	PVI-plus	RF	15.3
Abugattas [23]	PVI only	PVI	Cryo	12.0
Kautzner [24]	All patients underwent PVI first, and then additional left atrial linear lesions, coronary sinus ablation, or electrogram-guided ablations were performed empirically according to the clinical presentation and inducibility of the arrhythmia during the procedure	PVI-plus	RF	18.0–21.0
Bunch-2 [25]	All patients underwent PVI first, and then additional ablation beyond PVI was performed based upon individual operator choice	PVI-plus	RF	60.0
Lioni [26]	PVI only	PVI	RF	34.0 ± 15.1
Santangeli [27]	Isolation of all the pulmonary vein antra and the posterior wall contained between the pulmonary veins first; then the ablation catheter was positioned at right atrium–superior vena cava junction, where mapping and ablation was performed.	PVI-plus	RF	18.0 ± 6.0
Hao [28]	NA	NA	RF	1.0 W
Bunch-1 [29]	PVI with or without additional linear ablation based on decision	PVI-plus	RF	12.0
Kusumoto [30]	PVI with linear ablations (not routinely performed)	PVI-plus	RF	12.0
Bhargava [31]	PVI only	PVI	RF	14.7 ± 5.2
Liu [32]	PVI with or without additional linear ablation based on decision	PVI-plus	RF	12.0
Akhtar [33]	PVI first, then additional cavo-tricuspid isthmus ablation based on the discretion of the operator	PVI-plus	Cryo	12.0
Metzner [34]	Circumferential PVI was performed in all patients, then ablation of complex fractionated atrial electrograms and/or linear lesions were performed based on decision	PVI-plus	RF	37.0 ± 20.0
Corrado [35]	PVI and superior vena isolation	PVI-plus	RF	20.0 ± 14.0

AF: atrial fibrillation; PAF: paroxysmal atrial fibrillation; DM: diabetes mellitus; LVEF: left ventricular ejection fraction; LAD: left atrial diameter; AADs: antiarrhythmic drugs; PVI: pulmonary vein isolation; PVI-plus: PVI plus linear ablation and/or substrate ablation RF: radiofrequency; Cryo: cryoablation; NA: not available. Note: #, $, &, *, and £ represent the significantly higher proportion (elderly group vs. younger group) in terms of gender, hypertension, DM, LAD, and AF history duration, respectively. In the LAD column, cm^2 represents the unit of left atrial area; in the AF history duration column, M and Y represent months and years, respectively. In the Follow-up column, W represents week.

3.2. Rate of Freedom from AF between Elderly and Younger Groups

A total of 21 studies [6,10–17,19–27,29–31] on 18,608 AF patients in our meta-analysis reported rates of freedom from AF between elderly and younger groups. Compared with the younger group, the elderly group was significantly associated with a lower rate of freedom from AF (RR, 0.95; 95% CI, 0.92–0.99; p = 0.008; I^2 = 46.30%; Figure 2) via a random-effect model.

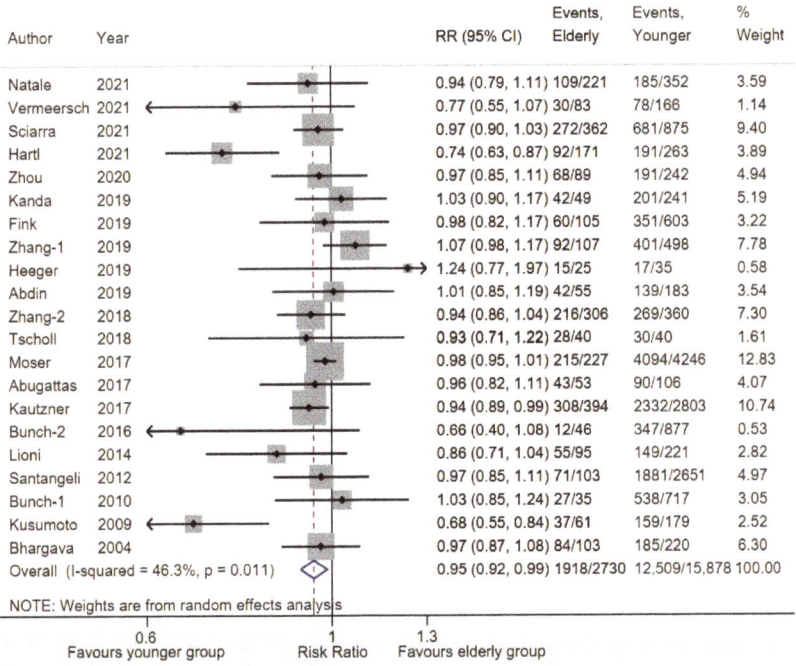

Figure 2. Forest plot of the freedom rate from AF between elderly and younger groups [6,10–17,19–27,29–31]. Comparison of the rates of freedom from AF between elderly and younger groups.

Subgroup analysis was performed with a total of 11 subgroup factors for the rate of freedom from AF, and the results are displayed in Figure 3. Elderly group sample size subgroup analysis showed a comparable rate of freedom from AF between the elderly group and the younger group: ≥100 subgroup (RR 0.96; 95% CI, 0.93–1.00; p = 0.054) and <100 subgroup (RR 0.92; 95% CI, 0.85–1.00; p = 0.050). Similar results were also shown in the LAD and AF history duration subgroups (Supplementary Figure S1). Compared with the younger group, the elderly group was significantly associated with a lower rate of freedom from AF in the single-center subgroup (RR 0.94; 95% CI, 0.89–0.99; p = 0.014), recently subgroup (RR 0.90; 95% CI, 0.80–1.00; p = 0.041), <75 years subgroup (RR 0.93; 95% CI, 0.88–0.98; p = 0.006), non-PAF subgroup (RR 0.95; 95% CI, 0.91–0.99; p = 0.012), higher female proportion subgroup (RR 0.94; 95% CI, 0.89–0.99; p = 0.022), higher hypertension proportion subgroup (RR 0.95; 95% CI, 0.91–1.00; p = 0.037), higher DM proportion subgroup (RR 0.95; 95% CI, 0.91–0.99; p = 0.010), PVI-plus subgroup (RR 0.93; 95% CI, 0.89–0.98; p = 0.010), and RF subgroup (RR 0.95; 95% CI, 0.91–0.99; p = 0.009), all of which were consistent with the pooled results, whereas no significant differences were found in the other subgroups. Importantly, the only potentially significant treatment–covariate interaction was identified in the follow-up time subgroups: ≥24 months (RR 0.87; 95% CI, 0.78–0.97; p = 0.015) and <24 months (RR 0.97; 95% CI, 0.94–1.00; p = 0.075) with p = 0.066 for interaction.

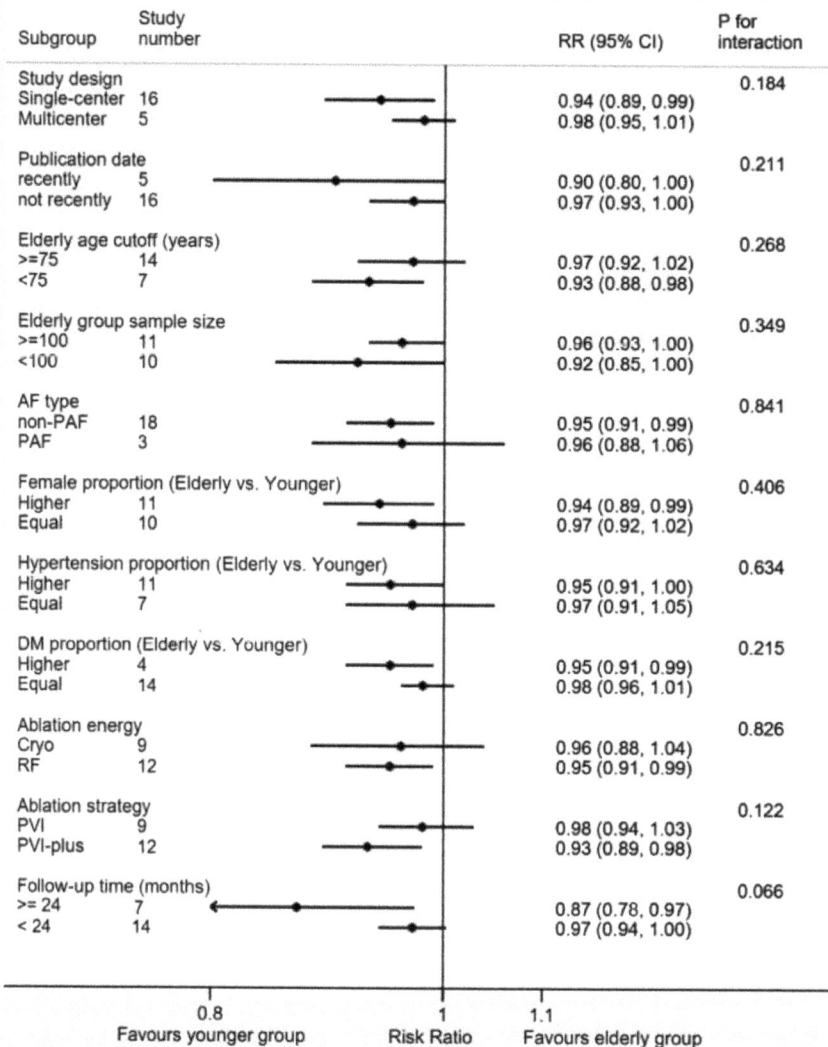

Figure 3. Forest plot of subgroup analysis of the freedom rate from AF between elderly and younger groups. Subgroup analysis of the rates of freedom from AF between elderly and younger groups. AF: atrial fibrillation; PAF: paroxysmal atrial fibrillation; RF: radiofrequency; Cryo: cryoablation; PVI: pulmonary vein isolation; PVI-plus: PVI plus linear and/or substrate ablation.

Sensitivity analysis was also performed, and the results showed no significant change, ranging from 0.94 (95% CI, 0.90–0.99) to 0.96 (95% CI, 0.93–1.00) in the overall combined proportion, which suggested that no single study dominated the combined proportion and heterogeneity. Moreover, no publication bias was presented in Begg's or Egger's test ($p = 0.174$ and $p = 0.115$, respectively).

In addition, TSA was used to assess whether there was adequate power for comparison of rates of freedom from AF between the elderly group and the younger group. The results showed that although the actual sample size (18,608) was smaller than the RIS (relative risk reduction, RRR = 35%; RIS = 25,240), the cumulative Z curve (Z = 2.55) crossed both the conventional boundary and the trial sequential alpha spending monitoring boundary (TSA monitoring boundaries = 2.49), suggesting firm evidence favoring the younger group in terms of the rate of freedom from AF (Figure 4).

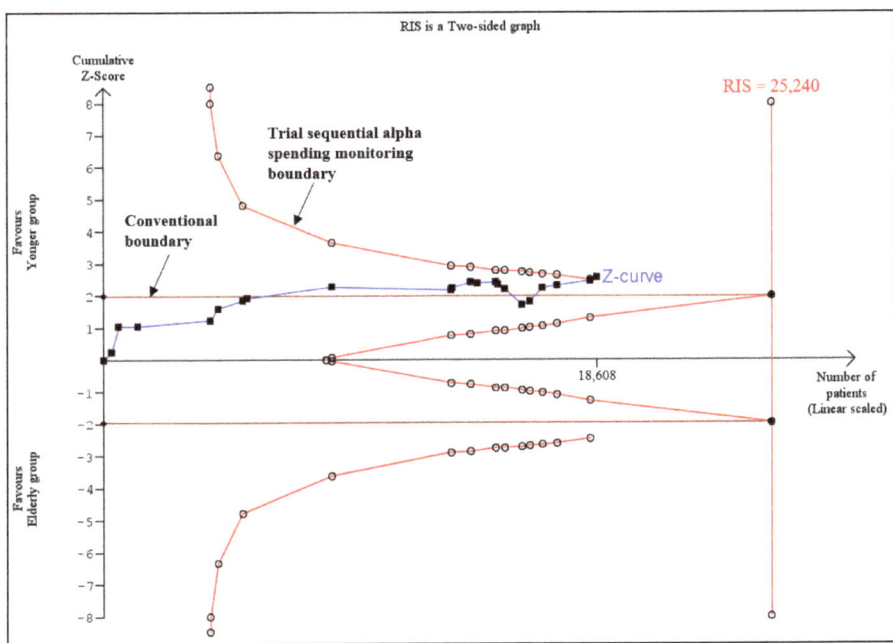

Figure 4. Trial sequential analysis of the rates of freedom from AF between elderly and younger groups. The results showed that the actual sample size (18,608) was smaller than the RIS (relative risk reduction, RRR = 35%; RIS = 25,240), and the cumulative Z curve (Z = 2.55) crossed both the conventional boundary and the trial sequential alpha spending monitoring boundary (TSA monitoring boundaries = 2.49). RIS: required information size.

3.3. Pooled Rate of Freedom from AF in Elderly Group

A total of 25 eligible studies (3879 elderly patients with AF) reported the rate of freedom from AF [6,10–17,19–27,29–35]. The pooled rate of freedom from AF was 0.69 (95% CI, 0.63–0.75; $p = 0.000$; $I^2 = 92.53\%$; Figure 5) with the random-effect model.

Subgroup analysis was performed with a total of eight subgroup factors for the rate of freedom from AF in the elderly group, and the results are shown in Table 2. Interestingly, in terms of follow-up time for elderly patients, a significantly lower rate of freedom from AF was shown in the ≥ 24 months subgroup (0.53; 95% CI, 0.43–0.62; $p = 0.000$; $I^2 = 85.67\%$) than in the <24 months subgroup (0.76; 95% CI, 0.71–0.81; $p = 0.000$; $I^2 = 86.11\%$) with $p = 0.000$ for interaction.

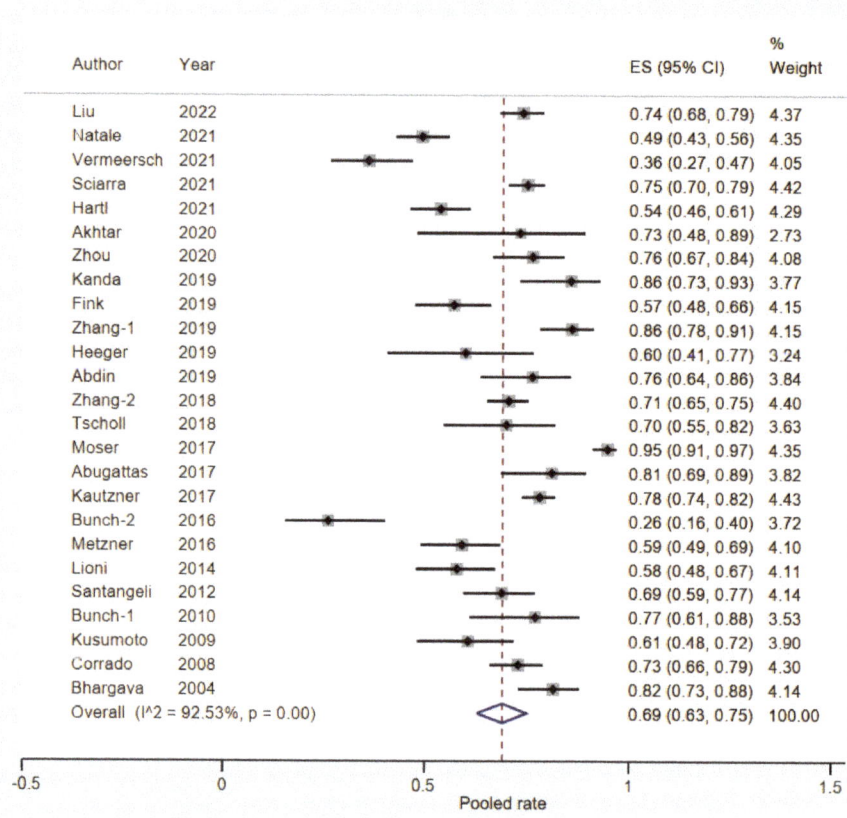

Figure 5. Forest plot of the pooled rate of freedom from AF in the elderly group [6,10–17,19–27,29–35]. The line of equity refers to the pooled result of eligible studies in the forest plots.

Table 2. Subgroup analysis of the rate of freedom from atrial fibrillation in the elderly group.

Subgroup Factors	Numbers in Study	Pooled Incidence	95% CI	I^2 (%)	p for Interaction
Study design					0.893
Multicenter	7	0.68	0.54–0.81	95.74	
Single-center	18	0.69	0.63–0.76	89.38	
Publication date					0.189
recently	7	0.63	0.51–0.74	93.52	
not recently	18	0.72	0.65–0.78	91.20	
Elderly age cutoff (years)					0.911
≥75	18	0.69	0.60–0.78	93.54	
<75	7	0.69	0.61–0.76	89.64	
Elderly group sample size					0.264
≥100	13	0.72	0.65–0.79	94.17	
<100	12	0.65	0.55–0.75	87.76	
AF type					0.484
PAF	3	0.75	0.56–0.91	-	
non-PAF	22	0.68	0.62–0.75	93.12	
Ablation strategy					0.771
PVI-plus	16	0.68	0.60–0.76	93.85	
PVI	9	0.70	0.60–0.80	89.60	

Table 2. Cont.

Subgroup Factors	Numbers in Study	Pooled Incidence	95% CI	I^2 (%)	p for Interaction
Ablation energy					0.765
RF	15	0.68	0.60–0.76	93.88	
Cryo	10	0.71	0.60–0.80	90.15	
Follow-up time (months)					0.000
≥24	8	0.53	0.43–0.62	85.67	
<24	17	0.76	0.71–0.81	86.11	

AF: atrial fibrillation; PAF: paroxysmal atrial fibrillation; PVI: pulmonary vein isolation; PVI plus: PVI plus linear and/or complex fractionated atrial electrogram ablations; CI: confidence interval.

Sensitivity analysis indicated that there was no significant change, ranging from 0.68 (95% CI, 0.62–0.74) to 0.70 (95% CI, 0.65–0.75), in the overall combined proportion, indicating that no single study dominated combined proportion and heterogeneity. No publication bias was shown in Begg's or Egger's test (p = 0.350 and p = 0.277, respectively). Therefore, the results were considered to be robust.

3.4. Relationship between Follow-Up Time and Rate of Freedom from AF

In terms of the elderly group, linear prediction fit and quadratic prediction fit plots with confidence intervals were constructed. The results showed that the correlation between the follow-up time and the rate of freedom from AF was significantly negative (quadratic prediction fit: R^2 = 57.10%, p = 0.000; linear prediction fit: R^2 = 55.90%, p = 0.000) (Figure 6). In addition, overlapping of the quadratic prediction fit plots with confidence intervals for elderly and younger groups was performed, and the result indicated that the rate of freedom from AF in the elderly group seemed to be consistently lower than in the younger group (Supplementary Figure S2). More interestingly, we took the quadratic prediction fit curve for the younger group minus the quadratic prediction fit curve for the elderly group, which calculated the difference in freedom from AF between the younger group and the elderly group. The result showed that the difference was monotonically decreased in the interval of 0 to 20.98 months, while the difference was monotonically increased in the interval of ≥20.98 months (Supplementary Figure S3).

3.5. Safety Outcomes between Elderly and Younger Groups

A total of 21 eligible studies [6,11–29,31] compared cerebrovascular events, including stoke or transient ischemic attack (TIA), between elderly and younger groups, whereas a total of 6 studies [6,14,15,19,23,27] were excluded because there were no events in either group. The result showed that the elderly group had a significantly higher incidence of cerebrovascular events than the younger group (RR, 1.64; 95% CI, 1.25–2.17; p = 0.000; I^2 = 0.00%) with a fixed-effect model (Figure 7). However, the pooled rate of the cerebrovascular events [6,11–29,31–33,35] in the elderly group was 0.00 (95% CI, 0.00–0.01; p = 0.000) (Supplementary Table S3).

A total of 19 eligible studies [6,11–17,19–23,26–31] reported serious hemorrhage complications (such as hemothorax, perforation, tamponade, or major bleeding) between the elderly and younger groups, whereas two studies [14,23] were excluded because of no events in either group. The result indicated that the elderly group had a significantly higher incidence of serious hemorrhage complications (RR, 1.50; 95% CI, 1.03–2.19; p = 0.035; I^2 = 0.00%) with a fixed-effect model (Figure 8). However, the pooled rate of serious hemorrhage complications [6,11–17,19–23,26–33,35] in the elderly group was 0.00 (95% CI, 0.00–0.01; p = 0.000) (Supplementary Table S3).

All-cause death was reported by 14 eligible studies [6,12–14,16–19,22–25,27,29] between elderly and younger groups. A total of five studies [6,14,19,23,27] without events in either group were excluded from the meta-analysis. The results also showed that the elderly group had a significantly higher incidence of all-cause death (RR, 2.61; 95% CI 1.38–4.93; p = 0.003; I^2 = 65.80%) with a random-effect model (Figure 9). The pooled rate of all-cause death [6,12–14,16–19,22–25,27,29,32,33] in the elderly group was 0.01 (95% CI 0.00–0.02; p = 0.050) (Supplementary Table S3).

In terms of phrenic nerve injury, 10 [6,11,12,16,17,19,21–23,28] of 12 eligible studies [6,11–13,16,17,19,21–23,28,29] were analyzed in our meta-analysis. The result showed there was no significant difference between elderly and younger groups (RR 0.90; 95% CI, 0.62–1.31; p = 0.587; I^2 = 0.00%) with a fixed-effect model (Figure 10). The pooled rate of phrenic nerve injury [6,11–13,16,17,19–23,28,29,32,33] in the elderly group was 0.01 (95% CI, 0.00–0.02; p = 0.011) (Supplementary Table S3).

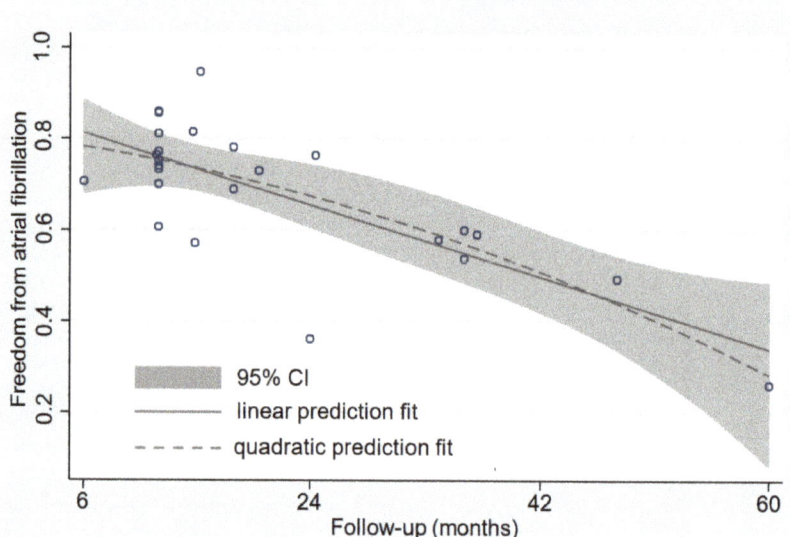

Figure 6. Linear and quadratic prediction fit plot with confidence interval between the follow-up time and the rate of freedom from AF for the elderly. The solid gray line represents the linear prediction fit. The dotted gray line represents the quadratic prediction fit. The gray area represents the 95% confidence interval for the quadratic prediction fit. Each dark blue circle represents a sample CI: confidence interval.

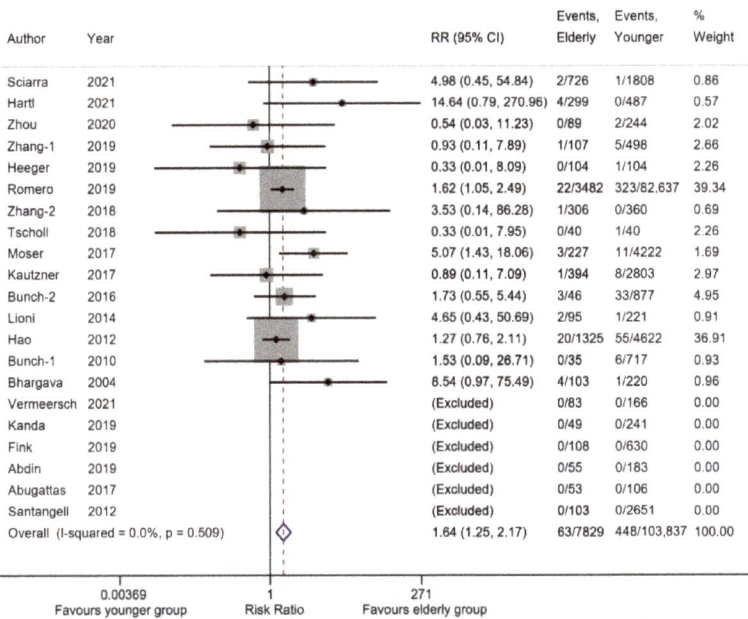

Figure 7. Forest plot comparing cerebrovascular events between elderly and younger groups [6,11–29,31]. The dotted red line represents the pooled risk ratio for cerebrovascular events between elderly and younger groups.

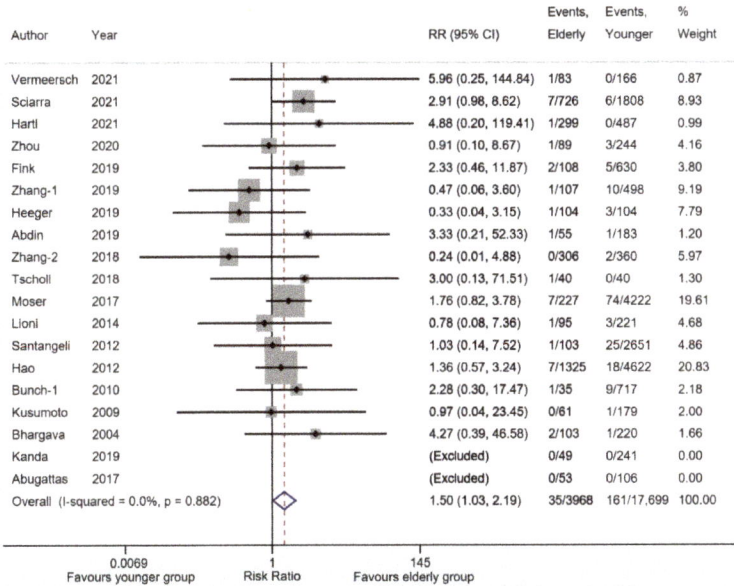

Figure 8. Forest plot comparing serious hemorrhage complications between elderly and younger groups [6,11–17,19–23,26–31]. The dotted red line represents the pooled risk ratio for serious hemorrhage complications between elderly and younger groups.

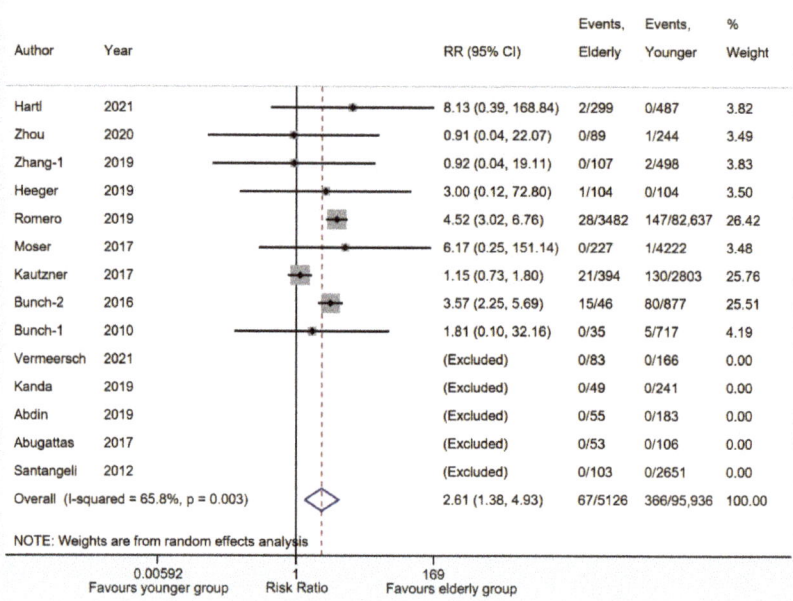

Figure 9. Forest plot comparing all-cause death between elderly and younger groups [6,12–14,16–19,22–25,27,29]. The dotted red line represents the pooled risk ratio for all-cause death between elderly and younger groups.

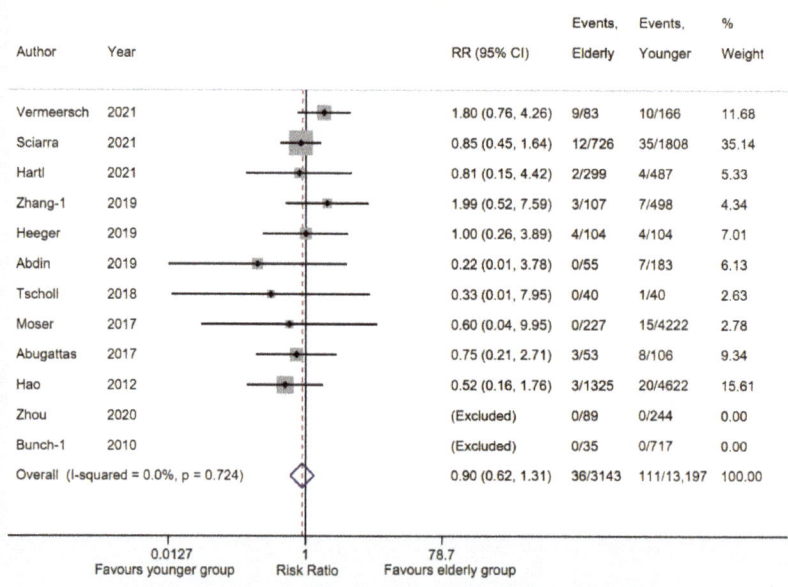

Figure 10. Forest plot comparing phrenic nerve injury between elderly and younger groups [6,11–13,16,17,19,21–23,28,29]. The dotted red line represents the pooled risk ratio for phrenic nerve injury between elderly and younger groups.

4. Discussion

We comprehensively evaluated a total of 113,106 AF patients (8686 elderly patients and 104,420 younger patients) from 27 original articles. To our knowledge, this study may be the first registered meta-analysis with a relatively large sample to compare the AF ablation outcomes between elderly patients and younger patients. Our main findings were as follows. (1) Elderly patients may have inferior efficacy and safety outcomes to younger patients with AF ablation. (2) Follow-up time may be a potential determinant of outcome impact on freedom from AF for elderly patients after AF ablation.

The prevalence of AF has been reported to increase with the aging progress, which leads to age as an independent risk factor of the progress and prognosis of AF [2,36]. At present, the diagnosis and management of AF guidelines recommend that catheter ablation should be considered in PAF and persistent AF patients for better symptom control (Class I) [3]. A prespecified age-subgroup analysis based on the CABANA trial also reported that AF recurrence rates were consistently lower with ablation than with drug therapy across three age subgroups, with adjusted hazard ratio (aHR) of 0.47 (95% CI, 0.35–0.62) for <65 years, aHR 0.58 (95% CI, 0.48–0.70) for 65–74 years, and aHR 0.49 (95% CI, 0.34–0.70) for $\geq$75 years, with p = 0.396 for interaction [37], indicating support for ablation without justification to discriminate by age. Several observational studies revealed a possible trend wherein elderly patients might be associated with a lower rate of freedom from AF and a higher rate of safety outcomes than younger patients [6,38], which meant that ablation outcomes between elderly and younger AF patients remain poorly understood. Therefore, a systematic review is needed to pool existing data and assess the AF ablation outcomes between elderly and younger patients.

In this meta-analysis, we compared the ablation outcomes between elderly and younger AF patients. For the rate of freedom from AF, the results indicated a pooled rate of freedom from AF in elderly patients of 0.69 (95% CI, 0.63–0.75; p = 0.000) and a significantly lower rate of freedom from AF in elderly patients than younger patients (RR, 0.95; p = 0.008), which was consistent with previous studies [6,32,33,38]. Moreover, the TSA result also showed firm evidence favoring the younger group in terms of the rate of freedom from AF, which further supported our pooled results. In terms of safety outcomes, we found a relatively low incidence (ranging from 0.00 to 0.01) of cerebrovascular events, serious hemorrhage complications, phrenic nerve injury, and all-cause death for elderly AF patients, whereas compared with younger ones, a significantly higher rate of cerebrovascular events, serious hemorrhage complications, and all-cause death was shown in elderly patients with AF, while a comparable rate of phrenic nerve injury was displayed in elderly patients. In summary, elderly patients may have inferior efficacy and safety outcomes to younger patients with AF ablation.

Previous studies revealed that the success rate of maintenance of sinus rhythm was progressively reduced as a function of follow-up time postablation, ranging from 75% to 93% and 63% to 74% for PAF and persistent AF, respectively, with 1-year follow-up, as well as ranging from 57% to 65% and <50% for PAF and persistent AF, respectively, with 5-year follow-up [39,40]. In our study, we found the rate of freedom from AF between elderly and younger groups in the $\geq$24 months subgroup (RR 0.87; p = 0.015) was lower in the <24 months subgroup (RR 0.97; p = 0.075) with p = 0.066 for interaction, which indicated a substantial potential trend between $\geq$24 months follow-up and <24 months follow-up. Meanwhile, a significantly lower rate of freedom from AF was shown in the $\geq$24 months subgroup (pooled rate: 0.53; p = 0.000) than in the <24 months subgroup (pooled rate: 0.76; p = 0.000) with p = 0.000 for interaction in terms of follow-up time for elderly patients, suggesting that extended follow-up time may be severely detrimental to freedom from AF for elderly patients after ablation. Similarly to previous studies [41–43], our quadratic prediction fit result for the elderly group showed that the correlation between the follow-up time and the rate of freedom from AF was significantly negative. In addition, we analyzed the difference in rates of freedom from AF between younger and elderly groups by means of the quadratic prediction fit curves. The result showed the rate of freedom from AF in the younger group seemed to be consistently higher than in the elderly group, as well as the difference between the rates of freedom from AF was increasing when the follow-up time was more than 20.98 months, which might provide a promising explanation for the potential trend in the follow-up time subgroup between elderly and younger groups.

Multiple risk factors, including unmodifiable risk factors (e.g., gender, age, and genetics) and modifiable risk factors (e.g., hypertension, DM, and obesity), played a significant role in contributing to the initiation and progression of AF. A growing number of clinical studies have suggested that female patients have a higher risk of AF recurrence than male patients after ablation, owing to more advanced atrial remodeling [44,45]. The recurrent AF subanalysis in the CABANA trial (NCT00911508) proved that the efficacy of ablation in the female subgroup was significantly inferior to that in the male subgroup when compared with the efficacy of drug therapy (HR: 0.64 vs. 0.46, p for interaction = 0.035) [46]. Similarly, compared with the younger group, the elderly group was significantly associated with a lower rate of freedom from AF in the higher female proportion subgroup, while a comparable rate of freedom from AF was found in the equal female proportion subgroup, which in part suggested that the higher the proportion of females, the lower the rate of freedom from AF. In addition, the latest subanalysis from the CABANA trial indicated that a superior result for reducing AF recurrence was displayed in the catheter ablation arm than in the drug therapy arm across age-groups [37]. Interestingly, our results showed that compared with the younger group, the elderly group was significantly associated with a lower rate of freedom from AF with the elderly age cutoff less than 75 years, while a comparable freedom rate from AF when the elderly age cutoff was more than 75 years. The reason might be the lower the elderly age cutoff and the higher the proportion of young patients in the younger group, ultimately contributing to a better prognosis in the younger group. Moreover, LAD, AF history duration, and AADs usage were also reported to affect the rate of freedom from AF ablation, whereas our results showed that subgroup analysis in terms of the LAD and AF history duration subgroups showed no significant difference between the equal and higher subgroups (p = 0.168 and p = 0.685, respectively), which might be attributed to the relatively small absolute difference between the two groups in the values of LAD and AF history duration, as well as there being fewer studies with higher LAD and AF history duration between elderly and younger groups. In addition, AADs usage was similar between the elderly and younger groups in most of the eligible studies.

Reportedly, hypertension and DM are the two most common cardiovascular risk factors and comorbidities, with a higher risk of developing AF and a lower rate of freedom from AF postablation than normotensives and non-DM patients, respectively [3,47]. Interestingly, the elderly group was significantly associated with a lower rate of freedom from AF in the higher hypertension proportion subgroup and the higher DM proportion subgroup, while comparable freedom rates from AF were found in the equal hypertension proportion subgroup and the equal DM proportion subgroup, respectively. A significant clinical implication underlying this result was that good management of hypertension and DM might be expected to extensively improve ablation efficacy for elderly patients with AF.

Additionally, our results indicated that compared with the younger group, the elderly group was significantly associated with a lower rate of freedom from AF in the single-center subgroup, recently subgroup, non-PAF subgroup, PVI-plus subgroup, and RF subgroup, while a comparable freedom rate from AF were found in the multicenter subgroup, not-recently subgroup, PAF subgroup, PVI subgroup, and Cryo subgroup, which indicated elderly patients might have benefits similar to younger patients in these subgroups. These results must still be demonstrated with more randomized controlled trials, which might play a guiding role on the optimal management of AF for elderly individuals.

5. Limitations

Several limitations in this meta-analysis should be highlighted. First, a major limitation is that all the eligible studies were observational studies without randomized controlled trials, which might restrict us from drawing a substantial conclusion. To the best of our knowledge, this study was the first registered meta-analysis with a relatively large sample to compare AF ablation outcomes between elderly and younger patients. The TSA result also indicated firm evidence supporting our pooled results. Second, consistently with previous meta-analyses, possible biases might have affected our results. In this study, sensitivity analysis and publication bias tests (e.g., Begg's and Egger's tests) both indicated that our results were robust. Third, similar to previous studies [18,25], our safety results showed higher rate of cerebrovascular events, serious hemorrhage complications, and all-cause death in the elderly group with AF ablation therapy than the younger group, but these results might be affected by potentially inherent confounding factors. The elderly might be associated with more frail profiles, higher stroke/bleeding risk, and a higher rate of comorbidities than younger individuals [3], which would overestimate our results owing to forward-causality bias. However, the pooled rates of safety outcomes in the elderly group were remarkably low, ranging from 0.00 to 0.01. Finally, the only potentially significant treatment–covariate interaction was identified in the follow-up time subgroup: ≥ 24 months and <24 months with $p = 0.066$ for interaction for the comparison of freedom rate from AF between elderly and younger groups. Meanwhile, important confounding factors, including LAD and AF history duration, showed no effect on the rate of freedom from AF ablation between elderly and younger groups, whereas the relatively few eligible studies are reason to interpret these results with more caution. Therefore, more studies with larger samples and longer follow-up are needed to confirm our results.

6. Conclusions

Our meta-analysis suggests that elderly patients may have inferior efficacy and safety outcomes to younger patients with AF ablation. Moreover, the follow-up time may be a potential determinant of outcome impact on freedom from AF for elderly patients after AF ablation. Additional randomized controlled trials are required for confirmation of our results.

Supplementary Materials: The following supporting information can be downloaded at: https://www.mdpi.com/article/10.3390/jcm11154468/s1. Table S1. Quality assessment of eligible studies according to the Newcastle-Ottawa Quality Assessment Scale [6,10–31]. Table S2. Quality assessment of the single-arm studies according to the Institute of Health Economics checklist [32–35]. Table S3. Pooled incidence of safety outcomes in the elderly group. Figure S1. Forest plot of subgroup analysis of the rates of freedom from AF between elderly and younger groups in terms of LAD and AF history duration ([6,10–14,16,17,19,20,23,24,26,27,29,31] for A and [6,11,13,19,26,27,31] for B). Figure S2. Quadratic prediction fit plot with confidence intervals between the follow-up time and the rates of freedom from AF for the elderly group and the younger group. Figure S3. The relationship of the follow-up time and the difference of freedom from AF between the younger group and the elderly group.

Author Contributions: R.-X.W. developed the concept of the study; F.L., L.Z., L.-D.W. and Z.-Y.Z. (Zhi-Yuan Zhang) designed this study and carried out the data analysis; F.L. wrote the manuscript with help from L.Z., L.-D.W., Z.-Y.Z. (Zhi-Yuan Zhang), H.-H.L. and Z.-Y.Z. (Zhen-Ye Zhang); and J.Z., R.-X.W. and L.-L.Q. provided critical reviews of the paper. All authors have read and agreed to the published version of the manuscript.

Funding: This research received no external funding.

Institutional Review Board Statement: Not applicable.

Informed Consent Statement: Not applicable.

Data Availability Statement: The data that support the findings of this study are available from the corresponding author upon reasonable request.

Acknowledgments: Feng Li sincerely acknowledges Jin-Yu Sun (from the Department of Cardiology, First Affiliated Hospital of Nanjing Medical University, Nanjing) for his valuable advice. Moreover, we would like show our sincere appreciation to the reviewers for critical comments on this article.

Conflicts of Interest: The authors declare no conflict of interest.

References

1. Lippi, G.; Sanchis-Gomar, F.; Cervellin, G. Global epidemiology of atrial fibrillation: An increasing epidemic and public health challenge. *Int. J. Stroke* **2021**, *16*, 217–221. [CrossRef] [PubMed]
2. Volgman, A.S.; Nair, G.; Lyubarova, R.; Merchant, F.M.; Mason, P.; Curtis, A.B.; Wenger, N.K.; Aggarwal, N.T.; Kirkpatrick, J.N.; Benjamin, E.J. Management of atrial fibrillation in patients 75 years and older: JACC state-of-the-art review. *J. Am. Coll. Cardiol.* **2022**, *79*, 166–179. [CrossRef]
3. Hindricks, G.; Potpara, T.; Dagres, N.; Arbelo, E.; Bax, J.J.; Blomström-Lundqvist, C.; Boriani, G.; Castella, M.; Dan, G.-A.; Dilaveris, P.E.; et al. 2020 ESC guidelines for the diagnosis and management of atrial fibrillation developed in collaboration with the European Association for Cardio-Thoracic Surgery (EACTS): The task force for the diagnosis and management of atrial fibrillation of the European Society of Cardiology (ESC) developed with the special contribution of the European Heart Rhythm Association (EHRA) of the ESC. *Eur. Heart J.* **2021**, *42*, 373–498. [PubMed]
4. Yang, P.S.; Sung, J.H.; Kim, D.; Jang, E.; Yu, H.T.; Kim, T.-H.; Uhm, J.-S.; Kim, J.-Y.; Pak, H.-N.; Lee, M.-H.; et al. Frailty and the effect of catheter ablation in the elderly population with atrial fibrillation-a real-world analysis. *Circ. J.* **2021**, *85*, 1305–1313. [CrossRef]
5. Kim, D.; Yang, P.-S.; You, S.C.; Jang, E.; Yu, H.T.; Kim, T.-H.; Pak, H.-N.; Lee, M.-H.; Lip, G.Y.H.; Sung, J.-H.; et al. Age and outcomes of early rhythm control in patients with atrial fibrillation: Nationwide cohort study. *JACC Clin. Electrophysiol.* **2022**, *8*, 619–632. [CrossRef]
6. Vermeersch, G.; Abugattas, J.-P.; Varnavas, V.; De Cocker, J.; Schwagten, B.; Sieira, J.; De Asmundis, C.; Chierchia, G.-B.; De Greef, Y. Efficacy and safety of the second-generation cryoballoon ablation for the treatment of persistent atrial fibrillation in elderly patients. *J. Arrhythm.* **2021**, *37*, 626–634. [CrossRef]
7. Furlan, A.D.; Pennick, V.; Bombardier, C.; van Tulde, M.; Editorial Board; Cochrane Back Review Group. 2009 updated method guidelines for systematic reviews in the Cochrane Back Review Group. *Spine (Phila Pa 1976)* **2009**, *34*, 1929–1941. [CrossRef] [PubMed]
8. Guo, B.; Moga, C.; Harstall, C.; Schopflocher, D. A principal component analysis is conducted for a case series quality appraisal checklist. *J. Clin. Epidemiol.* **2016**, *69*, 199–207.e2. [CrossRef]
9. Brok, J.; Thorlund, K.; Gluud, C.; Wetterslev, J. Trial sequential analysis reveals insufficient information size and potentially false positive results in many meta-analyses. *J. Clin. Epidemiol.* **2008**, *61*, 763–769. [CrossRef] [PubMed]
10. Natale, V.; Mohanty, S.; Trivedi, C.; Baqai, F.M.; Gallinghouse, J.; Rocca, D.G.D.; Gianni, C.; MacDonald, B.; Mayedo, A.; Burkhardt, J.D.; et al. Arrhythmia profile and ablation-outcome in elderly women with atrial fibrillation undergoing first catheter ablation. *Pacing Clin. Electrophysiol.* **2021**, *44*, 835–842. [CrossRef]
11. Sciarra, L.; Iacopino, S.; Arena, G.; Tondo, C.; Pieragnoli, P.; Molon, G.; Manfrin, M.; Curnis, A.; Russo, A.D.; Rovaris, G.; et al. Safety and efficacy of Cryoballoon ablation of atrial fibrillation in relation to the patients' age: Results from a large real-world multicenter observational project. *Cardiol. Res. Pract.* **2021**, *2021*, 9996047. [CrossRef]
12. Hartl, S.; Dorwarth, U.; Pongratz, J.; Aurich, F.; Brück, B.; Tesche, C.; Ebersberger, U.; Wankerl, M.; Hoffmann, E.; Straube, F. Impact of age on the outcome of cryoballoon ablation as the primary approach in the interventional treatment of atrial fibrillation: Insights from a large all-comer study. *J. Cardiovasc. Electrophysiol.* **2021**, *32*, 949–957. [CrossRef]
13. Zhou, G.; Cai, L.; Wu, X.; Zhang, L.; Chen, S.; Lu, X.; Xu, J.; Ding, Y.; Peng, S.; Wei, Y.; et al. Clinical efficacy and safety of radiofrequency catheter ablation for atrial fibrillation in patients aged ≥80 years. *Pacing Clin. Electrophysiol.* **2020**, *43*, 814–821. [CrossRef]
14. Kanda, T.; Masuda, M.; Kurata, N.; Asai, M.; Iida, O.; Okamoto, S.; Ishihara, T.; Nanto, K.; Tsujimura, T.; Okuno, S.; et al. Efficacy and safety of the cryoballoon-based atrial fibrillation ablation in patients aged ≥80 years. *J. Cardiovasc. Electrophysiol.* **2019**, *30*, 2242–2247. [CrossRef] [PubMed]
15. Fink, T.; Metzner, A.; Willems, S.; Eckardt, L.; Ince, H.; Brachmann, J.; Spitzer, S.G.; Deneke, T.; Schmitt, C.; Hochadel, M.; et al. Procedural success, safety and patients satisfaction after second ablation of atrial fibrillation in the elderly: Results from the German Ablation Registry. *Clin. Res. Cardiol.* **2019**, *108*, 1354–1363. [CrossRef]
16. Zhang, J.; Ren, Z.; Wang, S.; Zhang, J.; Yang, H.; Zheng, Y.; Meng, W.; Zhao, D.; Xu, Y. Efficacy and safety of cryoballoon ablation for Chinese patients over 75 years old: A comparison with a younger cohort. *J. Cardiovasc. Electrophysiol.* **2019**, *30*, 2734–2742. [CrossRef]
17. Heeger, C.-H.; Bellmann, B.; Fink, T.; Bohnen, J.E.; Wissner, E.; Wohlmuth, P.; Rottner, L.; Sohns, C.; Tilz, R.R.; Mathew, S.; et al. Efficacy and safety of cryoballoon ablation in the elderly: A multicenter study. *Int. J. Cardiol.* **2019**, *278*, 108–113. [CrossRef]
18. Romero, J.; Ogunbayo, G.; Elayi, S.C.; Darrat, Y.; Rios, S.A.; Diaz, J.C.; Alviz, I.; Cerna, L.; Gabr, M.; Chernobelsky, E.; et al. Safety of catheter ablation for atrial fibrillation in the octogenarian population. *J. Cardiovasc. Electrophysiol.* **2019**, *30*, 2686–2693. [CrossRef]
19. Abdin, A.; Yalin, K.; Lyan, E.; Sawan, N.; Liosis, S.; Meyer-Saraei, R.; Elsner, C.; Lange, S.A.; Heeger, C.; Eitel, C.; et al. Safety and efficacy of cryoballoon ablation for the treatment of atrial fibrillation in elderly patients. *Clin. Res. Cardiol.* **2019**, *108*, 167–174. [CrossRef]
20. Zhang, X.Y.; Yu, R.H.; Dong, J.Z. Clinical characteristics and efficacy of radiofrequency catheter ablation in the treatment of elderly patients with atrial fibrillation. *Am. J. Med. Sci.* **2018**, *355*, 357–361. [CrossRef]

1. Tscholl, V.; Lin, T.; Lsharaf, A.K.; Bellmann, B.; Nagel, P.; Lenz, K.; Landmesser, U.; Roser, M.; Rillig, A. Cryoballoon ablation in the elderly: One year outcome and safety of the second-generation 28mm cryoballoon in patients over 75 years old. *Ep Eur.* **2018**, *20*, 772–777. [CrossRef]
2. Moser, J.M.; Willems, S.; Andresen, D.; Brachmann, J.; Eckardt, L.; Hoffmann, E.; Kuck, K.; Lewalter, T.; Schumacher, B.; Spitzer, S.G.; et al. Complication rates of catheter ablation of atrial fibrillation in patients aged ≥75 years versus <75 years-results from the German ablation registry. *J. Cardiovasc. Electrophysiol.* **2017**, *28*, 258–265. [CrossRef] [PubMed]
3. Abugattas, J.P.; Iacopino, S.; Moran, D.; de Regibus, V.; Takarada, K.; Mugnai, G.; Ströker, E.; Coutiño-Moreno, H.E.; Choudhury, R.; Storti, C.; et al. Efficacy and safety of the second generation cryoballoon ablation for the treatment of paroxysmal atrial fibrillation in patients over 75 years: A comparison with a younger cohort. *Europace* **2017**, *19*, 1798–1803. [CrossRef] [PubMed]
4. Kautzner, J.; Peichl, P.; Sramko, M.; Cihak, R.; Aldhoon, B.; Wichterle, D. Catheter ablation of atrial fibrillation in elderly population. *J. Geriatr. Cardiol.* **2017**, *14*, 563–568.
5. Bunch, T.J.; May, H.T.; Bair, T.L.; Jacobs, V.; Crandall, B.G.; Cutler, M.; Weiss, J.P.; Mallender, C.; Osborn, J.S.; Anderson, J.L.; et al. The impact of age on 5-year outcomes after atrial fibrillation catheter ablation. *J Cardiovasc. Electrophysiol.* **2016**, *27*, 141–146. [CrossRef]
6. Lioni, L.; Letsas, K.P.; Efremidis, M.; Vlachos, K.; Giannopoulos, G.; Kareliotis, V.; Deftereos, S.; Sideris, A. Catheter ablation of atrial fibrillation in the elderly. *J. Geriatr. Cardiol.* **2014**, *11*, 291–295.
7. Santangeli, P.; Di Biase, L.; Mohanty, P.; Burkhardt, J.D.; Horton, R.; Bai, R.; Mohanty, S.; Pump, A.; Gibson, D.; Couts, L.; et al. Catheter ablation of atrial fibrillation in octogenarians: Safety and outcomes. *J. Cardiovasc. Electrophysiol.* **2012**, *23*, 687–693. [CrossRef]
8. Hao, S.C.; Hunter, T.D.; Gunnarsson, C.; March, J.L.; White, S.A.; Ladapo, J.A.; Reynolds, M.R. Acute safety outcomes in younger and older patients with atrial fibrillation treated with catheter ablation. *J. Interv. Card Electrophysiol.* **2012**, *35*, 173–182. [CrossRef]
9. Bunch, T.J.; Weiss, J.P.; Crandall, B.G.; May, H.T.; Bair, T.L.; Osborn, J.S.; Anderson, J.L.; Lappe, D.L.; Muhlestein, J.B.; Nelson, J.; et al. Long-term clinical efficacy and risk of catheter ablation for atrial fibrillation in octogenarians. *Pacing Clin. Electrophysiol.* **2010**, *33*, 146–152. [CrossRef]
10. Kusumoto, F.; Prussak, K.; Wiesinger, M.; Pullen, T.; Lynady, C. Radiofrequency catheter ablation of atrial fibrillation in older patients: Outcomes and complications. *J. Interv. Card Electrophysiol.* **2009**, *25*, 31–35. [CrossRef]
11. Bhargava, M.; Marrouche, N.F.; Martin, D.O.; Schweikert, R.A.; Saliba, W.; Saad, E.B.; Bash, D.; Williams-Andrews, M.I.C.H.E.L.L.E.; Rossillo, A.; Erciyes, D.; et al. Impact of age on the outcome of pulmonary vein isolation for atrial fibrillation using circular mapping technique and cooled-tip ablation catheter. *J. Cardiovasc. Electrophysiol.* **2004**, *15*, 8–13. [CrossRef] [PubMed]
12. Liu, Y.Y.; Du, X.; He, L.; Liu, T.; Chen, N.; Hu, R.; Ning, M.; Lv, Q.; Dong, J.; Ma, C. Evaluation of safety and effectiveness on catheter ablation of atrial fibrillation in patients aged ≥80 years. *Heart Lung Circ.* **2022**, *31*, 1006–1014. [CrossRef]
13. Akhtar, T.; Berger, R.; Marine, J.E.; Daimee, U.A.; Calkins, H.; Spragg, D. Cryoballoon Ablation of Atrial Fibrillation in Octogenarians. *Arrhythm. Electrophysiol. Rev.* **2020**, *9*, 104–107. [CrossRef] [PubMed]
14. Metzner, I.; Wissner, E.; Tilz, R.R.; Rillig, A.; Mathew, S.; Schmidt, B.; Chun, J.; Wohlmuth, P.; Deiss, S.; Lemes, C.; et al. Ablation of atrial fibrillation in patients ≥75 years: Long-term clinical outcome and safety. *Europace* **2016**, *18*, 543–549. [CrossRef]
15. Corrado, A.; Patel, D.; Riedlbauchova, L.; Fahmy, T.S.; Themistoclakis, S.; Bonso, A.; Rossillo, A.; Hao, S.; Schweikert, R.A.; Cummings, J.E.; et al. Efficacy, safety, and outcome of atrial fibrillation ablation in septuagenarians. *J. Cardiovasc. Electrophysiol.* **2008**, *19*, 807–811. [CrossRef]
16. Brunetti, N.D.; Santoro, F.; Correale, M.; de Gennaro, L.; Conte, G.; di Biase, M. Incidence of atrial fibrillation is associated with age and gender in subjects practicing physical exercise: A meta-analysis and meta-regression analysis. *Int. J. Cardiol.* **2016**, *221*, 1056–1060. [CrossRef] [PubMed]
17. Bahnson, T.D.; Giczewska, A.; Mark, D.B.; Russo, A.M.; Monahan, K.H.; Al-Khalidi, H.R.; Silverstein, A.P.; Poole, J.E.; Lee, K.L.; Packer, D.L. Association between age and outcomes of catheter ablation versus medical therapy for atrial fibrillation: Results from the CABANA trial. *Circulation* **2022**, *145*, 796–804. [CrossRef] [PubMed]
18. Liu, Y.; Huang, H.; Huang, C.; Zhang, S.; Ma, C.; Liu, X.; Yang, Y.; Cao, K.; Wu, S.; Wang, F. Catheter ablation of atrial fibrillation in Chinese elderly patients. *Int. J. Cardiol.* **2011**, *152*, 266–267. [CrossRef]
19. Latchamsetty, R.; Morady, F. Catheter ablation of atrial fibrillation. *Heart Fail. Clin.* **2016**, *12*, 223–233. [CrossRef] [PubMed]
20. Parameswaran, R.; Al-Kaisey, A.M.; Kalman, J.M. Catheter ablation for atrial fibrillation: Current indications and evolving technologies. *Nat. Rev. Cardiol.* **2021**, *18*, 210–225. [CrossRef]
21. Oral, H.; Pappone, C.; Chugh, A.; Good, E.; Bogun, F.; Pelosi, F., Jr.; Bates, E.R.; Lehmann, M.H.; Vicedomini, G.; Augello, G.; et al. Circumferential pulmonary-vein ablation for chronic atrial fibrillation. *N. Engl. J. Med.* **2006**, *354*, 934–941. [CrossRef] [PubMed]
22. Brooks, A.G.; Stiles, M.K.; Laborderie, J.; Lau, D.H.; Kuklik, P.; Shipp, N.J.; Hsu, L.; Sanders, P. Outcomes of long-standing persistent atrial fibrillation ablation: A systematic review. *Heart Rhythm.* **2010**, *7*, 835–846. [CrossRef] [PubMed]
23. Latchamsetty, R.; Morady, F. Long-term benefits following catheter ablation of atrial fibrillation. *Circ. J.* **2013**, *77*, 1091–1096. [CrossRef] [PubMed]
24. Chibber, T.; Baranchuk, A. Sex-related differences in catheter ablation for patients with atrial fibrillation and heart failure. *Front. Cardiovasc. Med.* **2020**, *7*, 614031. [CrossRef] [PubMed]

45. Wong, G.R.; Nalliah, C.J.; Lee, G.; Voskoboinik, A.; Chieng, D.; Prabhu, S.; Parameswaran, R.; Sugumar, H.; Al-Kaisey, A. McLellan, A.; et al. Sex-related differences in atrial remodeling in patients with atrial fibrillation: Relationship to ablation outcomes. *Circ. Arrhythm. Electrophysiol.* **2022**, *15*, e009925. [CrossRef] [PubMed]
46. Packer, D.L.; Mark, D.B.; Robb, R.A.; Monahan, K.H.; Bahnson, T.D.; Poole, J.E.; Noseworthy, P.A.; Rosenberg, Y.D.; Jeffries, N. Mitchell, L.B.; et al. Effect of catheter ablation vs. antiarrhythmic drug therapy on mortality, stroke, bleeding, and cardiac arrest among patients with atrial fibrillation: The CABANA randomized clinical Trial. *JAMA* **2019**, *321*, 1261–1274. [CrossRef]
47. Piché, M.E.; Tchernof, A.; Després, J.P. Obesity phenotypes, diabetes, and cardiovascular diseases. *Circ. Res.* **2020**, *126*, 1477–1500. [CrossRef]

MDPI
St. Alban-Anlage 66
4052 Basel
Switzerland
www.mdpi.com

Journal of Clinical Medicine Editorial Office
E-mail: jcm@mdpi.com
www.mdpi.com/journal/jcm

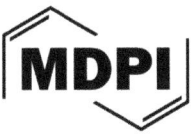

Disclaimer/Publisher's Note: The statements, opinions and data contained in all publications are solely those of the individual author(s) and contributor(s) and not of MDPI and/or the editor(s). MDPI and/or the editor(s) disclaim responsibility for any injury to people or property resulting from any ideas, methods, instructions or products referred to in the content.

www.ingramcontent.com/pod-product-compliance
Lightning Source LLC
LaVergne TN
LVHW070156120526
838202LV00013BA/1252